HYPERTENSION FLUID-ELECTROLYTES, AND TUBULOPATHIES
IN PEDIATRIC NEPHROLOGY

DEVELOPMENTS IN NEPHROLOGY

VOLUME 5

Also in this series:

1. Cheigh JS, Stenzel KH, Rubin AL eds: Manual of Clinical nephrology of the Rosogin Kidney Center. 1981. ISBN 90-247-2397-3
2. Nolph KD ed: Peritoneal dialysis. 1981. ISBN 90-247-2477-5
3. Gruskin AB, Norman ME eds: Pediatric Nephrology. 1981. ISBN 90-247-2514-3
4. Schuck O ed: Examination of the Kidney Function. 1981. ISBN 90-247-2609-3

HYPERTENSION, FLUID-ELECTROLYTES, AND TUBULOPATHIES IN PEDIATRIC NEPHROLOGY

Proceedings of Pediatric Nephrology
Seminar VIII, held at Bal Harbour,
Florida, January 25-29, 1981

Edited by

JOSÉ STRAUSS, MD

1982

MARTINUS NIJHOFF PUBLISHERS
THE HAGUE / BOSTON / LONDON

Distributors

for the United States and Canada
Kluwer Boston, Inc.
190 Old Derby Street
Hingham, MA 02043
USA

for all other countries
Kluwer Academic Publishers Group
Distribution Center
P.O. Box 322
3300 AH Dordrecht
The Netherlands

ISBN-13: 978-94-009-7543-9 e-ISBN-13: 978-94-009-7541-5
DOI: 10.1007/978-94-009-7541-5

FOREWORD

The thrust here is for those who want to know more than the answer to an exam question - an approach to disease diagnosis and treatment which emphasizes thoughtful consideration of alternatives, finding ones way through uncertainties and lack of knowledge. The annual seminar on which this volume is based has evolved into a forum for open discussion of puzzling questions - actually old questions in the light of new data.

To me, the adventure of life is in recognizing the openendedness of all things. So you thought that a certain disease was a settled question? In medicine a "settled" question is a transient conclusion. Even the solutions to the so-called simplest problems have another side.

Our aim this year was to air out concepts and conclusions about hypertension, fluid-electrolytes, and tubulopathies. The stars were Drs. Juan Rodriguez-Soriano, Alan Gruskin, and Donald Potter, along with Drs. Gustavo Gordillo, Ronald Kallen, and Antonia Novello as guest faculty. Local stars included Drs. Mary Jane Jesse, Jacques Bourgoignie, and Carlos Vaamonde. Their contributions added to those of the other faculty and registrants, coalesced into vibrant exchanges which are reproduced here for the reader's perusal.

José Strauss

CONTENTS

V. WORKSHOP

ACKNOWLEDGEMENTS

Those who must be recognized for outstanding contributions include (1) past registrants and faculty whose thoughts helped shape the Seminar VIII program on which this volume is based; (2) the authors who submitted their papers in the final form required by our publisher this year, and assume responsibility for all manuscript details (thereby complete uniformity of style has been lost but time has been gained which is a plus for the reader); (3) Pediatric Nephrology Division staff who responded to extra demands made by Seminar and book preparation, especially Pearl Seidler and Estela Garcia; (4) Louise Strauss who took responsibility for book details; and (5), the personnel of the following companies who are aware of the value of continuing education and gave financial support:

Abbot Laboratories Hospital Products Division
Beach Products, Inc.
Burroughs Wellcome Company
Ciba Pharmaceutical Company
Cordis Dow Corporation
Drake Willock
Eli Lilly and Company
E.R. Squibb & Sons, Inc.
Hoechst-Roussel Pharmaceuticals, Inc.
Lifemed/Division of Vernitron
Merck, Sharpe & Dohme
Roche Laboratories
Ross Laboratories
Schering Corporation
Smith Kline & French
Travenol Laboratories, Inc.
Upjohn Company
Willen Drug Company
William H. Rorer, Inc.

Finally, I acknowledge the approval and moral support of the University of Miami School of Medicine Acting Dean, Dr. Bernard Fogel, and Department of Pediatrics Chairman, Dr. William Cleveland.

José Strauss

I

FLUID-ELECTROLYTES

HIGHLIGHTS: A SYSTEMATIC APPROACH TO CLINICAL ACID-BASE DISORDERS USING ALGORITHMS

Ronald J. Kallen, M.D.

A systematic approach to clinical acid-base problems more consistently yields accurate solutions in comparison to intuitive methods based on an incomplete data base. Algorithms provide a schema for making a "decision-tree" analysis of such problems by systematically asking questions or making hypotheses, and then accepting or rejecting them based on the emerging data-base. These schemes are designed to translate intuitive mental processes to stereotypical deductive decision-making. The complete data-base incorporates information gleaned from the clinical history and physical examination which often suggests <u>primary processes</u>, such as: (1) bicarbonate loss, (2) increased acid production, (3) insufficient acid excretion by impaired kidneys, (4) clinical conditions of potassium or chloride loss, and (5) ineffective ventilation with retention of carbon dioxide.

In standard terminology, the major <u>primary</u> processes are metabolic acidosis, respiratory acidosis, metabolic alkalosis, and respiratory alkalosis. These processes include the usual physiologic adjustment aimed at restoring blood pH toward normal: (1) ventilatory adjustments of pCO_2 (metabolic acidosis and alkalosis), and (2) modulation of renal reabsorption of bicarbonate (respiratory acidosis and alkalosis).

In complex clinical disorders, multiple primary processes may coexist. Hence, acid base disorders are classified as simple and mixed. The net effect of multiple processes on blood pH may be described as acidemia (arterial pH < 7.35), and alkalemia (arterial pH > 7.45).

In addition to clinical history and physical examination, the complete data-base includes:

1. Blood pH (or $[H^+]$ in nanoequiv/L)
2. Plasma $[HCO_3^-]$, which is estimated roughly by plasma "total CO_2 content", or exactly by: Total CO_2 content - 0.03 x pCO_2
3. pCO_2 (most reliably estimated in an arterial sample obtained during a state of "usual" ventilation, i.e., neither crying nor breath-holding)
4. Anion gap, estimated as: $[Na^+] - [HCO_3^-] + [Cl^-]$
   Normal anion gap is 8-16 mEq/L

Given the complete data-base, one may proceed as follows in cases of suspected metabolic acidosis:

1. Are the blood acid-base data internally consistent or is there lab error?
   a. check by means of <u>nomogram</u>
   b. use Kassirer-Bleich equation: $[H^+] = 24 \times \frac{pCO_2}{[HCO_3^-]}$

where,

pCO_2 is arterial carbon dioxide in mm Hg

$[HCO_3^-]$ is plasma bicarbonate in mEq/L

$[H^+]$ is in nanoequiv/L, and may be estimated from:

$$[H^+] = 80 - 100 \text{ (actual pH - 7.00)}$$

This estimate is approximate in the pH range, 7.15 - 7.50; outside this range, accuracy falls off.

2. Are we dealing with a pure primary process (i.e., metabolic acidosis) or is there a superimposed process?
   a. Review history and physical
   b. Is the ventilatory adjustment for metabolic acidosis appropriate?
3. What is the anion gap? Is the result consistent with the above data-base?

A similar approach, using algorithms, may be used for other clinical acid-base disorders. This approach aims to uncover unsuspected concurrent acid-base disorders frequently encountered as complex, mixed acid-base disturbances in clinical practice. Some of the mixed disorders are indicated in Tables 1 and 2.

Table 1. Mixed Acid-base Disorders

PRIMARY	SUPERIMPOSED	CLINICAL DISORDER
Metabolic acidosis	Acute respiratory acidosis	Cardiopulmonary arrest
	Respiratory alkalosis	Salicylate intoxication
Chronic respiratory acidosis	Acute respiratory acidosis	COPD with acute deterioration
	Metabolic acidosis Acute respiratory acidosis	COPD with acute hypoxemia
	Metabolic alkalosis	Loop diuretic, vomiting

Table 2. Mixed Acid-base Disorders

PRIMARY	SUPERIMPOSED	CLINICAL CONDITION
Metabolic alkalosis	Underlying chronic respiratory alkalosis	COPD with sudden ↑ ventilation
	Acute respiratory alkalosis	Sepsis, ↑ ventilation pulmonary embolism
Acute respiratory alkalosis	Underlying chronic metabolic acidosis	Too rapid administration of bicarbonate
Chronic respiratory alkalosis	Metabolic alkalosis	Hepatic insufficiency with diuretic or vomiting

FLUID BALANCE IN THE NEWBORN

Eduardo Bancalari, M.D.

The balance of fluids and electrolytes is easily disturbed in the neonate because of the anatomical and functional peculiarities of the newborn (1-2). Some of these disturbances may lead to serious complications such as intracranial hemorrhage, persistent ductus arteriosus or chronic lung disease.

The following are some of the characteristics that make the neonate more susceptible to disturbances of water and electrolyte balance.

1) The total body water is proportionally more in the neonate and increases at lower gestational ages. The total water content decreases from 88% of the fat free weight at 23 weeks gestation to 82% at term, still high compared with 72% in the adult. The distribution of the body water is also different in the newborn than in the adult. While the extracellular water in the neonate corresponds to 45% of the body weight, in the adult it is only 16%.

2) The intake of water and electrolytes is not controlled by the normal physiological mechanism, but it is determined by the amount given to the infant by the caretaker.

3) Insensible water losses are higher because of the larger surface area in relation to body mass and because of the increased skin water permeability in the premature (3,4,5). The higher minute ventilation and basal metabolism also increase the water losses.

4) The capacity of the kidney to maintain a normal homeostasis is limited, especially in the small preterm infant.

Normal Requirements

In order to maintain a normal balance the intake of water and electrolytes must necessarily be equal to the losses. Water loss through the skin, respiration and retained for growth ranges from 30 to 100 ml/kg/day. This amount varies depending on the gestational age, the ambient temperature and the humidity. The lower the gestational age, the larger is the water loss through the skin due to evaporation (3). While the transcutaneous water loss in a 27 week gestation infant can be 50 $g/m^2/hr$, in the same environment at 37 weeks gestation it is less than 10 $g/m^2/hr$. These losses increase several times at higher ambient temperatures or at lower humidities. The use of a radiant warmer or phototherapy can also increase the insensible water losses while the use of clothing or a plastic shield around the infant can reduce evaporative losses through the skin (6,7).

The water eliminated in the urine and stool is usually 30-100 ml/kg/day, but obviously the urine output varies depending on the state of hydration. Under normal conditions then total water losses range from 60 to 200 ml/kg/day with an average of 150 ml/kg/day. The requirements are lower during the first 2-4 days of life because of the larger extracellular water content of the newborn and the reduced urinary output during the first few days of life.

The electrolyte needs in the newborn range between 2-4 mEq/kg/day for Na^+ and Cl^- and between 2-3 mEq/kg/day for K^+. Urine sodium losses can be much higher in small preterm infants in whom it may reach values of 10 mEq/kg/day or more.

Negative Water Balance

This occurs when losses of water are larger than normal and the intake is not increased proportionally. Increased insensible water losses may occur secondary to increased minute ventilation, use of radiant warmers, phototherapy or low ambient humidity. Diarrhea may also increase considerable water and electrolyte losses.

Excessive urine losses may occur in cases of osmotic diuresis or secondary to the use of diuretics. The first occurs frequently in the small premature infant secondary to hyperglycemia and glucosuria.

The consequences of negative water balance are dehydration, hypernatremia with increased serum osmolarity and hypovolemia. This may lead to arterial hypotension, shock and renal failure. Hyperosmolarity may also increase the risk of CNS hemorrhage especially in the very small premature.

Positive Water Balance

This occurs as a result of excessive water intake in relation to the losses. While the healthy full-term infant can handle a water load by increasing his diuresis, the sick premature frequently is not able to eliminate the excess water resulting in an increase in his total body fluids. This leads frequently to decompensation of cardiopulmonary function. The risk of overhydration is increased in cases of renal failure or inappropriate ADH secretion or in situations when insensible losses are markedly reduced. This can occur in infants who are mechanically ventilated in whom the inspired gas is saturated with water vapor or when the environment is highly humidified.

Excessive fluid intake in the premature infant has been associated with an increased incidence of patent ductus arteriosus and heart failure (8), and in infants who require mechanical ventilation with increased incidence of bronchopulmonary dysplasia (9). It has also been suggested that overhydration may predispose prematures to the development of necrotizing enterocolitis. Because of the possible association between excess fluid intake and these life-threatening complications, it is essential to avoid fluid overload in the premature infant.

Evaluation of Water Balance

Because of the large variations in water and electrolyte requirements in different patients or even in the same infant under different environmental conditions, it is difficult to use a predetermined schedule to adjust the required water intake. It is crucial then to evaluate continuously the state of hydration and adjust the fluid intake according to the needs of each infant. The following are some of the indicators that can be used to evaluate the state of hydration in the newborn.

1) Body weight: When done repeatedly, this is the simplest and most accurate indicator of the state of hydration in the newborn.

2) Diuresis: This is also a very valuable indicator of fluid balance assuming renal function is normal and no drugs that influence diuresis are given. Under normal conditions a newborn passes between 2-3 ml/kg/hr of urine.

3) Urine specific gravity and osmolarity: Again, if renal function is normal, urine density and osmolarity are useful in determining water balance status. With adequate hydration and a normal renal function, one can expect a urine osmolarity between 150-400 mOsm/l. An exception is the case of inappropriate ADH secretion when the urine is concentrated, but the patient may be overhydrated. It is important then to evaluate all these factors simultaneously and not guide the management of fluids following a single parameter.

4) Serum osmolarity and electrolyte concentration: These values will only change if water or electrolytes vary independently, but when both water and electrolytes are retained or lost together, their plasma concentration may remain normal even when the total balance is altered. Also, the changes in serum electrolyte concentration occurs relatively late in these disturbances and one should make the diagnosis early by using the more sensitive indicators mentioned before.

5) Physical signs: These are also late signs and include edema, heart failure and increased venous pressure as signs of overhydration. Dehydration is characterized by dryness of the skin and mucous membranes, sunken fontanel and eyes, low central venous pressure and arterial hypotension in severe cases.

In conclusion, water balance in the sick neonate is difficult to maintain because of his anatomical characteristics and functional limitations. Because of the large individual variability and environmental influences, it is difficult to anticipate the fluid requirements for each infant, and therefore, it becomes critical to continuously evaluate the state of hydration in these infants. Alterations in water and electrolyte balance can have serious consequences in the neonate and for this reason every effort should be made to maintain a normal state of hydration in this age group.

REFERENCES

1. Bell, E.F., Oh, W.: Fluid and electrolyte balance in very low birth weight infants. Clin in Perinatol 6:139, 1979.

2. Roy, N.R., Sinclair, J.C.: Hydration of the low birth weight infant. Clin in Perinatol 2:393, 1975.

3. Hammarlund, K., Nilsson, G.E., Oberg, P.A., Sedin, G.: Transepidermal water loss in newborn infants. Acta Paediatr Scand 66:553, 1977; Acta Paediatr Scand 68:371, 1979.
4. Wu, P.Y.K., Hodgman, J.E.: Insensible water loss in preterm infants: Changes with postnatal development and nonionizing radiant energy. Pediatrics 54:704, 1974.
5. Fanaroff, A.A., Wald, M., Gruber, H., et al.: Insensible water loss in low birth weight infants. Pediatrics 50:236, 1972.
6. Bell, E.F., Weinstein, M.R., Oh, W.: Heat balance in premature infants: Comparative effects of convectively heated incubators and radiant warmer, with and without plastic heat shield. J Pediatr. 96:460, 1980.
7. Marks, K.H., Gunther, R.C., Rossi, J.A., Maisels, J.: Oxygen consumption and insensible water loss in premature infants under radiant heater. Pediatrics 66:228, 1980.
8. Bell, E.F., Warburton, D., Stonestreet, B.S., et al.: Effects of fluid administration on the development of symptomatic patent ductus arteriosus and congestive heart failure in premature infants. N Engl J Med 302:598, 1980.
9. Brown, E.R., Stark, A., Sosenko, I., et al.: Bronchopulmonary dysplasia: Possible relationship to pulmonary edema. J Pediatr 92:982, 1978.

METABOLIC ALKALOSIS OF INFANCY

Alan B. Gruskin, M.D., Martin S. Polinsky, M.D., H. Jorge Baluarte, M.D., James W. Prebis, M.D. and Howard W. Rosenblum, M.D.

Metabolic alkalosis is a subject which tends to be under-emphasized in pediatric medicine because it occurs less frequently than other acid-base disturbances. Consequently, its presence is often overlooked and its pathophysiology inadequately understood. The purpose of this presentation will be to consider 1) definitions involved with the evaluation of patients with metabolic alkalosis; 2) factors which enable metabolic alkalosis to be generated, as well as those factors which permit metabolic alkalosis to persist and 3) a discussion of the pathophysiology of diseases associated wtih metabolic alkalosis, stressing disorders which occur during infancy. Therapy will not be considered.

DEFINITIONS

Biochemical evidence for metabolic alkalosis should be sought when the history and physical exam suggest the presence of a disorder known to be associated with metabolic alkalosis. Basic laboratory studies should include a measurement of the serum concentrations of sodium, potassium, chloride, CO_2 content, BUN and creatinine. Additional help can be obtained by determining blood pH, pCO_2 and HCO_3^-, the pH of the urine, and the urinary concentrations of sodium and chloride. Different disorders are associated with low or high urinary concentrations of chloride (Table 1). A urine pH above 6.0 suggests that excessive quantities of bicarbonate are being filtered and not reabsorbed by the tubule. When the urine pH is less than 5.5 one may conclude that the metabolic alkalosis is associated with an excessive secretion of hydrogen ions by the distal tubule, and that any bicarbonate reaching the distal tubule has been reabsorbed. The determination of the urinary concentrations of sodium and chloride are helpful in deciding whether volume contraction is present and whether the development of chloride deficiency has been a major factor leading to metabolic alkalosis.

Table 1. Urinary Chloride Concentration in Disorders With Metabolic Alkalosis

Urinary Chloride Concentration	
<10 mEq/L	>10 mEq/L
Loss of stomach contents	Primary mineralocorticoid excess
Chloride losing diarrhea	Bartter syndrome
Diuretic administration	Glucocorticoid excess
Ingestion low chloride formula	Hypercalcemia
Cystic fibrosis	Severe potassium depletion
Post hypercapnea	
HCO_3^- loading in renal failure	

Metabolic alkalosis may be operationally defined as a primary physiologic process characterized by either a gain of bicarbonate and/or loss of non-volatile acid from the extracellular fluid (1,2). Metabolic alkalosis by definition is associated with alkalemia or a blood pH which is elevated because of the serum bicarbonate being disproportionately elevated in relation to the pCO_2. Primary uncomplicated metabolic alkalosis is easily recognized because blood pH and serum HCO_3^- are elevated while the pCO_2 is either normal or high depending upon the degree of compensation. Compensation in a primary acid base disturbance may be defined as being absent, partial, or complete (3). These terms refer to the degree of return of blood pH toward a normal pH. The degree of compensation depends upon two factors. The first is the length of time a particular disturbance has been present while the second reflects the ability of the compensating organ, i.e. the lungs, to maximally alter pCO_2 and permit the pH to return towards normal. Maximal compensation may be recognized as being present when the acid-base parameters which indicate compensation fall within the previously established 95% confidence limits determined experimentally, and blood pH approaches normal. The presence of metabolic alkalosis need not preclude the simultaneous occurrance of another acid-base disorder. For example, if the value for pCO_2 in a patie with a primary metabolic alkalosis did not fall within the 95% confidence ban for metabolic alkalosis despite adequate time to do so, the presence of a com plicating disorder, i.e. a mixed acid-base disturbance should be sought (4). Respiratory compensation for metabolic alkalosis should occur in 12-24 hours. The 95% confidence limit for changes in pCO_2 in patients with metabolic alkalosis may be approximated by the following formula (4,5):

$$\Delta pCO_2 = \Delta HCO_3^- \times 0.9 \pm 5 \text{ or } pCO_2 = 0.95(HCO_3^-)+14.5$$

The question arises as to how to recognize the presence of metabolic alkalosis when a primary respiratory acid-base disturbance is also present. Disorders associated with a metabolic alkalosis should be sought whenever the blood pH and/or serum bicarbonate exceeds values known to define the 95% confidence limits for changes in pCO_2 occurring as a result of chronic respiratory alkalosis and acidosis (1).

It is possible that the two primary disorders of metabolic alkalosis and metabolic acidosis may occur simultaneously in the same patient. Blood studie will reflect the more severe of the two disorders, although the degree of dev ation from normal will be less than expected were only one disorder present. Only by recognizing that a child has two distinct clinical diseases will one deduce that the pathophysiologic processes of both metabolic alkalosis and acidosis may be operative.

Other important terms requiring definition are renal bicarbonate threshold and "effective" volume (6,7). The renal bicarbonate threshold may be defined as the serum level of bicarbonate at which free bicarbonate ions appear in the urine. Normally the serum level of bicarbonate exists at a level 2-3 mM/L below that at which free bicarbonate will appear in the urine, assuming the patient is normovolemic. Unfortunately, the renal threshold is not a fixed level of serum bicarbonate and it can be altered by a number of factors which influence the tubular reabsorption of bicarbonate. Bicarbonate is reabsorbed primarily, i.e. 80-85% of filtered bicarbonate, in the proximal tubule secondarily to the secretion of hdrogen ion (6,7). As regards bicarbonate reabsorption, the pH in the proximal tubule does not fall to values less than 6.0-6.2. The remaining 15-20% of the filtered bicarbonate is reabsorbed by the distal tubule,which is apparently limited in the quantity of bicarbonate which it can reabsorb,even though it can reduce the lumen concentration of bicarbonate to zero and permit the urinary pH to fall to levels of less than 5.5. Thus, the distal tubule, as regards its capacity to reabsorb bicarbonate, functions as a high gradient, low capacity system. It apparently cannot reabsorb more bicarbonate than an amount corresponding to a load of 15-20% of a normally filtered quantity of bicarbonate (0.15 x 24 mM/100 ml GFR). Free bicarbonate ions will be found in the urine when either the proximal reabsorption of bicarbonate is depressed, or the capacity of the proximal and distal tubule to reabsorb bicarbonate is exceeded.

The term "effective" volume refers to an immeasurable quantity of extracellular volume capable of eliciting a response by the kidney, primarily the proximal tubule (8,9). When extracellular volume is "effectively" diminished, the kidney behaves as if it were receiving a signal that the patient has a reduced extracellular volume, similar to that which occurs when a loss of sodium chloride has occurred. When the extracellular fluid compartment is either "effectively" or actually decreased, the proximal tubule will respond by increasing its reabsorption of glomerular filtrate. For example, 90-95% of the glomerular filtrate including its accompanying solutes might be reabsorbed rather than 80-85%. The concentration of solute, including bicarbonate, returned to the circulation would of course parallel that within the glomerular filtrate. "Effective" reductions of extracellular fluid occur in patients who have heart failure, cirrhosis and perhaps nephrosis. Real reductions occur in patients who sustain losses of sodium and water.

GENERATION AND PERSISTENCE OF METABOLIC ALKALOSIS

Because metabolic alkalosis may persist even though the original cuase of the metabolic alkalosis has been removed, it is helpful to view the pathophysiology of metabolic alkalosis as occurring in two discrete phases - a generation and a persistance phase (1,2,6,7,10). The physiologic processes occuring in these two aspects of metabolic alkalosis in most of the clinical disorders occurring in infants involve changes from normal in the renal handling of hydrogen ion and/or bicarbonate ion, sodium, potassium and chloride. Although the pathophysiology of the metabolic alkalosis in many of the disorders involving infants has not been specifically studied,it may be assumed that similar processes are operative in both adults and infants. Specific pediatric data when available will be mentioned.

Metabolic alkalosis is generated by either a net body gain of base or loss of acid. Alkalosis develops at least transiently when bicarbonate is added to the extracellular space in the form of bicarbonate containing salts or when citrate and/or lactate salts are metabolically converted to bicarbonate. Bicarbonate is added to extracellular fluid when hydrogen ion is lost from the gastrointestinal tract, or when hydrogen ions move into cells. Loss of acid, i.e. hydrogen ions, may occur via the kidney and/or gastrointestinal tract.

When the kidney is the organ responsible for generating metabolic alkalosis an increased quantity of bicarbonate is added to the extracellular space in response to a net loss of acid. The kidney generates metabolic alkalosis when the distal tubule increases its excretion of hydrogen ions. Specific factors influencing distal hydrogen secretion include the rate of delivery of sodium to the distal tubule (6), circulating levels of mineralocorticoids (10), distal transtubular potential difference, and distal intracellular potassium concentration (6).

An increased delivery of sodium to the distal tubule occurs when the intake of sodium is increased, when less sodium is reabsorbed in either the proximal tubule and/or ascending limb of henle, and when sodium salts of poorly reabsorbed anions (phosphates, sulfates) are administered. Aldosterone per se apparently does not directly affect hydrogen or potassium secretion in the distal tubule (1). However, if sodium delivery to the distal tubule is increased and is in excess of that required for bicarbonate regeneration, the presence of aldosterone enhances and increases potassium and hydrogen ion secretion (1).

The administration of sodium salts of nonreabsorbable anions increases the degree of distal intraluminal negativity, increases hydrogen ion secretio and thereby promotes bicarbonate generation (6,11). The degree to which hydr gen ion is secreted depends upon the level of stimulus for the sodium moiety the salt to be absorbed.

When the intracellular potassium concentration of the tubular cells is lowered, hydrogen ion secretion increases. The rate of hydrogen ion secretio depends upon sodium delivery, and the effect of circulating mineralocorticoid (1,6).

The generation of metabolic alkalosis and an increased serum bicarbonate concentration does not imply that metabolic alkalosis will persist. If an ex trarenal external source of bicarbonate is continuously available metabolic alkalosis will persist. However, in most disorders associated with metabolic alkalosis persistance of the alkalemia occurs because of functional changes occurring in the kidney. In normal individuals an increase in serum bicarbonate would be accompanied by an increased filtered load of bicarbonate. Onc the renal threshold for bicarbonate was exceeded,bicarbonaturia would ensue and the concentration of bicarbonate would return to normal. Therefore, in order for the serum bicarbonate to remain elevated, there must be a net increase in the tubular reabsorption of bicarbonate above that normally operati Three factors which enable more bicarbonate to be absorbed and/or hydrogen io to be secreted in the proximal tubule,and thus permit metabolic alkalosis to maintained include the quantity and quality of the extracellular fluid, i.e. the state of sodium balance and "effective" volume (9,12,13), potassium depletion (14), especially if severe, and hypocapnea (15). Both hypokalemia and changes in the pCO_2 content of blood can apparently alter the proximal tubule reabsorption of bicarbonate by altering hydrogen ion secretion independently of the effect of extracellular volume. The distal tubule also continues to participate in the maintenance phase of metabolic acidosis by continuing to secrete hydrogen ions for reasons similar to those just discussed. Once many of the renal factors become operative alkalemia will persist despite removal of those factors which originally enabled a metabolic alkalosis to occur. Steps must be undertaken to correct those factors enabling the metabolic alkalosis to persist before alkalosis can be corrected.

In short, the factors enabling metabolic alkalosis to develop in patient are often different from those which permit metabolic alkalosis to persist. A appropriate understanding of the influence of these many factors involving multiple organ systems should lead to easier identification of affected patie and provide a rational basis upon which appropriate therapy may be planned.

CLINICAL DISORDERS ASSOCIATED WITH METABOLIC ALKALOSIS

A large number of disorders may be associated with metabolic alkalosis. Complete lists of disorders and detailed reviews can be found elsewhere (1,6,7). This review, as mentioned will focus on providing a pathophysiologic overview of those disorders (Table II) which occur during infancy.

Table II: Classification of Infantile Metabolic Alkalosis

I. External loss of H^+ and Cl^-

A. Gastrointestinal
1. Drug induced gastric hypersecretion
2. Familial chloride losing disorders
3. Gastric drainage without appropriate electrolyte replacement
4. Pyloric stenosis
5. Vomiting secondary to either obstruction above the entrance of the bile duct, or to increased intracranial pressure

B. Renal
1. Bartter syndrome
2. Congenital renal alkalosis
3. Diuretic administration
4. Excessive glucocorticoids
5. Gittleman syndrome-hypomagnesemia, hypokalemia
6. Hypercalcemia
7. Hypermineralocorticoidism
8. Liddle syndrome
9. Potassium losing nephropathy
10. Renal tubular acidosis with metabolic alkalosis

C. Skin
1. Cystic fibrosis - sweat losses

II. Altered intake or production of Base

A. Chronic ingestion of low chloride formula containing a bicarbonate precursor

B. Metabolic compensation for respiratory acidosis

C. Oral and/or IV administration of bicarbonate or metabolic precursors of bicarbonate, i.e. citrate, lactate

III. Extracellular fluid contraction

A. Loop diuretics

B. Distal tubule diuretics - Thiazides

1. Disorders Associated With an External Loss of H^+ and Cl^-

a. Gastrointestinal losses of H^+ and Cl^-

The pathogenesis of metabolic alkalosis associated with the loss of stomach contents has been intensively studied. The effect on acid-base and electrolyte balance of the loss of stomach contents, including sodium, potassium, hydrogen ion, chloride and water, as well as the selective loss of HCl achieved by gastric drainage and replacement of all of the electrolytes except HCl has been investigated(16).The isolated loss of HCl will be considered first. The ongoing loss of HCl results in an increase in serum HCO_3^-, and a decrease in serum chloride concentration. A greater quantity of bicarbonate is filtered and the bicarbonate threshold is exceeded, so more sodium bicarbonate is delivered to the distal tubule. Because of the increased distal delivery of sodium bicarbonate, K^+ exchange is increased and H^+ secretion suppressed. Urine pH and bicarbonate excretion increases. In these patients urine pH should exceed 6.0; urinary bicarbonate, sodium and potassium concentrations may be high while that of chloride is low. But, in most clinical disorders associated with the loss of HCl from the gut, such as pyloric stenosis, water loss and extracellular volume contraction occur simultaneously. Also, sodium and potassium chloride are lost from the stomach. This increase aldosterone secretion and further augments distal tubule potassium secretion and increases distal sodium reabsorption and hydrogen ion secretion. In these patients urine pH should be less than 5.5 and the urine relatively free of bicarbonate, sodium and chloride. These findings reflect volume contraction superimposed upon the loss of stomach contents.

In short, the generation of metabolic alkalosis due to vomiting is due to a combination of three factors: 1) the loss of hydrochloric acid, 2) the development of contraction alkalosis becuase of the concomittant loss of sodium chloride and water without any loss of serum bicarbonate and 3) the movement hydrogen ions into cells in exchange for intracellular potassium. Maintenance depends upon the proximal tubule reabsorbing most of the filtered bicarbonate as a consequence of potassium deficiency, an increase in pCO_2, and volume contraction. Also, the occurrence of secondary hyperaldosteronism will result in an increase in the distal secretion of hydrogen and potassium ions.

Familial chloride losing diarrhea is a rare disorder in which chronic diarrhea is accompanied by metabolic alkalosis rather than metabolic acidosis (17,18). These infants have a defect in the chloride-bicarbonate pump in the ileum and are unable to transport chloride across the bowel wall (18). As a consequence of this transport defect stool losses of both chloride and hydrogen ion are increased. Extracellular volume contraction also develops. The net result is the development of metabolic alkalosis and a chloride free urine for reasons similar to those already discussed.

Treatment of an infant with tolazoline for persistant fetal circulation has been associated with the development of metabolic alkalosis (19). The reason for the generation of the metabolic alkalosis is that tolazoline, similar to histamine, increases both the free and total acidity as well as the volume of gastric secretions. Maintenance of metabolic alkalosis occurs because of chloride depletion and volume contraction.

b. Renal losses of H^+ and Cl^-

A number of transport defects involving renal tubular cells result in metabolic alkalosis. The Bartter syndrome is felt by some to be associated with a transport defect of chloride in the ascending limb of Henle (20,21). Salt wasting leads to ECF volume contraction, hyperreninemia and hyperaldosteronism and hypokalemia. Congenital renal alkalosis is another syndrome whose clinical features are similar in appearance to those of Bartter syndrome differing in that hypertrophy of the juxtaglomerular apparatus is absent and the transport defect may be in the distal tubule (22).

Transport defects involving an increased excretion of potassium may result in the development of hypokalemic alkalosis. Liddle syndrome or pseudoaldosteronism is a familial disorder consisting of hypertension, hypokalemia, alkalosis, failure of the kidney to conserve potassium and low aldosterone excretion (23,24). The hypokalemic alkalosis may be corrected by administering triamterene, a diuretic which specifically blocks potassium secretion. Also, idiopathic hypomagnesemia, Gitelman syndrome, may be associated with renal potassium wasting, hypokalemia, metabolic alkalosis, increased plasma renin activity and normal aldosterone levels (25).

The generation of metabolic alkalosis in these disorders may reflect increased chloride loss with its concomittant effect on extracellular volume, and the effect of potassium depletion on the proximal reabsorption of bicarbonate. Hypokalemia also alters acid excretion in the distal tubule and the ability of mineralocorticoids to stimulate the reabsorption of chloride (1). Maintenance of alkalosis is due to volume contraction and the persistant effect of hypokalemia on hydrogen ion secretion by the cells located in the proximal and distal tubule.

A few patients with proximal renal tubular acidosis who have had large defects in proximal bicarbonate reabsorption have been documented as having metabolic alkalosis (26). In such patients the generation of alkalosis is due to the delivery of excessively large quantities of $NaHCO_3$ to the distal tubule. Some of the Na^+ is exchanged for K^+ and H^+ while some escapes reabsorption leading to excessive loss of glomerular filtrate, ECF contraction, and secondary hyperaldosteronism. The secondary hyperaldosteronism leads to further renal losses of potassium and hydrogen ion. The net result is metabolic alkalosis. It is probable that excessive amounts of sodium bicarbonate are continuously delivered to the distal tubule because of the magnitude of the proximal defect. Correction of the metabolic alkalosis and the emergence of proximal RTA occur when sufficient quantities of sodium and potassium chloride are provided.

Most clinical disorders associated with mineralocorticoid excess are associated with metabolic alkalosis (27) (Table III).

Table III: Disorders Associated with Metabolic Alkalosis, Hypertension, Mineralocorticoid Excess and Volume Expansion, adapted from Seldin, D.W., Metabolic Alkalosis in Brenner, B.M. and The Kidney, W.B. Saunders, Phila. 1976, p.686.

Table III Continued

I Low renin, low aldosterone

1. DOC excess
   a. 11-hydroxylase deficiency+
   b. 17-hydroxylase deficiency+
   c. adrenal carcinoma

2. Hydrocortisone+

3. Liddle syndrome+

4. Licorice ingestion

II Low renin, high aldosterone

1. Adrenal carcinoma
2. Dexamethasone suppressible hyperaldosteronism
3. Primary hyperaldosteronism+

III High renin, high aldosterone

1. Juxtaglomerular cell tumor+
2. Secondary hyperaldosteronism-edema absent

   a. Intrarenal vasculitis+
   b. Malignant hypertension+
   c. Renal artery obstruction+

+occurs in infants

These disorders have many features in common (6). They include: 1) a variety of stimuli leading to mineralcorticoid excess; 2) the excessive mineralocorticoid activity is continuous; 3) distal sodium delivery is excessive unless dietary sodium is severely restricted; 4) an increase in "effective" volume occurs and 5) the distal tubular secretion of potassium and hydrogen ion is increased (6). Chloride deficiency is not an essential feature. Excessive mineralocorticoid activity alone will not cause metabolic alkalosis. It appears that potassium depletion as well as ECF volume expansion is required in addition to excess mineralocorticoid activity for metabolic alkalosis to occur and persist.

Many of the adrenal hormones manufactured in inborn errors of metabolism, including those associated with either adrenal enzyme defects or glucocorticoid excess do have mineralocorticoid effect. Although the mineralocorticoid activity of these hormones is substantially less than that of aldosterone, it is felt that the extremely high quantities present in these disorders exert sufficient mineralocorticoid activity to generate metabolic alkalosis (27). A simplistic view of the generation and persistance phases of this form of metabolic alkalosis follows (28,29,30); mineralocorticoid excess enhances potassium excretion and sodium reabsorption in the distal tubule. Subsequently, ECF volume expansion ensues and proximal bicarbonate reabsorption is depressed leading to an increased delivery of sodium to the distal tubule. Sodium is exchanged for potassium and hydrogen ion further augmenting the renal excretion of potassium and hydrogen ion. Noteworthy is the observation that potassium depletion (1) in the presence of mineralocorticoid excess augments the capacity of the distal tubule to lower the pH of the urine. Hypokalemic metabolic alkalosis ensues in those infants who also have mineralocorticoid excess and persistant volume expansion when their sodium intake is normal.

Maintenance of the metabolic alkalosis in patients with mineralocorticoid excess is primarily due to the distal tubule effect of mineralocorticoids and hypokalemia on hydrogen ion secretion. Also, hypokalemia may alter the proximal reabsorption of bicarbonate. It is possible that the tendency of hypokalemia to raise the bicarbonate threshold, through its effect on the proximal reabsorption of bicarbonate may be offset in affected infants by a mineralocorticoid-induced increase in extracellular volume, which in turn would depress proximal tubular reabsorption of bicarbonate. When a volume effect is present its influence on tubular function usually suppercedes that which is due to changes in serum concentrations of electrolyte. Most patients with disorders associated with metabolic alkalosis and excessive mineralocorticoid activity have hypertension (6). Levels of plasma renin activity and of aldosterone will vary depending on the disease involved.

Hypercalcemia may lead to metabolic alkalosis (10). The generation phase of metabolic alkalosis is poorly understood. Maintenance of this form of metabolic alkalosis has been attributed to the suppressive effect of hypercalcemia on circulating levels of parathyroid hormone level, which in turn permits more bicarbonate to be reabsorbed in the proximal tubule.

c. Skin losses of chloride

Metabolic alkalosis may develop in children with cystic fibrosis (31, 32,33). Excessive skin losses of chloride as well as sodium may occur in these children especially when active sweating is present. Infants with cystic fibrosis have been reported to lose more than 80 mEq of chloride and 40 mEq of potassium in a day during periods of excessive sweating (33). Unless adequate sodium, chloride, and water replacement is provided, hypochloremic metabolic alkalosis, hyponatremia, and volume contraction will occur. Also, infants with cystic fibrosis ingesting formulas with a low content of sodium and chloride may present with metabolic alkalosis because they are not ingesting quantities of chloride sufficient to replace skin losses. Noteworthy is the fact that the sodium chloride content of infant formulas and baby food has been reduced in the past few years (34).

2. Altered Intake of Base

An increased rate of intake of bicarbonate or bicarbonate precursors will elevate serum bicarbonate and, therefore, generate metabolic alkalosis. Assuming the presence of euvolemia and normokalemia, the degree to which the alkalosis will persist depends on a sustained intake which is greater than the ability of the kidney to excrete bicarbonate as the serum level of bicarbonate exceeds the renal threshold for bicarbonate. Because of the ability of the normal kidney to excrete large quantities of bicarbonate, sustained metabolic alkalosis because of the ingestion of exogenous bicarbonate does not often occur unless the patient has a low GFR (35). In patients with a low GFR, i.e. renal failure, and perhaps neonates with a physiologically low GFR, smaller doses of bicarbonate may generate metabolic alkalosis because of the limitatio placed by a low GFR on the filtered load of bicarbonate. Tubular mechanism fo handling bicarbonate remain intact even at low levels of GFR. Maintenance in these patients would then depend on the ongoing ingestion of bicarbonate.

During the past few years there has been a number of reports of infants who developed metabolic alkalosis in association with the ingestion of infant formula containing almost no chloride (36,37). The ingestion of a low chlorid formula containing less than 2-3 mEq/L, together with ongoing losses of chlori from the body via stool, sweat, regurgitation, intercurrent illness associated with vomiting, etc. resulted in a combination of hypochoremic alkalosis and volume contraction, factors necessary to generate and sustain metabolic alkalo sis. In addition to the low chloride intake, the formula primarily involved contained citrate, a bicarbonate precursor. Thus, bicarbonate loading as well as chloride and volume depletion may have been involved in both the generation and persistance phases of the metabolic alkalosis which developed in these infants.

The kidney responds to chronic retention of CO_2, i.e. respiratory acidosi by increasing its excretion of chloride and acid. Simultaneously the proximal reabsorption of HCO_3^- is increased. The combination of these factors results i the development of an appropriate compensatory metabolic alkalosis. When such patients are maintained on either diuretics and/or a low chloride intake, the correction, especially if rapid, of the respiratory acidosis will leave the patient with a persistant metabolic alkalosis whose correction requires chloride (38).

Another potential source of an abnormal intake of bicarbonate is the combined administration of Kayexalate and phosphate binding gels to infants with advanced renal failure (39). Antacids such as Amphojel interact with HCl in t stomach to form CO_2, H_2O, and aluminum chloride ($AlCl_3$). Subsequently, the $AlCl_3$ combines with $NaHCO_3$ to form NaCl, $Al_2(CO_3)_3$, CO_2, and H_2O. Thus, when antacids alone are ingested there is no $NaHCO_3$ left over in the small bowel. When Kayexalate is also given the $AlCl_3$ and the sodium resin interact to form NaCl and $Al(resin)_3$ because of the high affinity of resin for aluminum. The bicarbonate normally secreted into the small bowel is no longer able to be neutralized by H^+ from the stomach and is reabsorbed into the body generating a metabolic alkalosis. Persistance of a metabolic alkalosis is maintained by a constant absorption of bicarbonate from the intestine.

3. Contraction Alkalosis

Diuretic administration may lead to metabolic alkalosis by two mechanism The administration of loop diuretics such as Lasix$^{(R)}$ or ethacrynic acid blocks chloride reabsorption in the loop of Henle. Equivalent amounts of sodium are lost. Since most of the filtered bicarbonate has been reclaimed in th proximal tubule, an acute depletion of ECF occurs without the loss of ECF bicarbonate. The result is "contraction" alkalosis (40). The alkalosis may develop over a period of a few hours. In one study involving adults with congestive heart failure treated with loop diuretics, the loss of each liter o ECF was associated with an increase of serum bicarbonate of approximately 1.4 mEq/L (1).

The chronic administration of diuretics which inhibit chloride and sodium reabsorption prior to the hydrogen ion secreting site in the distal tubule increases the intratubular negativity in the distal tubule. This leads to an increase in hydrogen ion secretion and the generation of a metabolic alkalosis. The increase in distal sodium delivery will also enhance potassium secretion, as well as enable a natriuresis and ECF volume contraction to occur. Secondary hyperreninemia and hyperaldosteronism ensue and further losses of potassium and hydrogen ion occur. Such a combination of factors enable metabolic alkalosis to persist. The chronic administration of thiazide as well as loop diuretics has been associated with the development of metabolic alkalosis. It is probable that the maintenance of metabolic alkalosis in patients who initially develop contraction alkalosis depends upon these factors.

REFERENCES

1. Sebastian, A., Halter, H.N., and Rector, F.C.,Jr.: Metabolic alkalosis in acid base and potassium homeostasis. Contemporary Issues in Nephrology 2, ed. Brenner, B.M. and Stein, J.H., Churchill Livingstone, New York, Edinburgh and London, 1978, pp. 101-136.
2. Coe, F.L.: Metabolic alkalosis (Special Communication). JAMA 238:2288,1977.
3. Winters, R.W., Engle, K. and Dell, R.B.: Acid-Base Physiology in Medicine, Westlake, Ohio, London Co., 1968.
4. van Ypersele de Strihou, C., and Frans, A.L The respiratory response to chronic metabolic alkalosis and acidosis in disease. Clin.Scien.& Mol.Med. 43:439, 1973.
5. Carroll, H.J. and Oh, M.S.: Water, electrolyte and acid base metabolism: Diagnosis and management. Phila., Lippincott, 1978.
6. Seldin, D.W.: Metabolic alkalosis. In The Kidney, ed. Brenner, B.M. and Rector, F.C.,Jr., W.B. Saunders, Philadelphia, Ch.17, 1976.
7. Seldin, D.W. and Rector, F.C.,Jr.: The generation and maintenance of metabolic alkalosis. Kid.Int. 1:305, 1972.
8. Kunau, R.T., Jr., Frick. A., Rector, F.C.,Jr. and Seldin, D.W.: Effect of extracellular fluid (ECF) volume expansion, K^+ deficiency and pCO_2 on bicarbonate reabsorption in the rat. Clin.Res. 14:380, 1966.
9. Kurtzman, N.A.: Regulation of renal bicarbonate reabsorption by extracellular volume. J.Clin.Invest. 49:586, 1970.
10. Kurtzman, H.A.: Metabolic alkalosis. The Kidney. National Kidney Foundation 9:27, 1976.
11. Clapp, J.R., Rector, F.C.,Jr. and Seldin, D.W.: Effect of unreabsorbed anions on proximal and distal transtubular potentials in rats. Am.J.Physiol. 202:781, 1962.
12. Purkerson, M.L., Lubowitz, H., White, R.W. and Bricker, N.S.: On the influence of extracellular fluid volume expansion on bicarbonate reabsorption in the rat. J.Clin.Invest.48:1754, 1969.
13. Slatopolsky, E., Hoffsten, P., Purkerson, M. and Bricker, N.S.: On the influence of extracellular fluid volume expansion and of uremia on bicarbonate reabsorption in man. J.Clin.Invest. 49:988, 1970.

14. Kunau, R.T.,Jr., Frick, A., Rector, F.C.,Jr. and Seldin, D.W.: Micropuncture study of the proximal tubular factors responsible for the maintenance of alkalsois during potassium deficiency in the rat. Clin.Sci.34:223, 1968.
15. Relman, A.S., Etsten, B. and Schwartz, W.B.: The regulation of renal bicarbonate reabsorption by plasma carbon dioxide tension. J.Clin.Invest.32:972, 1953.
16. Kassirer, J.P. and Schwartz, W.B.: The response of normal man to selective depletion of hydrochloric acid. Am.J.Med.40:10, 1966.
17. Evanson, J.M. and Stanbury, S.W.: Congenital chloridiarrhea or so-called congenital alkalosis with diarrhoea. Gut.6:29, 1965.
18. Bieberdorf, F.A., Gorden, P. and Fordtran,J.S.: Pathogenesis of congenital alkalosis with diarrhea. Implications for the physiology of normal ileal electrolyte absorption and secretion. J.Clin.Invest.51:958,1972.
19. Adams, J.M., Hyde, W.H., Procianoy, R.S. and Rudolph, A.J.: Hypochloremic metabolic alkalsois following tolazoline-induced gastric hypersecretion. Pediatrics 65:298, 1980.
20. Cannon, P.J., Leeming, J.M., Sommers, S.C., Winters, R.W. and Laragh, J.H Justzglomerular cell hyperplasia and secondary hyperaldosteronism (Bartter syndrome): a re-evaluation of the pathophysiology. Medicine 47:107, 1968.
21. Bardgette, J.J. and Stein, J.H.: Pathophysiology of Bartter syndrome. In Acid-Base and Potassium Homeostasis, Brenner, B.M. and Stein, J.H. (eds.) Churchill Livingstone 1978, p.269.
22. Calcagno, P.L.: A short communication. Congenital renal alkalosis. Pediatr. Res. 13:1379, 1979.
23. Liddle, G.W., Bledsoe, T. and Coppage, W.S.,Jr.: A familial disorder simulating primary aldosteronis but with negligible aldosterone secretion. Trans.Assoc.Am.Physicians 76:199, 1963.
24. Liddle, G.W., Bledsoe, T. and Coppage, W.S.: A familial renal disorder simulating primary aldosteronism but with negligible aldosterone secretion. In Baulieu, E.E. and Robel, P., eds. Aldosterone, Philadelphia, F.A. Davis Company, 1964. pp.353-368.
25. Gitelman, H.J., Graham, J.B. and Welt, L.G.: A new familial disorder characterized by hypokalemia and hypomagnesemia. Trans.Assoc.Am. Physicians 79:221, 1966.
26. Houston, I.B., Boichis, H., and Edelmann, C.M.,Jr.: Fanconi syndrome with renal sodium wasting and metabolic alkalosis. Am.J.Med.44:638, 1968.
27. Schambelan, M., Sebastian, A. and Hulter, H.N.: Mineralocorticoid excess and Deficiency Syndromes. In Acid-Base and Potassium Homeostasis, Brenner B.M. and Stein, J.H. (eds.) Churchill Livingstone, 1978, p.232.
28. Kassirer, J.P., London, A.M., Goldman, D.M. and Schwartz, W.B.: On the pathogenesis of metabolic alkalosis in hyperaldosteronism. Am.J.Med. 49:306, 1970.
29. Seldin, D.W., Welt, L.G. and Cort, H.J.: The role of sodium salts and adrenal steroids in the production of hypokalemic alkalosis. Yale J.Biol.Med. 29:229, 1956.
30. Mills, H.N., Thomas, S. and Williamson, K.S.: The acute effect of hydrocorticisone, deoxycorticosterone and aldosterone upon the excretion of sodium, potassium and acid by the human kidney. J.Physiol.151:312, 1960.
31. Beckerman, R.C. and Taussig, L.M.: Hypoelectrolytemia and metabolic alkalosis in infants with cystic fibrosis. Pediatrics 63:580, 1979.

32. Gottlieb, R.P.: Metabolic alkalosis in cystic fibrosis. J.Pediatr. 79:936, 1971.
33. Arvanitakis, S.N. and Lobeck, C.C.: Metabolic alkalosis and salt depletion in cystic fibrosis. J.Pediatr. 82:535, 1973.
34. Stewart, B.A.: Salt in the infant dietary, editorial in Pediatric Basics, Issue 21, Gerber Products ompany, 1978.
35. Husted, F.C., Nolph, K.D. and Maher, J.F.: $NaHCO_3$ and NaCl tolerance in chronic renal failure. J.Clin.Invest.56:414, 1975.
36. Linshaw, M.A., Harrison, H.L., Gruskin, A.B. et al: Hypochloremic alkalosis in infants associated with soy protein formula. J.Pediatr. 96:635, 1980.
37. Grossman, H., Duggan, E., McCamman, S. et al: The dietary chloride deficiency syndrome. Pediatrics 66:366, 1980.
38. Schwartz, W.B., Hays, R.M., Polack, A. and Haynie, G.D.: Effects of hyper capnia on electrolyte and acid-base equilibrium. II. Recovery, with special reference to the influence of chloride intake. J.Clin.Invest.40:1238, 1961.
39. Baluarte, H.J., Prebis, J., Goldberg, M. and Gruskin, A.B.: Metabolic alkalosis in an anephric child caused by the combined use of Kayexalate and Basaljel. J.Pediatr. 92:237, 1978.
40. Cannon, P.J., Heinemann, H.O., Albert, M.S., Laragh, J.H. and Winters, R.W.: "Contraction" alkalosis after diuresis of edematous patients with ethacrynic acid. Ann.Intern.Med. 62:979, 1965.
41. Support in part by NIH Grants RR-75,HL23511 and the Hoechst Roussel Pharmaceutical Co.

HIGHLIGHTS: EVALUATION OF SELECTED FLUID AND ELECTROLYTE DISORDERS

Ronald J. Kallen, M.D.

A number of fluid and electrolyte disorders are frequently encountered in clinical practice. The focus here is on diarrheal dehydration, metabolic acidosis, late metabolic acidosis of premature infants, metabolic alkalosis, acute oliguria, and Syndrome of Inappropriate ADH Secretion (SIADH).

DIARRHEAL DEHYDRATION

After obtaining the history, each patient should be evaluated in terms of a 5-point assessment:

1. Extent of volume depletion (as % of pre-illness body weight)
   a. Recent acute weight loss
   b. Physical examination. Is peripheral circulatory collapse impending?
2. Is there an osmotic disturbance of the body fluids?
3. Is there an acid-base disturbance?
4. Renal functional status?
5. Potassium (if anuric or markedly azotemic).

While awaiting laboratory results, parenteral rehydration may begin with an initial "pulse" of volume expansion, 10-20 ml/kg over 30-60 min, with either of the two solutions shown in Table 1.

Table 1. Initial Phase of Rehydration

10-20 ml/kg, 30-60 min

Age < 6 mo Doughy skin turgor BP maintained	Tenting of skin Shock Pallor Cold skin
↓	↓
Half-isotonic saline (Na^+ = 77 mEq/L)	Isotonic saline (Na^+ = 154 mEq/L) or Colloid

The subsequent rate of replacement of volume deficit should be for isotonic dehydration: 75%, over first 24 hours; hypertonic dehydration: 50%, over first 24 hours; hypotonic dehydration: 75-100% in first 12 hours. The total volume of parenteral fluid should include maintenance fluid requirement (modify for fever, anuria, etc.), deficit replacement, and an estimate of continuing losses, replaced volume-for-volume. The type of solution to administer may be determined from the scheme shown in Table 2.

In general, potassium chloride should not be added to parenteral fluids until it is clear that renal function is intact. The amount of potassium administered should not exceed 4-5 mEq/kg/day, over the first 24 to 48 hours. The potassium concentration in final solution should not exceed 40 mEq/L.

Recovery from diarrheal dehydration is indicated by progressive weight gain, declining specific gravity of urine and increasing urinary output, and declining BUN, with half-time of 24-30 hours and progressive improvement on physical examination.

METABOLIC ACIDOSIS

Treatment of metabolic acidosis is rarely indicated in acute, self-limited disorders provided the primary condition is adequately treated (e.g. gastroenteritis, diabetic ketoacidosis, etc.). Indications for sodium bicarbonate include (1) blood pH <7.10, (2) blood $[HCO_3^-]$ 6-7 mEq/L, (3) $PaCO_2 < 14$ mm Hg, (4) anuria (with above acid-base parameter), and (5) coma (with above acid-base parameters).

Table 2. Type of Solution to Administer

Serum $[Na^+]$			
150 mEq/L	130-150 mEq/L	120-130 mEq/L	120 mEq/L
Sodium concentration in final solution			
30-40 mEq/L	50-60 mEq/L	70-80 mEq/L	80-100 mEq/L
0.2% NaCl/5% D	0.33% NaCl/5% D	0.45% NaCl/5% D	0.45% NaCl/5% D + Bicarbonate*
(Na^+ = 34 mEq/L)	(Na^+ = 56 mEq/L)	(Na^+ = 77 mEq/L	(Na^+ = 100 mEq/L

*0.45% NaCl/5% (1000 ml) + $NaHCO_3$, 23 mEq

Metabolic acidosis should never be corrected *completely* or *rapidly* by $NaHCO_3$ administration. The serum $[HCO_3^-]$ should only be "nudged" up about 5 mEq/L. The appropriate dose for *partial* correction is 2.5 mEq/kg, administered slowly (over 2-3 hours) as 0.5 *M* solution. This is based on an assumed distribution factor of 50% of body weight (in newborns or prematures, an appropriate distribution factor is 30% of body weight). Do not administer $NaHCO_3$ to asphyxiated newborns for presumptive hypoxemic metabolic acidosis without first assuring adequate mechanical ventilation. There are no advantages in using THAM (Tris buffer) for the treatment of metabolic acidosis.

LATE METABOLIC ACIDOSIS OF PREMATURE INFANTS

This is a self-limited condition that ordinarily does not require treatment. If indicated, a few doses of sodium bicarbonate, 2-4 mEq/kg may be given on one or two occasions.

METABOLIC ALKALOSIS

It is important to establish the presence of *saline-responsive* metabolic alkalosis (urinary chloride <10 mEq/L). Treatment is effectively accomplished with either NaCl or KCl. Potassium should not be given as a salt other than KCl. Gradual correction will occur with intakes of NaCl or KCl that approximate usual daily requirements.

ACUTE OLIGURIA

Review the history from the standpoint of possible insults (including nephrotoxic agents) causing acute renal failure. The physical examination should aim at establishing state of hydration and circulatory status (blood pressure, pulse, orthostatic hypotension, etc.). If the patient is palpably overhydrated (edema, pulmonary congestion or edema, etc.), then it is unlikely that oliguria is on the basis of volume depletion. An analysis of the urine in relation to the history and physical examination should help differentiate prerenal oliguria from oliguria consequent to acute renal failure:

1. Specific gravity or urine osmolality
2. Fractional excretion of sodium index (FE - Na) where

$$FE - Na = \frac{\dfrac{U_{Na}}{P_{Na}}}{\dfrac{U\ creat}{P\ creat}}$$

FE - Na $\leq$ 0.01 suggests prerenal oliguria

FE - Na $\geq$ 0.025 suggests intrinsic acute renal failure

In the instance of prerenal oliguria, judicious volume expansion (saline, colloid, etc.) should be attempted. In the instance of intrinsic acute renal failure (acute tubular nephropathy), fluid intake should be restricted to replacing insensible loss and urine output.

SYNDROME OF INAPPROPRIATE ADH SECRETION (SIADH)

SIADH is generally a hyponatremic syndrome in the presence of an apparently normal state of hydration accompanied by inappropriately high urinary osmolality despite dilute body fluids. Appropriate measures include fluid restriction, declomycin, and furosemide with 3% NaCl (Hantman-Schrier method). In general 3% NaCl alone should be avoided unless there is severe hyponatremia with consequent seizures. In the latter instance, temporary benefit may be gained by administering 3% NaCl in an amount appropriate to raising the serum sodium concentration by 10 mEq/L which may be calculated as: 10 mEq/L x 0.6 x Body Weight (kg)= mEq of NaCl desired; 3% NaCl is approximately 0.5 mEq Na^+ per ml. Therefore, the actual volume to infuse is 20 ml of 3% NaCl x 0.6 x Body Weight (kg) = ml of 3% NaCl.

DISCUSSION

José Strauss, M.D., Moderator

MODERATOR: This is an open discussion. Questions may be submitted in writing or using the microphones. I wonder whether the panel would like to comment about the concentrating ability of patients with dehydration. We have observed in this country that infants with diarrhea do not necessarily concentrate their urine. I have stopped paying attention to that as a measure of functional ability or to differentiate between renal organic damage and functional disability. Would anyone care to comment on these points? Dr. Yuceoglu, Dr. Kaplan and I did a study (Brooklyn, N.Y., 1957-1959) in babies with diarrhea. At that time, our conclusion was that these babies did not concentrate their urine because they had decreased total body potassium and related functional disturbances. Earlier in this Seminar, somebody referred to the concentrating ability of diarrheic infants from a population which includes many malnourished children; I was surprised that they had good concentrating capacity. In addition to the potassium deficiency in diarrhea and malnutrition, we tend to expect some difficulties in urinary concentration, presumably due to the depletion of urea in the renal papilla. Can we touch on that subject? It is of great interest to us.

COMMENT: Many patients have a defect in renal concentrating capacity. When they become dehydrated, we have to consider this aspect, not only from the clinical findings point of view but from the type of dehydration that they are going to get and from the therapeutical aspects. We compared the neonatal patients with malnourished patients. They reach about the same maximal capacity of concentrating ability. We have only seen that with malnourished patients; they only reach at most about 600 mOsm/kg. You must see many of these patients with sickle cell anemia; they also have the same problem. With this particular group we found a great variability in its degree of malnutrition. They did not have third degree malnutrition as we call those patients that have a weight loss higher than 40% of body weight, according to age and height. We have some cases of malnutrition but not very severe in this group of infants. So, we have an average of 450 mOsm/kg of urine for most of these patients. But there were some that reached figures higher than 800 mOsm/kg and others that had only about 250 mOsm/kg. Those figures are daily averages.

MODERATOR: Was there any difference, any clinical history that would have separated those patients that had a urinary osmolality of about 800 mOsm/kg versus the ones that had about 200-300 mOsm/kg?

RESPONSE: Not in these cases. When we were looking particularly at this aspect (maximal concentrating ability) and malnutrition problems, we found that there was a good correlation: with more severe malnutrition, we reached lower values of renal concentrating capacity.

COMMENT: I want to mention that malnutrition may be different in different countries. What was just mentioned happens in some European and Latin American countries, namely hypertonic dehydration. This occurs because infants receive formulas with concentrated milk. We had a child who was given this formula as his usual formula. The mother thought that by using more of the powder--a very heavy powder--that the child would get bigger and healthier than the neighborhood children. This happened because at that time we didn't have evaporated milk. At that time the companies made only powdered milk. This situation became very common. We got a lot of hypertonic dehydration. Fortunately, now the occurrence of hypertonic dehydration has decreased at the same time that the sodium content of formulas was decreased, and the mothers' knowledge of the situation increased. The point is, these patients with severe hypertonic dehydration, very severe hypernatremia--as much as 180-190 mEq/L--despite this amount of protein load they had received before, despite this amount of urea they had before, when they came in with severe hypertonic dehydration, they had a concentrating defect in the urine. They were concentrating less than children with hypertonic dehydration whose problem was only due to fluid deprivation. This was very interesting.

In addition, they had a lot of sodium in the urine, a higher amount of sodium than in pure renal failure but the urine concentration was very low and the index of renal failure was quite similar to that in organic renal failure. We waited and this functional state disappeared; it was not real renal failure. But it took several days to bring the sodium down to normal. We got the impression that it was not good for the child--high serum sodium--for more than a few hours or one or two days. And the cause of this functional defect? I don't have the explanation as to why hypernatremia per se was blocking the urinary concentrating mechanism but that was so. We spent a lot of time designing special solutions for peritoneal dialysis to treat these children with severe hypertonic dehydration due to excessive ingestion of concentrated milk without a true organic renal failure. We obtained very good results --as did another group--and concluded that children with hypertonic dehydration due to excessive solute intake should be treated with peritoneal dialysis as are the cases of true salt intoxication. I think it's a point to make because though you don't have this problem in the States, somebody in the audience may.

QUESTION: I would like to hear an expanded comment on the use of oral solutions for rehydration containing glucose.

RESPONSE: Apparently the studies that have been presented have very good results. I haven't any question about this possibility but as the problem exists, we would like to know if by changing the glucose or giving other carbohydrates we may get better results. So far, they have not posed the question from the clinical results (the people who have been using oral rehydration), but I think there could be some changes if we used one or another carbohydrate. Theoretically, there can be some changes. So, it is a point that should be studied in a small group of infants. Most of the people who have a lot of experience have used oral rehydration in massive programs. They cannot give too much attention to these small details.

COMMENT: This way of using oral rehydration, it is not necessary to use glucose. You can use sucrose or saccharose. It has been proved that sucrose may facilitate overgrowth of bacteria in a small bottle. This sucrose is metabolized to lactic acid, the lactic acid then acts on the bicarbonate, and the bicarbonate disappears. People have tried it and found that if there is increased CO_2 in the urine, if you can determine the content of the feces, you will not find bicarbonate in the feces because of the lactic acid produced from action of the bacteria on the sucrose given to rehydrate the patient. The fact that you have or don't have bicarbonate in the feces does not mean that you are or are not producing bicarbonate. It depends on the overgrowth of the bacteria and the formation of lactic acid.

COMMENT: I was going to raise the question of the initial hydrating solution mentioned. If I understood correctly, it was said that a one to one solution (which should be about 75 mEq sodium/L) was being used. Do you include 5% dextrose in that solution as well?

RESPONSE: Yes. We use one part of saline and one part of 5% glucose in water.

QUESTION: Some individuals recommend that the initial hydrating solution for fluid and electrolytes deprivation, if the patient is in shock, contain albumin. They state that the most physiological approach is to administer something like albumin so that all the administered volume stays intravascularly. Although that makes physiologic sense, my impression has been that if you give balanced salt solution and you give enough of it rapidly, you accomplish the same thing. I am not aware of anybody running into complications from the rapid change of sodium in that first hour or two until you know what the serum sodium is. What has your experience been?

RESPONSE: We have been using for many years this one to one solution and we have found that it works very, very well. No complications except in some circumstances where they have been very worried because the infant does not start urinating and so they repeat the same load two or three times and then they get into trouble. Doing this in the first hour never seems to cause any complications. Now we haven't used albumin for obvious reasons. It's very expensive and we have had very good results just with the one to one solution. So we don't think it's necessary to go into another type of treatment.

MODERATOR: One of the panelists wants to say something but I don't want to leave this subject yet. Are you going to modify the question?

COMMENT: I am going to modify the treatment! I think the question of the bolus to be given to dehydrated children coming to the Emergency Room or Pediatric Walk-In Service is a question which depends on each place. Any child who is dehydrated has a depletion of the extracellular volume. When the child comes to the Emergency Room, you don't need to give a solution adapted to the type of dehydration because you want to expand the volume, to better perfuse the tissues. I disagree with the speakers that earlier presented their schemes of treatment. I always use isotonic saline to produce the expansion, whatever the type of dehydration. The Pediatric Resident doesn't care. Here comes the child and he/she puts the isotonic saline infusion. You have time--about one hour--to figure out the type, evaluate the signs, etc. It's a routine. The thing that changes is the amount of fluid; initially, we give 20-40 ml/kg if he is severely dehydrated, with marked signs of extracellular depletion. We give less, 10-20 ml/kg if the child is hypertonic. But always the same solution. There may be only two differences: if the child is very severely acidotic because he looks very severely acidotic, we replace the isotonic saline with isotonic bicarbonate solution - 1/6 molar bicarbonate solution. We do the same expansion at the same time. We don't put chloride, we just put bicarbonate and we have the same results. After this first hour the child has some correction of the acidosis. If after one hour of 10 ml/kg in the very hypernatremic or 40 ml/kg in the very severely hypovolemic child, if we don't have correction of the shock, then we proceed in another hour with oncotic solutions as was suggested just a while ago. If you infuse with isotonic solution a child who has a serum sodium of 175 mEq/L, you are diluting his serum; you don't need to use a solution of 30 mEq/L with the risk of convulsions due to a very sudden drop in plasma osmolality. I can also tell you that for many years this scheme has worked and continues to work well. Each one should stick to one scheme and evaluate the results until the best one for him/her is found.

MODERATOR: Our experience was similar in working with those babies from Brooklyn that I mentioned earlier. We had no problems in following such an approach.

COMMENT: The decision as to what initial expanding solution one should use, at one time I was conservative and did use a half-isotonic solution as a hedge against the possibility that we might be dealing with a hypernatremic infant. We didn't know at the time the infant presented what the serum sodium was, but it seemed prudent to provide a solution that had some free water as a hedge against the possibility of hypernatremia. I've tended to adopt basically the position of one of the members of the Panel, in that an isotonic solution is perfectly satisfactory because, as has been pointed out, the possibility of hypotensive shock in an infant with hypernatremia is practically nonexistent. The pathogenesis of that form of dehydration is such that there is a shift in water into the extracellular fluid so they are, in a sense, somewhat less extracellularly volume depleted than the patient who has isonatremia or hypotonic dehydration. I think the ones who in fact do present critical emergencies in terms of intravascular volume depletion are the occasional patients with isotonic or hypotonic dehydration. As a matter of fact, an isotonic expanding fluid, a pulse type infusion, would probably cover most of the situations.

COMMENT: I agree and would like to add a few words more in favor of the last scheme which is also the last one of many we have used at my hospital. It's not my scheme but I say the last one because we have passed through all these experiences before and we have seen the problem of the scleredema that develops in many of the small infants - particularly those with malnutrition. In those cases we have seen that, if we start by giving too much sodium, then the total amount allowed in these children has been administered rapidly and we have very little sodium we can give to them afterwards. That is one of the reasons we stopped using the half-strength saline which is not needed for expanding the extracellular fluid and increases the risks by giving more sodium.

COMMENT: When you give a bolus or a high rate infusion in a hyponatremic child, or in an isotonic child, you want to treat volume depletion, but why give it in a hypernatremic child? You say it is not necessary; it is necessary because if not, the child takes many,many hours to put urine because he is very hypernatremic. Your plan of hydration being two or three days, that will take a very long time to put urine. If you expand extracellular volume despite this hypernatremia, you will go slowly with hydration and you will get the urine much faster. You will have the stimulus of hypernatremia, but you will not have anymore the stimulus of hypovolemia. I think the aim is different for the expansion in the severely volume depleted child than in the less volume depleted child. The volume administered should be smaller in the less volume depleted but in every case you have benefits from this systematic approach.

COMMENT: I think it is more risky to try to correct very quickly the depleted volume in the hypernatremic child because the risk in hypernatremia is that you may cause acute changes in sodium concentration or in fluid concentration. That is one of the reasons why the treatment of hypernatremic dehydration has switched through the years from a time when we used to give only a glucose solution to the time when we are now giving more and more sodium in the solution in order not to make these big changes in the patients. They can get cerebral damage either by sodium excess or by changes from sodium excess to fluid excess.

COMMENT: In view of the outline presented about the type of solutions to use in rehydration, does Ringer's lactate have a place in this kind of therapy?

RESPONSE: I am sure you are now referring to replacement over the first 24 hours or so. Lactate Ringer's is an isotonic solution and on the average most children with isotonic dehydration require some of a more dilute solution in the area of the sodium concentration in the final solution of around 50-60 mEq/L. Lactate Ringer's, being an isotonic solution, does not have the free water that the other types of solution have. I think that since most of the time we deal with isotonic dehydration as we work it out on the average, that seems to be a very sterotypical solution that we come up with: 0.33% saline and 5% dextrose.

QUESTION: It surprised me that you used the 0.3% saline. I don't quite understand the role of hypo-osmotic solutions in hypernatremic dehydration. I also wanted to ask over how long a period do you try to protract your rehydration of an infant with hypernatremic dehydration.

COMMENT: We work things out as exercises with our students. I have been through this many times. If you analyze a child with hypernatremic dehydration, the solution they really need is practically 25% dextrose but you can't give that. That will drop the serum sodium too rapidly. You must have some sodium in the solution. Following the recommendation of Finberg and others we decided on the quarter isotonic saline as being good all around to use as a replacement solution in the hypernatremic dehydrated patient. But again, on the basis of calculations, it could turn out that they would practically not need any sodium at all. But, to prevent too rapid a fall in extracellular sodium, this is the amount that Finberg seems to use.

QUESTION: Do you know for how long a period do you protract...

RESPONSE: Again, Finberg's recommendation is to replace the volume deficit in hypertonic dehydration more gradually than in isotonic dehydration, to take about two days for total correction. So, you correct about 50% of the deficit on the first day but include with the deficit the usual maintenance requirement.

COMMENT: If I can go back to the bolus correction for a minute, I think that everybody sitting at the table is correct. There is a multiplicity of different ways of approaching it. I don't want to give anybody the impression that I particularly feel that albumin is the therapy of choice. In my simplistic view the body is compartments and vascular volume, etc., the simple goal of bolus initial therapy is to place enough osmols into the intravascular compartment to correct shock. I would point out that a half-normal dilution with 5% dextrose is a hyperosmotic solution because of the dextrose and consequently it will tend to pull some volume into the interstitial compartment. Except for albumin, any other solution that you put in, despite the fact that we talk about flat boxes, the solution rapidly diffuses out of the intravascular and into the interstitial compartments. As long as you give enough back into the intravascular compartment you will stay ahead and you will end up with intravascular expansion and correction of shock. In terms of the hypernatremic individual, my view is somewhat similar to that of one of the Panelists in that, by correcting intravascular volume and interstitial volume, you will begin to see some urine output if you push a little quickly. Actually although I've talked about it for ten years, I've never seen shock in hypernatremic dehydration because the patient will die. I have had two experiences in the last couple of years of children with hypernatremic dehydration in shock who have survived which is indeed very unusual. The comment about hypernatremic dehydration and the reason as to why one wishes to correct in 48 to 72 hours, is that it appears that with the development of persistent hyperosmolality irrespective of the cause, one develops something in the intracellular compartment of the brain called idiogenic osmols, perhaps tertiary amino acids such as taurine which is released with time and that, unless you drop the serum osmolality slowly, apparently these idiogenic osmols cannot fold back into the tertiary protein structures. So, if you drop the osmolality too quickly, you now create a reverse gradient. That is one view of the pathogenesis of the seizures that occur with the rapid dropping of serum sodium. One final comment about the correction of hypernatremic dehydration, at least from our experience. Oftentimes, everything with the child will proceed very nicely and will get down to a sodium between 145 and 150 mEq/L and the treating physician will say, "I'm home free, things are going well, let us begin to refeed the child". In most places people don't think much about it and they will give as the first feeding, dextrose and water. You've got a starving hungry child and he will gobble down eight ounces and the sodium will drop from 147 to 132 mEq/L. Although it is all "in the normal range", he will have seizures. So, what we have done with the initial oral hydration is to make sure that there are some electrolytes in it. I would also like to ask the people in the panel what they do in terms of potassium. No one has mentioned potassium.

COMMENT: This was precisely what I wanted to say in the treatment of hypernatremic dehydration, starting with a very dilute fluid of 0.2% normal saline. The way Finberg suggests is to give potassium chloride so that the solute content would be about 70-80 mEq/L. The only problem would be if there is no urine production at the time. I would be very scared to give a solution of 0.2% sodium chloride as the treatment.

QUESTION: Without potassium or with potassium?

RESPONSE: If I give with potassium, then there is no problem. Then I am reaching 70-80 mEq/L as suggested by Finberg.

COMMENT: In the scheme that is in the handout, I neglected potassium only because I was assuming that that would be the normal replacement. We give 4 mEq/kg/day if there is urine output; it works for all the types of dehydration.

COMMENT: I forgot to mention that we start giving potassium as soon as we see that the infant has started voiding and then, for eutrophic infants, we give 3 mEq/kg/day. We have repeated Dr. Darrow's studies in malnourished children and we have found that in order to have a positive potassium balance it is necessary to give 6 mEq/kg/day. So, we add this amount to the solution we are giving as soon as we see that the infant has started urinating.

QUESTION: My question is to the panelist who advocated giving physiological saline as initial fluid. Do you suggest any modification for neonates? This is a problem one comes across, especially when one wants to differentiate between dehydration and acute renal shut-down.

RESPONSE: In neonates, in our experience, in the first few days of life, the problem is not dehydration; they are very sick, on the respirator, have hyaline membrane disease, or some other problem and the neonate does not put out urine. You have a two-three week old coming up with dehydration because of diarrhea; the approach will not be very different. But the question that was asked refers to the neonate who has oliguria. The question is what to do because the renal situation and the treatment should be completely different. You need to evaluate the clinical status of the patient. In addition, you should determine urine osmolality and probably indexes we are using to rule out acute renal failure. Let us say the child looks dehydrated, you have the history that the child has some weight loss and the urine osmolality is concentrated (on the range you would expect of a neonate); then, we use a hydration technique. After that, if the patient doesn't put urine, then we use a furosemide test of 1-2 mg/kg given intravenously. In this manner we can separate the organic from the functional acute renal failure. But, always making sure the hydration is correct, evaluate the clinical status, the urine output as far as it relates to urine osmolality and the age of the patient, and the response to furosemide. We are just completing a study, just getting the results of the value of tests to separate functional from organic renal failure in the premature and neonatal age in general. The results are not yet complete but I would say that the index of fractional sodium excretion which was mentioned earlier is good but there are some overlapping results of pre-renal and renal failure. This separation is dependent on the response to furosemide. Furosemide sensitive and furosemide resistant will be similar to pre-renal and renal causes, respectively. Just now we have the best index in the neonate; it is the urine creatinine to plasma creatinine ratio. For the time being, I don't have the data completely evaluated but it seems there is no overlapping on this ratio.

QUESTION: So, would you suggest before furosemide physiological (normal 0.9 %) saline 20 ml/kg/hr or half strength saline in the neonate?

RESPONSE: We don't use isotonic saline generally in these cases. I would say that it is not a child with acute dehydration. Generally we use a two to one solution to hydrate those patients.

QUESTION: What is your experience with glucose containing oral fluids in diarrhea? In my experience, abdominal distension has been a big problem; it is invariably present in these children with diarrhea and dehydration.

QUESTION: You mean only glucose, no electrolytes?

RESPONSE: No. Glucose-containing fluids with electrolytes.

RESPONSE: That is the usual formula that has been advised for oral rehydration. The glucose helps the sodium and chloride to be absorbed in the intestine, it's a good combination.

COMMENT: I was saying initially, it generally causes more distension. It is my experience that one has to go to intravenous therapy and then come to oral.

RESPONSE: It depends on the severity of the dehydration. If the patient is in shock, you are right. You have to start with intravenous fluid. It is not good to start with oral rehydration because in shock states the absorption of these fluids in the intestine is not very good. But, if the patient is not in shock, even if he's severely dehydrated but not in shock, you can start directly with an oral glucose and electrolyte solution. There are studies which indicate that there are good results even with more than 10% body weight reduction.

QUESTION: Could you comment on calcium metabolism in hypernatremic dehydration?

RESPONSE: All I can say is that there is a commonly observed phenomenon which is hypocalcemic tetany as referred to here earlier. For that reason, as a precaution, it is advisable to add calcium gluconate to the parenteral fluid. I'm not aware that the mechanism is understood but there seems to be that association. It's also Finberg's recommendation to include calcium in the replacement fluid.

COMMENT: I would like to comment about the fluid administration in newborn infants. I think it's important to make a distinction as to which newborn infant we are talking about. Also, we have to keep in mind that the therapy we use needs to take into account the increased insensible water loss using an artificial way to keep the infant's temperature.

QUESTION: I have a question about a problem we got into with an infant with hypernatremic dehydration that also had severe metabolic acidosis. Because of all the sodium we had to give with the sodium bicarbonate (without meaning to), we ended up pushing the sodium up even higher. How do you go about preventing this type of complication?

RESPONSE: I think it is a matter of balance - which one is higher or lower. For instance, if the hypernatremia is more than 170 mEq/L, we would be very careful but we can give some small amount of sodium bicarbonate to move from the risky levels. We don't routinely use sodium bicarbonate but if the CO_2 content is less than 5 mM/L, we can give 1-3 mEq/kg of sodium bicarbonate and then move to safer levels. Then we start to treat the hypernatremia in the usual way. So, it's a matter of making an evaluation of the risk factors and then to go into priorities - which one is more risky than the other.

COMMENT: I would tend to avoid the administration in bolus form of sodium bicarbonate in the usual one molar preparation, especially in an infant like that, and would take pains to give it more gradually over several hours, perhaps in the overall replacement fluid so that it is relatively dilute. The instances where you have to give sodium bicarbonate are fairly limited. If this child has acute renal failure on top of everything else, your hand may be forced. Whatever sodium you may give to a hypernatremic infant could all be accompanied by bicarbonate rather than by chloride as the anion. I think there are ways you can minimize getting into further hypernatremia.

QUESTION: What is the experience of the panel in treating metabolic alkalosis with intravenous hydrochloric acid? At what pH level do they institute that or is it based on some clinical signs or symptoms that would make one want to use it? Do you use it at all?

RESPONSE: I've given arginine hydrochloric acid once. The rest of the time by dealing with volume and chlorides, in our experience we have been able to avoid giving intravenous hydrochloric acid. The particular situation that we ran into was a child with cystic fibrosis who was in heart failure, on a ventilator, had post hypercapnic metabolic alkalosis, was on diuretics, did not want to give him any chloride etc., whose pH was so high we wanted to bring it down. That's the only personal experience I've had. I think in pediatric medicine, most of the time by tending to the other issues you can avoid having to give things such as intravenous hydrochloric acid.

COMMENT: I have never given hydrochloric acid. I don't think I've ever seen a clinical situation where it was really necessary although I can conceive of extremely alkalotic situations where you might be worried about hypocalcemia, the effect of alkalemia on cardiac function, etc. I agree with what was just said. If the alkalosis is the consequence of protracted vomiting or GI drainage where the patient continued to lose hydrochloric acid, one of the tricks the adult medicine people use is to give cymetidine; then it's a little easier to keep up with those losses.

QUESTION: In relation to the former question about the situation in which one has to give so much sodium bicarbonate to combat the acidosis and in a setting of hypernatremia, I think that doing a peritoneal dialysis is the answer. Is that not right?

COMMENT: When you get involved with the newborn in giving all these boluses of bicarbonate, I think the first question you should ask is "Should I have done it more slowly and kept something running into the IV drip?" The other thing is, occasionally you get yourself backed into the corner where you will have hypernatremia as a result of your therapy. We use two different approaches for dealing with that. One is to give Lasix, get a sodium diuresis, and then replace those losses with something that is a little more hypotonic. The other is to consider a peritoneal dialysis. One of the problems, if you get involved with peritoneal dialysis, is that many such infants who require that much bicarbonate have a lactic acidosis to begin with. If you use the normal lactate containing peritoneal dialysis solution you won't get anywhere. You have to make up a bicarbonate containing peritoneal dialysis solution. At 3 a.m. in the morning, that's usually a pain in the neck for most people. So, you really don't have many choices.

Another issue which we ought to address and about which I rarely hear anybody talk is just how much acidosis is bad. What is it about acidosis that is so bad? We all say that it's bad. Can you have a child with a blood pH of 7.2, 7.1, and not correct it? At what point is there agreement that they ought to be treated; what would I really treat? Although we all say we should treat, when you go and find out what is bad about acidemia - there's a bunch of theoretical reasons of course, but it's very hard to find facts.

MODERATOR: That's a good but too complicated question. For that we should ask for written answers. We are running out of time and there are more questions. Don't let that one go; we will get to it another time.

QUESTION: We found in many infants with hypernatremic dehydration a significant increase in the fibrin degradation products in urine. What is the reason for this finding?

RESPONSE: In our experience with hypernatremic dehydration, we have had quite an important number of cases with renal vein thrombosis. It is demonstrated that hypernatremia increases the viscosity of the blood. In some way this viscosity leads to some disseminated intravascular coagulation. It, in turn, leads to increased products of fibrin in the urine. Hypernatremic dehydration has this risk but to find increased fibrin products in the urine is not by itself the problem. The risk of renal vein thrombosis is a very important complication of hypernatremic dehydration - especially with an overloading of formula before the hypernatremic dehydration develops. It is more risky (when preceded by ingestion of hyperconcentrated milk) than the pure water loss hypernatremia.

QUESTION: Clinically did you have any indication of there being a renal vein thrombosis?

RESPONSE: No. It was found in the kidney biopsy of some of the children--intracapillary coagulation.

QUESTION: I would like to reiterate the question about acidosis, especially in the acidosis with hypernatremic dehydration. I agree that with this kind of dehydration we should begin treatment with isotonic sodium but at the risk of cerebral edema. But, I don't agree that the use of bicarbonate solution is necessary especially with the risk of rapid correction of acidosis. The first question is: if you use bicarbonate you will correct the blood pH, but not the spinal fluid pH. So, the brain still will have lower pH than the blood. Because of the shift in the oxygen dissociation curve, there still will be cerebral hypoxia and an increased risk of cerebral edema. The second question is: if you use bicarbonate, you increase $PaCO_2$ and then brain circulation will be higher and again, you have the risk of cerebral edema. This question we demonstrated there in the treatment of diabetic acidosis in dogs some months ago. I would like to hear the panel's opinion about the use of bicarbonate in this kind of dehydration.

MODERATOR: I might expand the question to the possibility of using THAM in situations where you are concerned about worsening the CSF pH by administration of large amounts of sodium bicarbonate.

RESPONSE: I didn't understand your question.

MODERATOR: I will not attempt to re-state the Registrant's question. I believe that what he is referring to is the information about sodium bicarbonate producing a decrease in the CSF pH as you correct the blood pH. This is something that has been confirmed in different studies; presumably it occurs because of the greater ease of diffusion of CO_2 formed in the blood than the blood bicarbonate ion. My question pertains to comparisons that were made between sodium bicarbonate and tris THAM. They showed that you do not get that decrease in the CSF pH because THAM diffuses much more rapidly into spinal fluid and inside cells than the bicarbonate ion; in addition, THAM does not generate CO_2 (it may actually decrease $PaCO_2$).

RESPONSE: I have had no experience with THAM. I would point out, as I recall, that it can be rather hepatotoxic. To come back to the original point about the correction, I think there's another point we are making. That is, if you raise the pH too quickly with the sodium bicarbonate solution, you alter the 2-3 DPG red cell level, the oxygen release, etc., in addition to cerebral blood flow problems and so on. A point which no one has mentioned is that when you are treating a number of these disorders, the ongoing production of acid is immense. Unless you can really do something about it, almost all of the bicarbonate you can give is going to be consumed. We come back again to the basics of trying to support circulation and oxygenation. Certainly, if you do that in infantile gastroenteritis, you can then raise serum bicarbonate quite slowly. Recently in our own institution we talked about raising serum bicarbonate one to two mEq/hour. If someone comes in with a bicarbonate of four, perhaps raise it up to eight in an hour or two and then try and go from quite slowly. The advantages of going slowly in terms of pH changes, CSF pH changes, cerebral blood flow, etc., far outweigh the disadvantages of giving hypertonic sodium. You add it all together, pay your money and take your options. The more we learn about acute anything in medicine, the more we learn it pays to go slow. That's where I would leave it.

MODERATOR: For the record, the information on the hepatotoxicity of THAM is based on one paper from London which was poorly designed and dogmatic in its conclusions. We had incomplete studies which did not confirm that statement even in neonates with intra-arterial or intravenous catheter. So that question has remained open at least in my mind. If I thought it was a desirable substance to use, I would not stop using it because of that unconfirmed and poorly documented statement about hepatotoxicity.

RESPONSE: I would agree. All drugs that are worth anything have toxicity. You always weigh the toxic-therapeutic ratio. That was not meant to imply not to use it. I am talking about its overall end result as a physiologic tool.

QUESTION: Did everyone understand my explanation about the decrease of bicarbonate in acute respiratory acidosis or should I explain it again? The speaker on that subject was right. When you add buffer to CO_2, you are increasing the amount of bicarbonate. Then, you should have to increase the bicarbonate when PCO_2 goes up. When you do your determination, this thing happens. But the things you compare in your results in the normogram don't take into account the diffusion of bicarbonate into interstitial fluids. The normogram was constructed having blood exposed to several levels of PCO_2, and shaking the chamber; in this manner, all the bicarbonate formed stays there. The normal line is built with this curve. When you get the blood from your patient and you put it in the machine, you get his curve. Then, when you put it in the normogram you get a negative difference. In the normal, say -4, -3, you get a minus base excess over lower bicarbonate not because the reaction is not taking place when bicarbonate decreases with acute acidosis but because the normogram is built from an in vitro titration and the blood you are taking is from an in vivo titration. In the latter all the bicarbonate has diffused to the interstitial fluid and you don't get it with your blood determination. I thought this question was not correctly answered. Now, it has been.

MODERATOR: With that optimistic note we must end this Panel Discussion. Thank you.

II

TUBULOPATHIES AND FLUID-ELECTROLYTES

CLEARANCE METHODOLOGY IN THE STUDY OF TUBULAR HANDLING OF WATER AND SODIUM

Juan Rodriguez-Soriano, M.D. and Alfredo Vallo, M.D.

The study of tubular reabsorption of water and sodium becomes very important in the functional examination of patients with renal tubular disorders. These human studies are limited to the application of clearance methods, which although less sophisticated than modern experimental techniques, retain the unique advantage of being relevant to the whole kidney "in situ" rather than to an isolated population of nephrons. When fractional clearances are calculated under conditions of hypotonic saline diuresis, a functional assessment of tubular handling of water and sodium becomes possible (1,2). This brief review examines the physiological basis of such clearance methodology, describes the experimental protocol and summarizes results in health and disease.

PHYSIOLOGICAL BASIS

The experiment should be performed during production of maximally diluted urine; that is, a situation when the rate of urine flow (V) greatly exceeds the value of osmolar clearance (Cosm). The difference between these values (V - Cosm) is called free water clearance (C_{H_2O}) and expresses the volume of tubular fluid which is "cleared" of solute during formation of hypotonic urine. The production of diluted urine is schematized in Figure 1. Normally about two-thirds of glomerular filtrate is reabsorbed isotonically along the proximal tubule whereas the remaining third becomes progressively hypertonic in the descending loop of Henle due to water outflow and solute inflow. At some point of the ascending loop of Henle which is impermeable to water reabsorption, the intratubular fluid again reaches isotonicity due to solute reabsorption. From this point beyond, in the so-called "diluting segments", almost no water reabsorption will be present in the absence of antidiuretic hormone (ADH), and continuous solute reabsorption will lead to the formation of hypotonic urine. Since maximal free water clearance is used as an index of NaCl reabsorption in the diluting segments, it is important to consider the factors upon which such large water diuresis is dependent (3).

1. Impermeability of the diluting segments to water. This condition is best accomplished by complete endogenous ADH suppression, as obtained by an oral water load and subsequent infusion of hypotonic fluids. Direct stimuli of ADH release such as stress, painful procedures, etc. should be avoided. It must be understood, however, that even in the absence of circulating ADH, the distal

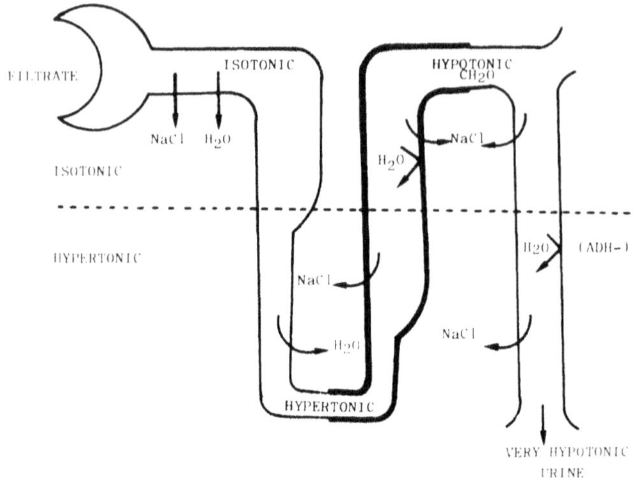

FIGURE 1. Representation of renal diluting mechanism.

nephron is not completely watertight and some ADH-independent water reabsorption is impossible to quantitate or prevent. The error introduced by that phenomenon in the estimation of distal NaCl reabsorption is probably small, providing that a minimal urinary osmolality of about 50 mOsm/L is present. The measurement of plasma arginine-vasopressin is a useful tool to validate that a higher urinary osmolality is due to a defect in distal NaCl reabsorption rather than to a situation of incomplete ADH suppression (4).

2. Adequate delivery of tubular fluid to the diluting segments. Adequate volume of fluid must be filtered and escape proximal reabsorption to allow for maximal water diuresis. To obtain such increased distal delivery of filtrate, a small degree of extracellular fluid volume expansion becomes necessary since other maneuvers such as infusion of hypotonic mannitol or administration of osmotic diuretics are not properly physiological.
3. Adequate reabsorption of solute in the diluting segments. Continuous reabsorption of NaCl is necessary to bring about the formation of free water. This is the tubular function we intend to explore by this experimental technique. To ascertain the validity of the results, it is important to be sure that all filtered NaCl leaving the proximal nephron and reaching the diluting segments is available for reabsorption and can serve as substrate for free water formation.

INTERPRETATION OF DATA

When all previous requirements for maximal water diuresis are accomplished, some derived terms based on the measurement of fractional clearances can be used to assess the proportion of glomerular filtrate being reabsorbed along either the proximal or the distal part of the nephron. The terms "proximal" and "distal" do not have a topographic meaning and refer to the parts of the nephron up to or beyond the point of the ascending loop of Henle where the tubular fluid starts to become hypotonic.

Assessment of proximal tubular function

Several terms can be used to express distal delivery of filtrate to the diluting segments; that is, the proportion of the filtered load escaping reabsorption in the "proximal" -in the functional sense- part of the nephron (2).

"Volume" term (V/GFR). The fractional urine volume approximates distal delivery of filtrate providing there is almost complete impermeability to water of the distal diluting segments of the nephron. This term reflects more precisely the functional ability of the proximal nephron when water diuresis is achieved by a pure water load since extracellular fluid volume expansion and osmotic diuretics (glucose, mannitol) will necessarily increase the proportion of glomerular filtrate entering the distal tubule.

"Sodium" term ($C_{H_2O} + C_{Na}$/GFR). This expression of distal sodium delivery, widely used since it was proposed by Seldin and Rector (1), is based on the assumption that all NaCl leaving the proximal nephron either is reabsorbed along the diluting segments and leads to the formation of free water (C_{H_2O}) or escapes reabsorption and appears in the urine (C_{Na}), Although this term is not altered by the presence of osmotic diuresis, it does not take into account the sodium reabsorbed distally by exchange with potassium and hydrogen ion. The degree of such exchanges is probably small under the conditions of the experiment since extracellular fluid volume expansion will inhibit aldosterone release, but under particular circumstances the following considerations should be taken into account: 1) exchange of sodium with potassium decreases the value of C_{Na} but does not change the value of C_{H_2O}. Distal delivery of sodium is therefore underestimated. When a high potassium clearance is present, the term $C_{H_2O} + C_{Na+K}$ is more reliable and closely approximates the value of the "chloride" term (5); 2) exchange of sodium with hydrogen ion will not change the value of distal sodium delivery since the decrease in C_{Na} will be compensated by a simultaneous increase in C_{H_2O}. When an important bicarbonaturia is present, this exchange plays little role in distal sodium reabsorption, but the increased amount of bicarbonate reaching the distal segments makes difficult sodium reabsorption and free water formation since the bicarbonate behaves as a poorly reabsorbable anion and obligates the excretion of proportionate quantities of sodium (6). As pointed out by Danovitch (2), the "sodium" term is not suitable for studies in which significant amounts of bicarbonate are present in the urine, as is the case in patients with renal tubular acidosis (7).

"Chloride" term ($C_{H_2O} + C_{Cl}$/ GFR). This term has been recently proposed (2,6) to avoid the previously discussed disadvantages of the "volume" and "sodium" terms. It is based on the assumption that all chloride leaving the proximal segment either is reabsorbed with sodium or it appears in the urine. It retains also the important property of being unaltered by the presence of bicarbonate in the urine and thus is completely reliable in the presence of bicarbonate diuresis (2,6). When fractional clearances during hypotonic saline diuresis are calculated in normal individuals, all terms ($C_{H_2O} + C_{Na}$, $C_{H_2O} + C_{Na+K}$, $C_{H_2O} + C_{Cl}$)

are of similar value, but distinctions are important when the investigator is confronted with pathological situations such as Bartters syndrome, where the "chloride" term gives the more reliable assessment of both proximal and distal tubular functions (5).

Assessment of distal tubular function

As already discussed, the value of maximal free water clearance expresses the ability of the distal diluting segments to reabsorb the NaCl leaving the proximal segment. A meaningful interpretation of such distal ability must necessarily take into account the value of distal sodium delivery; that is, the proportion of the load being offered for reabsorption (Fig. 2). The ratios, $C_{H_2O}/C_{H_2O} + C_{Na} \times 100$, $C_{H_2O}/C_{CH_2O} + C_{Cl} \times 100$, represent, therefore, the percentage of the distal load being reabsorbed distally and examine functionally the adequacy of such reabsorption in function of the load. In Figure 2, these ratios are expressed by the broken diagonal lines. It can be observed that low or high values of C_{H_2O} do not necessarily represent an abnormal situation since they can be proportional to a low or high distal delivery, respectively. We should only refer to a defect in distal NaCl reabsorption when the value of free water clearance, even related to distal load, is significantly lower than values found in normal subjects studied under identical experimental conditions.

EXPERIMENTAL PROTOCOL OF HYPOTONIC SALINE DIURESIS

We use a modification of the protocol given by Chaimovitz et al. (8). In the morning of the test, each subject receives an oral water load of 20 ml/kg body weight over a 30 minute period. This is followed by the intravenous infusion of 0.45 percent saline at a rate of 1,000 ml/hr/1.73 m^2 body surface, over a period of two hours. We do not adjust the rate of infusion to urinary flow to avoid dangerous extracellular fluid volume expansion in patients with renal disease. In our opinion such a maneuveris not necessary providing minimal urinary

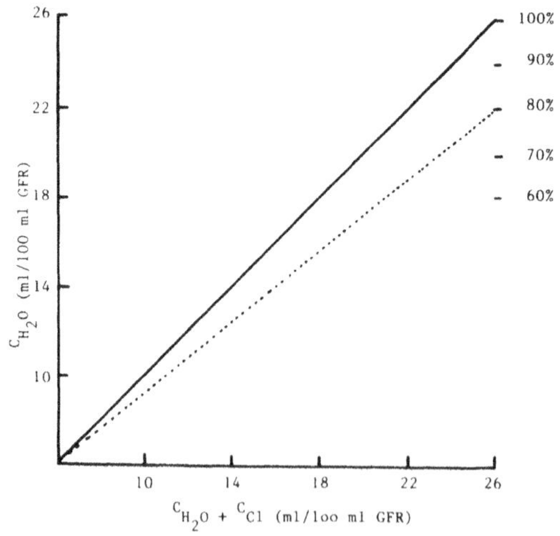

FIGURE 2. Free water clearance (C_{H_2O}) is plotted as a function of distal delivery, represented here by the "chloride" term ($C_{H_2O} + C_{Cl}$). The broken diagonal line indicates the normal relationship between both variables.

osmolalities are reached; only the period of maximal free water clearance is taken into consideration for calculation of results. A unique advantage of the test is that bladder catheterization is unnecessary since results of each period of spontaneous urine collection are factored by GFR so that accuracy in such urine collections is not required. To calculate GFR, however, and to obviate such inaccuracy of individual collection periods, the average value of all collection periods should be considered. Specimens of urine are obtained at 20 minute intervals, and blood samples are drawn between urine collections from an indwelling needle that is flushed with slightly heparinized isotonic saline solution after each sampling. An estimated serum value at the midpoint of each urine collection is used for clearance calculations.

CLEARANCE CALCULATIONS

The following calculations are used to derive the values of fractional clearances, all expressed in ml/100 ml GFR.

$$V / GFR : \frac{P_{Cr}}{U_{Cr}} \times 100$$

$$C_{Osm} / GFR : \frac{V/GFR \times U_{Osm}}{P_{Osm}}$$

$$C_{Na} / GFR : \frac{V/GFR \times U_{Na}}{P_{Na}}$$

$$C_{Cl} / GFR : \frac{V/GFR \times U_{Cl}}{P_{Cl}}$$

$$C_{K} / GFR : \frac{V/GFR \times U_{K}}{P_{K}}$$

$$C_{H_2O} / GFR : V/GFR - C_{Osm} / GFR$$

RESULTS IN NORMAL INFANTS AND CHILDREN

We have recently studied with this technique a group of normal infants and children (9). The study included 22 infants aged one week to 15 months and 17 children aged two to 12 years. All had normal growth and development and in no case were renal abnormalities present. A summary of results is presented in Table 1. Infants showed significantly higher values for osmolar, sodium, potassium and chloride clearances, but urinary osmolality was identical in both groups. Fractional urine volume (V), and fractional distal NaCl delivery ($C_{H_2O} + C_{Na}$, $C_{H_2O} + C_{Cl}$)

Table 1. Summary of Data from Period of Maximal Free Water Clearance Obtained in Normal Subjects (Mean ± SD) (9).

	Infants (n = 22)	Children (n = 17)	p
U_{Osm}, mOsm/kg	51.8 ± 12.8	54.1 ± 13.3	NS
V, ml/100 ml GF	22.8 ± 3.6	17.2 ± 2.7	< 0.0005
C_{Osm}, ml/100 ml GF	4.3 ± 1.3	3.2 ± 0.7	< 0.0025
C_{H_2O}, ml/100 ml GF	18.5 ± 2.9	14.0 ± 2.6	< 0.0005
C_{Na}, ml/100 ml GF	1.9 ± 0.8	1.4 ± 0.4	< 0.01
C_{Cl}, ml/100 ml GF	2.7 ± 1.1	2.1 ± 0.7	< 0.05
C_K, ml/100 ml GF	19.9 ± 12.0	12.9 ± 5.2	< 0.025
$C_{H_2O} + C_{Na}$, ml/100 ml GF	20.4 ± 2.9	15.3 ± 2.3	< 0.0005
$C_{H_2O} + C_{Cl}$, ml/100 ml GF	21.2 ± 3.1	15.9 ± 2.6	< 0.0005
$C_{H_2O} / C_{H_2O} + C_{Na}$ x 100, %	90.8 ± 4.5	90.9 ± 3.3	NS
$C_{H_2O} / C_{H_2O} + C_{Cl}$ x 100, %	87.2 ± 5.3	86.7 ± 4.1	NS
C_{Cr}, ml/min 1.73/m^2	88.5 ± 27.1	124.8 ± 25.2	< 0.0005

Abbreviations: U_{Osm}, urine osmolality; V, urine volume; C_{Osm}, osmolar clearance; C_{Na}, C_{Cl}, C_K, sodium, chloride and potassium clearances, respectively; $C_{H_2O} + C_{Na}$, $C_{H_2O} + C_{Cl}$, distal NaCl delivery; $C_{H_2O}/ C_{H_2O} + C_{Na}$, $C_{H_2O} / C_{H_2O} + C_{Cl}$, percentage of distal NaCl reabsorption; C_{Cr}, creatinine clearance; NS = not significant.

were significantly higher in infancy. Since no important hyperkaliuria nor bicarbonaturia were present, the values of distal delivery calculated by either the "sodium" or the "chloride" terms were almost identical. Sodium chloride reabsorption at the diluting segments, estimated by the value of C_{H_2O}, was significantly higher in infants than in children. This finding implies an important compensatory distal reabsorption of the proportionally higher amount of filtrate escaping proximal reabsorption in infancy. As a consequence, the proportion of the load reabsorbed distally, estimated by the ratios $C_{H_2O}/C_{H_2O}+C_{Na}$x 100 or $C_{H_2O}/C_{H_2O}+C_{Cl}$x 100, was identical in both groups. When distal NaCl reabsorption was correlated with the age of the subject, no significant correlation was present beyond two years of age, but it was present in infancy: the younger the infant, the higher the value of fractional distal delivery; that is, the lower the proportion of filtered load reabsorbed proximally. The same negative correlation existed in infancy, but not in childhood, between the value of free water clearance and age.

The previous data in normal subjects indicate that, at least under conditions of extracellular fluid volume expansion, proximal sodium reabsorption lags behind glomerular filtration during the first year of life but an exaggerated sodium loss is not present because of the existence of a compensatory increase in distal sodium reabsorption during that age span.

RESULTS IN SOME RENAL DISORDERS

In our hands the study of fractional clearances during hypotonic saline diuresis has become a very useful tool in the functional examination of various tubular disorders. We shall briefly discuss results in patients with renal tubular acidosis, Bartter's syndrome and nephrogenic diabetes insipidus.

Renal tubular acidosis

We have recently published the results obtained in 14 patients with renal tubular acidosis (RTA): nine patients had proximal RTA, secondary to Fanconi syndrome, and five patients had primary distal RTA (7). Data are summarized in Figure 3. It can be observed that patients with proximal RTA presented mainly an impaired reabsorption of sodium in the proximal segment, which although in part was compensated by an absolute increase in distal sodium reabsorption, did oblige to the excretion of an excessive fraction of the filtered NaCl. In patients with distal RTA, proximal tubular reabsorption was not impaired but there did exist an incapacity to reabsorb adequately the normal distal sodium load due to an isolated defect of sodium reabsorption in the distal diluting segments. These results are in agreement with findings by other authors using similar or different techniques (10, 11), and are compatible with the current concepts on the localization of the tubular pathology in each type of renal tubular acidosis.

Bartters syndrome

The more proximal defect in Bartters syndrome is believed to be an impaired chloride reabsorption in the thick ascending loop of Henle. The increased arrival of NaCl to more distal segments will lead sequentially to increased potassium secretion, plasma and cellular potassium depletion, increased renal and vascular prostaglandin production, increased activity of the axis renin-angiotensin-aldosterone and increased peripheral resistence to the pressor effects of angiotensin and norepinephrine (12). The test of hypotonic saline diuresis becomes a necessary tool to establish the diagnosis since the demonstration of a defect in distal chloride reabsorption is a constant finding in this disease (4,5,8,13,14). When such finding is absent, a syndrome mimicking but

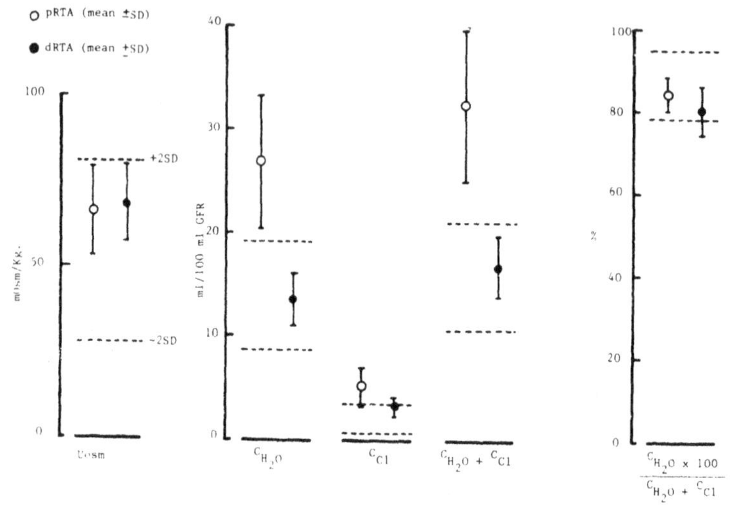

FIGURE 3. Results in 14 children with renal tubular acidosis (RTA): 9 patients with proximal RTA (pRTA) and 5 patients with distal RTA (dRTA). Broken horizontal lines represent range of values in normal children (9).

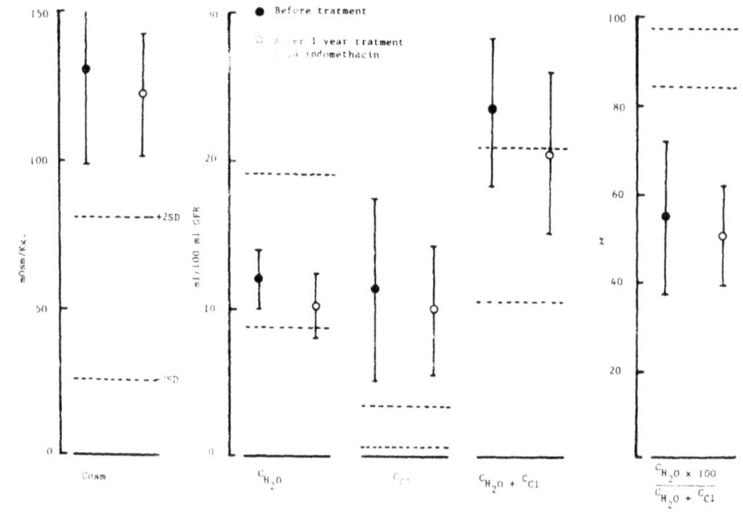

FIGURE 4. Results in 4 children with Bartter's syndrome, before and after one year of treatment with indomethacin. (Mean ± SD). Broken horizontal lines represent range of values in normal children (9).

different from Bartters syndrome must be suspected, either secondary to subreptitious vomiting (5,15) or representing a pathogenically different familial entity (16).

In Figure 4 we report data in four children with Bartters syndrome, before and one year after therapy with indomethacin. It can be observed that the percentage of distal chloride reabsorption is below normal values in all cases, and that it is not modified by treatment with indomethacin. The modest increase in distal NaCl delivery found in our patients before treatment occasionally has been observed by other authors (5), and since there is progressive normalization with indomethacin therapy, it represents probably a secondary proximal defect which is variably demonstrated depending on the state of sodium balance, GFR, and the balance of action between the vasoactive hormones: angiotensin, bradykinin and prostaglandins (14).

Nephrogenic diabetes insipidus

The finding by Crawford and Kennedy (17) that administration of thiazides to patients with nephrogenic diabetes insipidus is followed by a diminution of urinary volume has greatly facilitated the management of such patients, especially during infancy. The beneficial action of the diuretics is believed to be secondary to a contraction of extracellular fluid volume which leads to an increased reabsorption of filtrate in the proximal tubule (18). This hypothesis is graphically demonstrated in Figure 5. Data correspond to two infants with hereditary nephrogenic diabetes insipidus, before and after treatment

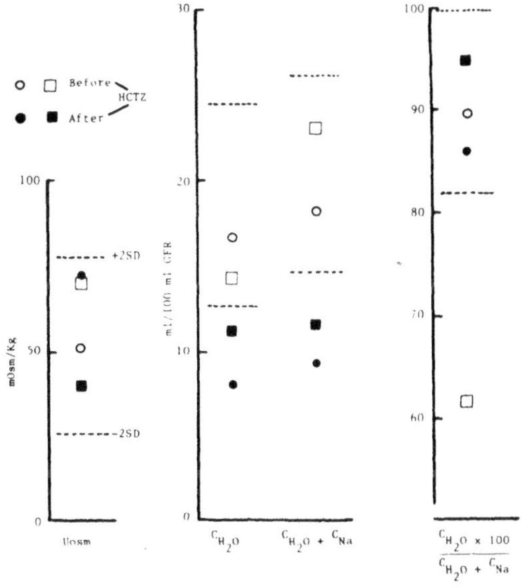

FIGURE 5. Results in 2 infants with hereditary nephrogenic diabetes insipidus, before and after treatment with hydrochlorothiazide (HCTZ). Broken diagonal lines represent range of values in normal infants (9).

with hydrochlorothiazide. Following treatment with the diuretic, a marked decrease in the values of distal sodium delivery is observed, indicating increased reabsorption of filtrate in the proximal tubule. The decrease in urinary volume will represent a necessary consequence. Similar findings after hydrochlorothiazide therapy have been reported in two patients with cystinosis (10), indicating that the beneficial action of this therapy in patients with proximal tubular disorders is also probably mediated by an increase in the proximal tubular reabsorption of filtrate.

CONCLUSIONS

The study of fractional clearances during hypotonic saline diuresis provides useful information about the function of specific segments of the nephron. It is easy to perform technically and has the special advantage of making unnecessary the catheterization of the patient, since all results are factored by GFR. The interpretation of the results, however, should always be regarded with the limitations derived from the physiological assumptions upon which the test is based. Although in experimental investigation more sophisticated and reliable techniques are available, in human studies the conclusions provided by clearance studies have greatly contributed to the understanding of renal tubular function in health and disease.

REFERENCES

1. Seldin, D.W. and Rector, F.C.: Evaluation of clearance methods for localization of the site of action of diuretics in modern diuretic therapy in the treatment of cardiovascular and renal disease. In Modern Diuretics Therapy in the Treatment of Cardiovascular and Renal Disease. Amsterdam: Excerpta Medica, 1972, p. 97.
2. Danovitch, G.M.: Clearance methodology in the study of the function of the distal tubule. Renal Physiol. 1:56, 1978.
3. Hays, R.M. and Levine, S.D.: Pathophysiology of water metabolism. In Brenner B.M. and Rector, F.C. (eds.): The Kidney. Philadelphia, W.B. Saunders, 1976, vol. 1, p. 553.
4. Baehler, R.W., Work, J., Kotchen, T.A., et al.: Studies on the pathogenesis of Bartter's syndrome. Am. J. Med. 69:933, 1980.
5. Gill, J.R. Jr. and Bartter, F.C.: Evidence for a prostaglandin-independent defect in chloride reabsorption in the loop of Henle as a proximal cause of Bartter's syndrome. Am. J. Med. 65:766, 1978.
6. Danovitch, G.M. and Bricker, N.S.: Influence of volume expansion on NaCl reabsorption in the diluting segments of the nephron: A study using clearance methods. Kidney Int. 10:229, 1976.
7. Rodriguez-Soriano, J., Vallo, A., Castillo, G. et al.: Renal handling of water and sodium in children with proximal and distal renal tubular acidosis. Nephron 25:193, 1980.
8. Chaimovitz, C., Levi, J., Better, O.S., et al.: Studies on the site of renal salt loss in a patient with Bartter's syndrome. Pediat. Res. 7:89, 1973.

9. Rodriguez-Soriano, J., Vallo, A., Castillo, G. et al.: Renal handling of water and sodium in infancy and childhood: A study using clearance methods during hypotonic saline diuresis. Kidney Int. (In press).
10. Callis, L., Castello, F., Vila, A. et al.: Studies on the site of renal sodium loss in two patients with cystinosis. Nephron 18:35, 1977.
11. Sebastian, A., McSherry, E., and Morris, R.C. Jr.: Impaired renal conservation of sodium and chloride during sustained correction of systemic acidosis in patients with type 1, classic renal tubular acidosis. J. Clin. Invest. 58:454, 1976.
12. Bartter, F.C.: On the pathogenesis of Bartter's syndrome. Mineral Electrolyte Metab. 3:61, 1980.
13. Rodriguez-Soriano, J., Vallo, A. and Oliveros, R.: Bartter's syndrome presenting with features resembling renal tubular acidosis. Improvement of renal tubular defects by indomethacin. Helv. Paediat. Acta 33:141, 1978.
14. Delaney, V.B., Oliver, J.F., Simms, M., et al.: Bartter's syndrome. Physiological and pharmacological studies. Quart. J. Med., New Series, 198:213, 1981.
15. Veldhuis, J.D., Bardin, C.W. and Demers, L.M.: Metabolic mimicry of Bartter's syndrome by covert vomiting. Utility of urinary chloride determinations. Am. J. Med. 66:361, 1979.
16. Güllner, H.G., Gill, J.R. Jr., Bartter, F.C., et al.: A familial disorder with hypokalemic alkalosis hyperreninemia, aldosteronism, high urinary prostaglandins and normal blood pressure that is not "Bartter's syndrome". Trans. Ass. Am. Physns.92:175, 1979.
17. Crawford, J.D. and Kennedy, G.C.: Chlorothiazide in diabetes insipidus. Nature 183:891, 1959.
18. Martinez-Maldonado, M., Eknoyan, G. and Suki, W.N.: Diuretics in nonedematous states. Physiological basis for the clinical use. Arch. Intern. Med. 131:797, 1973.

SICKLE CELL NEPHROPATHY

Carlos A. Vaamonde, M.D.

Herrick in 1910 gave the first known published description of renal involvement, although sickle cell disease had long been recognized in West Africa (1,2). He described "peculiarly elongated and sickle-shaped" red blood cells in a young black student from Grenada with anemia, white blood cells and casts in the urine, slightly increased urine output, and low urinary specific gravity. In the following years, a number of studies described the renal functional and structural abnormalities in such patients. Although the term sickle cell nephropathy has been used to describe many of the renal lesions found in patients with sickle cell disorders, recently it has been most often limited to the setting of proteinuria with predominantly glomerular lesions; Friedman et al. (3) imply that it may represent a state of life-threatening renal failure. It is only recently that the study of these lesions gained momentum in comparison to the massive body of literature related to hematuria and the disordered concentrating ability and hemodynamics. Excellent reviews of the general and renal aspects of these disorders have been published (2,4-6).

The following definitions are currently accepted and will be used throughout this review: Sickle cell disease involves the possession of two abnormal allelomorphic genes related to hemoglobin formation, with at least one of them being the gene for hemoglobin S. The genotypes that constitute sickle cell disease are thus sickle cell anemia (HbSS), sickle cell-hemoglobin C disease (HbSC), sickle cell-thalassemia disease (HbSThal), and so on. Therefore, although often used as a synonym for sickle cell anemia, the term sickle cell disease does not necessarily imply the presence of the homozygous HbSS state. The term trait is reserved for the heterozygous state involving a normal gene (A) with an abnormal gene: sickle cell trait (HbAS), hemoglobin C trait (HbAC), and so on.

Although accurate statistics are not available, the relative incidences of the various sickle cell hemoglobinopathies in the black population in the United States are approximately 8% for HbAS, 0.2% for HbSS, 2% for HbAC, and 0.04% for HbSC. There are no accurate data for the incidence of the various renal abnormalities.

Certain hematologic considerations related to hemoglobin S are important in understanding the pathophysiology of the renal abnormalities in sickle cell disease. Hemoglobin S polymerizes during deoxygenation, increasing its internal viscosity and forming a gel, which causes the irregular, sickled shape of the red blood cells and their loss of the flexibility needed for normal, free circulation. The polymerization of the hemoglobin S requires certain conditions, among which are low oxygen tension, hypertonicity, and low pH (2). Since these conditions exist in the renal medulla, sickling should be expected in this location. Indeed, renal functions requiring a normal medulla and papilla (e.g., concentrating ability, acidification) are perturbed in sickle cell disease, and medullary and papillary necrosis, focal scarring, and interstitial fibrosis have been described (2,4,5). Thus, medullary and papillary dysfunction and anatomic distortion have a predominant role in determining the renal abnormalities in sickle cell disease.

In this chapter, we will discuss the most important renal morphologic and clinical abnormalities of sickle cell disease and only some selected functional abnormalities (Table 1). We will omit the description of the altered renal hemodynamics and renal concentrating ability since these can be found in many published reviews and articles (2,4-6). Likewise, the few functional perturbations that we have chosen are those less well known or recognized more recently.

TABLE 1. Renal Abnormalities in Sickle Cell Disease

Functional	
1.	Perturbed renal hemodynamics
2.	Renal concentrating defect
3.	Impaired renal acidification
4.	Uric acid metabolism
5.	Others (Na,K)
Clinical	
6.	Hyposthenuria. Enuresis
7.	Hematuria
8.	Papillary necrosis
9.	Glomerulonephritis, Nephrotic syndrome
10.	Renal failure

SICKLE CELL NEPHROPATHY

Morphologic findings

The first description of the histologic changes in the kidneys of patients with sickle cell anemia seems to be that of Sydenstricked et al. (7), who found distended glomeruli and necrotic tubules containing deposits of pigments. In 1934, Diggs and Ching reported congestion of the small renal blood vessels, pigmentation, and scarring (8). Subsequently, renal medullary infarctions (9); hemorrhage in the interstitium, tubules, and pelvis without glomerular involvement (10); and glomerular enlargement, congestion, and fibrosis (11,12) were described. Glomerular basement membrane changes were first reported in detail in 1969 by McCoy (13) and more recently by others (14,15). Similar findings were subsequently reported by Strauss et al. (16), Pardo et al. (17), and other investigators (18,19).

Gross changes. Macroscopic examination typically reveals kidneys of normal or increased size (5,20). The external surface is often irregularly and finely scarred. Hemorrhage is common, particularly under the mucosa of the pelvis (10), as are white subcapsular infarcts (10) and papillary necrosis. Radiologic examination may reveal papillary necrosis, caliectasis, and renal vein thrombosis (20a).

Microscopic changes. In general, the congested, often enlarged glomeruli and interstitium of patients with sickle cell nephropathy have distended capillaries, sometimes filled with closely packed aggregates of sickled red blood cells; the juxtamedullary glomeruli appear to be particularly affected (11,14). There may be dilatation of the afferent and efferent arterioles. Glomerular fibrosis may be lobular and either focal or diffuse (11), and periglomerular fibrosis may be seen (21). In some patients (mainly older children and adults) obsolescence of glomeruli is noted, along with interstitial fibrosis (11,22), cortical infarcts and proximal tubular deposits of iron pigment. Tubules are often dilated and atrophic and contain large, pigmented casts (12). The medulla and papilla show edema, capillary and vasa recta congestion, interstitial fibrosis, medullary infarcts, papillary necrosis, and areas with lesions indistinguishable from those of chronic pylonephritis.

Recently, much interest has centered on the glomerular alterations, with the recognition that some patients demonstrate changes characteristic of membranoproliferative glomerulonephritis with capsular adhesions, basement membrane thickening and splitting (with partial circumferential mesangial interposition [23], cellular proliferation, and an increase in mesangial matrix).

Electron and immunofluorescent microscopy. (12,13,17,22) Electron microscopy has demonstrated focal fusion of the epithelial foot processes (14,16,18,19). The basement membrane may show focal thickening, occasional duplication due to mesangial interposition, and, rarely, small granular deposits. The mesangial matrix may be increased and may contain fibrillar material. The mesangial cell cytoplasm may reveal prominent homogeneous to granular, occasionally lamellated, electron-dense material (Fig. 1), some of which has been thought to represent accumulations of iron-protein complexes. Immunofluorescent evaluation has demonstrated the localization of renal proximal tubular epithelial (RTE) antigen in association with immunoglobulins G and M and the C1q fraction of the first and third component of complement arranged in a granular pattern along the glomerular basement membrane (16,17).

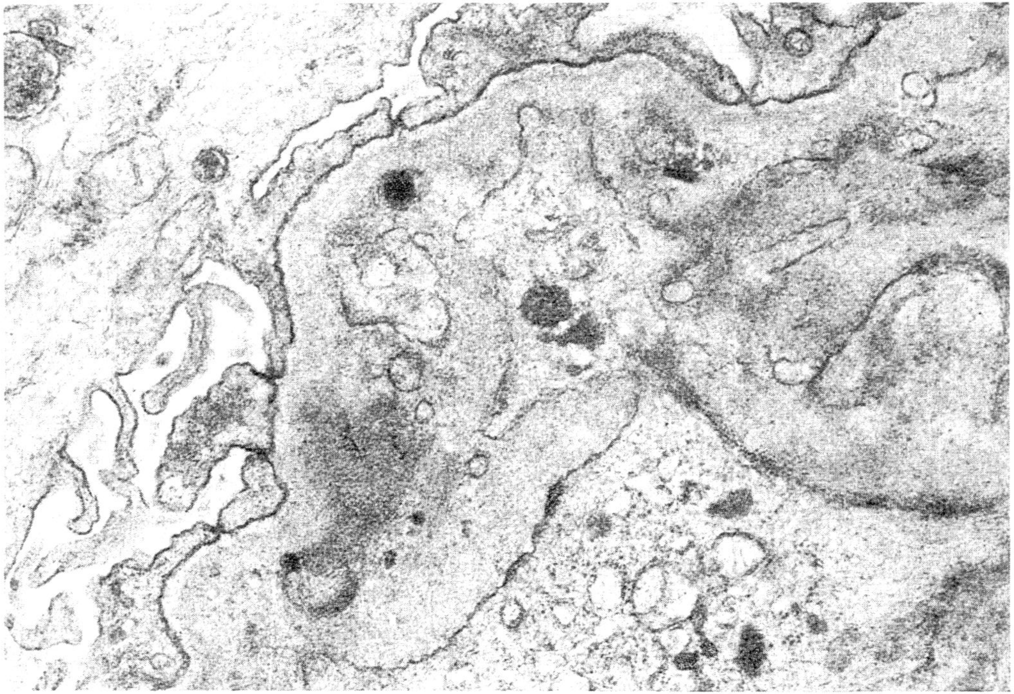

Figure 1. Representative findings of a renal biopsy obtained from a patient with HbSS and immunocomplex glomerulonephritis. Small electron dense deposits are seen in the inner aspect of the lamina densa of the capillary wall. There is splitting of the glomerular basement membrane. Stain is uranyl acetate and lead citrate: original magnification x 5,250. (Reproduced with the permission of Pardo et al., Ref. 17, and the editors of the American Journal of Medicine.)

Clinical features of sickle cell nephropathy

Proteinuria. The incidence of proteinuria in patients with sickle cell disorders is unknown, and to our knowledge there have been no systematic evaluations conducted. Proteinuria, however, appears to be relatively common in cases of sickle cell disorders. Margolies, in a review of sickle cell anemia (24), stated that many patients have "albuminuria" of some degree without antecedent nephritis or hypertension. Henderson (25) noted proteinuria in 17 of 54 patients with sickle cell anemia. In only four of these subjects, however, was the level greater than 2+. Halankar et al. (26) reported that 20 of 30 randomly studied patients attending their sickle cell clinic had protein excretion rates of 0.5 g/day or higher.

Glomerulonephritis, nephrotic syndrome. With the exception of lesions of apparently minor clinical significance, such as glomerular enlargement and mild hypercellularity (11), information on the glomerular involvement in patients with overt renal disease such as the nephrotic syndrome is limited. Berman and Schreiner, who (27) reported on a patient whose nephrotic syndrome was associated with sickle cell disease, were the first to postulate a causal relationship. Subsequently, additional instances of this association have been reported (12,20a,22,28-33). However, in these investigations the nature of the glomerular lesions was not clearly defined, because of the limitations in defining the structural changes using only light microscopy or of studying advanced stages at autopsy.

In a report that included electron microscopic examination of three patients with sickle cell disease and the nephrotic syndrome, McCoy (13) demonstrated mesangioproliferative glomerulonephritis with circumferential mesangial extension into the capillary loops (membranoproliferative glomerulonephritis). Similar findings were reported by Antonovych (15) and Elfenbein et al. (18) in ten additional patients.

The relationship between glomerulonephritis and sickle cell disease is still unclear. Recently, Strauss et al (16) described a patient with sickle cell disease and immune-complex glomerulonephritis and presented evidence that the immune deposit nephropathy was secondary to circulating complexes of RTE antigen and specific antibody deposited in the renal glomerulus. It was postulated that the release of antigen was triggered by tubular damage secondary to hemodynamic or renal oxygenation abnormalities related to sickle cell disease. Subsequently, a clinicopathologic study of seven additional proteinuric patients was reported (17), which also demonstrated an immune deposit normocomplementemic nephritis (Table 2). These findings further support the hypothesis that the syndrome is mediated by glomerular deposition of immune complexes of RTE antigen-antibody (16).

Several alternative pathogenic mechanisms can be postulated to explain the presence of the immune complex nephritis observed in patients with sickle cell disease (16): (a) sensitization to erythrocyte antigens released by hemolysis in these patients or received by blood transfusion with subsequent development of complexes of the antigen and specific antibody;

TABLE 2. Clinical and Morphologic Manifestations in 7 Patients with Sickle Cell Nephropathy (University of Miami School of Medicine)*

Patient population	Mean	Range
Age at time of renal biopsy (yr)	17.9	10-28
Age at diagnosis of HbSS (yr)	3.7	0.5-9
Sex	4M , 3F	
Clinical findings		
Proteinuria (g/day)	1.2-20	
Nephrotic syndrome	4/7	
Hematuria	5/7	
Renal failure	4/7	
Hypertension	3/7	
Morphologic findings		
GBM splitting	7/7	
Glomerular sclerosis	5/7	
Interstitial fibrosis	5/7	
E M deposits	4/7	
Tubular atrophy	5/7	
Hemosiderin in tubules	7/7	
C_3	4/4	
RTE antigen	2/2	

* Adapted from Pardo et al (17).
GBM = Glomerular basement membrane.

(b) undue susceptibility to infection and inadequate host defense mechanisms, leading to chronic or recurrent infection and formation of immune complexes of microbial antigen and antibody; (c) an altered immune response leading to the constant presence of pathogenic immune complexes in a critical antigen-antibody ratio; (d) sensitization to homologous antigens or hepatitis-associated antigen by repeated transfusions, leading to the production of antigen-antibody complexes; (e) inadequate phagocytic mechanisms limiting the clearance of immune complexes, or other host abnormalities leading to an abnormal glomerular response to or recovery from an immunologic injury. Pardo et al. (17) believed that these mechanisms were less likely to be operative in their patients than the mechanism they had postulated (16,17). These authors also pointed out that the proposal of McCoy (13)--that deposits of iron complexes in the mesangial region have a pathogenic role in the production of the nephrotic syndrome--could be related to their own theory if tubular iron deposits could be shown to alter cellular constitutents in such a way as to render them antigenic.

Despite these data suggesting a direct relationship between sickle cell disease and the nephrotic syndrome, it should be emphasized that it remains unclear whether the histologic changes are specific or merely coincidental. Alleyne et al. (5) have stated that their experience in Jamaica indicates a close association among proteinuria, chronic ulceration of the legs, and streptococcal infection. It should also be pointed out that there are rare reports of poststreptococcal acute glomerulonephritis in patients with sickle cell disorders (34-36). Since it is believed that the prognosis in children for recovery from post-streptococcal glomerulonephritis is generally more favorable than that for sickle cell nephropathy (13,17,21), the differentiation of the two disorders is clinically important.

Chronic renal failure. Until recently it has been accepted that renal failure is a rare complication of sickle cell anemia. That this may not be the case is evident from the data of Alleyne (37), which indicate that renal failure may be the most common cause of death in Jamaican blacks, older than 40 years, with sickle cell anemia. The newly recognized increased longevity of patients with sickle cell disease may well be an important factor in this regard.

Henderson (25) had noted that each of his 4 patients with greater than 2+ proteinuria had BUN values in the range of 90 to 150 mg/100 ml. In the study of Halankar et al. (26), 15 of the 30 patients evaluated showed a mild to moderate decrease in creatinine clearance. Of the eight patients with proliferative glomerulonephritis studied by Walker and his associates (22), two died of uremia. In addition, two of McCoy's three patients died in renal failure despite treatment with corticosteroids (13), and 4 of the 7 patients reported by Pardo et al. rapidly developed severe renal insufficiency (Table 2). Friedman's group (3), has reported four sickle cell patients with renal failure, at least two of whom had glomerulonephritis. Of note is a recent report by Avram (39) of seven subjects with sickle cell trait who were receiving chronic maintenance hemodialysis, whose course had been characterized by hematuria and progressive renal failure from no apparent cause. Furthermore, uremic sickle cell nephropathy has been reported in patients with alleged sickle cell trait (19).

It is still not clear if the severity of renal involvement can be related to age, hematocrit values, or the number or severity of sickle cell crises, or to the presence of extrarenal complications. In sickle cell patients older than 40 years Alleyne (37) has noted a close association of renal failure with the presence of leg ulcers.

It is obvious that several renal complications of sickle cell disorders other than sickle cell nephropathy, such as bilateral renal vein thrombosis (20), infarction, papillary necrosis (40), pyelonephritis (41,42) or occlusion of glomeruli by sickled cells (43), might lead to chronic renal failure.

Decreasing renal function was recently described in one third of 25 patients with sickle cell disorders older than 40 years (age range 40-64) studied in Jamaica by Morgan (44). Sex distribution, radiological findings (IVP), leg ulcerations or number of sickle cell crisis were not different from those aged patients without renal failure. Although they did not have history of nephrotic syndrome their proteinuria was greater, and an early indicator of failing renal function was a worsening of the anemia. The cause of this progressive decline in renal function was not apparent.

Acute renal failure. Acute renal insufficiency has been rarely reported in patients with sickle cell disease secondary to bilateral papillary necrosis and in subjects with HbAS after renal vein thrombosis or exercise-induced muscle injury (45,46).

Dialysis and transplantation in sickle cell disorders. Several sickle cell anemia patients with end-stage renal failure have undergone chronic maintenance hemodialysis (3,17,38,47-50). In their review of the renal manifestations of sickle cell disease, Buckalew and Someren (4) have expressed concern that the performance of long-term hemodialysis in these patients might be complicated by many problems, particularly those related to vascular access, thrombotic, hemolytic, and acid-base disturbances. Friedman et al. (3,38) have not observed an inordinate number of such difficulties. In addition, these and other authors (47,49,50) have noted that dialysis per se does not produce an increase in transfusion requirements. In recent reports, however, Manis and Friedman (38) and Rao (51) have noted that all four of their patients died, two probably of cardiac causes and two of severe infections.

At the University of Miami six patients with sickle cell disorders and chronic uremia have been maintained on chronic hemodialysis for three to 48 months without an inordinate number of vascular access complications, enhanced transfusion requirements, or precipitation of sickle cell crisis (Table 3).

Although most investigators have not reported an apparent adverse effect of hemodialysis or uremic acidosis on the incidence of sickle cell crisis, Smith et al. (52) recently described a patient with dialysis-induced crisis, which they attributed to decreased tissue perfusion and hypoxia. Overall, the experience with hemodialysis in HbSS patients is encouraging, although the extrarenal complications of sickle cell disease impose serious limitations on rehabilitation and longevity.

Although the experience with renal transplantation in sickle cell disorders is limited (38,53,54), a recent report reveals that 34 renal transplants were performed in 30 patients in the U.S.A. (55). Nine patients had sickle cell disease and 21 trait. At one year the reported graft survival was 76% for living related donors and 64% for cadaveric donors. Thus, it can only be concluded that there appears to be no major contraindications for the procedure, except for the report of Spector et al. (54), who noted that the increase in hematocrit values subsequent to transplantation was associated with the reemergence of numerous severe, painful crises. This complication responded to a program of prophylactic exchange transfusions.

TABLE 3. Patients with Sickle Cell Disorders and End Stage Renal Disease Maintained on Hemodialysis at the University of Miami Medical Center

Patient	Hb	Age, Sex	Total months of dialysis	Sickle Crisis	Status at 1/1981
1	SS	22, F	35	1	alive
2	SS	40, F	30	0	alive
3	SC	29, F	10	0	alive
4	SS	13, M	48	0	died, sepsis
5	SS	17, F	30	0	died, CVA
6	Sthal	19, M	3	0	alive

1 crisis in 156 months-dialysis. No unusual vascular access problems. Some patients have low Hb. CVA = cerebro vascular accident.

In summary, it is obvious that neither the pathologic changes nor the pathogenesis of sickle cell nephropathy are clear at the present time. Several hypotheses have been advanced but additional experimental and clinical work must be done to establish the sequence of events leading to the various changes observed in patients with sickle cell nephropathy and to decide on appropriate therapy, particularly when the nephropathy has progressed to end-stage kidney disease.

OTHER CLINICAL CONSIDERATIONS

Hyposthenuria, enuresis

Loss of the ability to concentrate the urine is compatible with a normal life under most circumstances. However, there may be situations during the lifespan of patients with sickle cell disease when the characteristic concentrating defect may increase the risk of dehydration. Most patients are only minimally polyuric, although on occasion they may excrete large volumes of dilute urine. Nevertheless, Hatch and Diggs (56) frequently found negative water balances in many adult patients with sickle cell disease, despite increased daily fluid intake. When fluid intake was restricted in these patients it was poorly tolerated, with the appearance of dehydration, loss of weight, and symptoms suggesting impending sickle cell crisis. Similar findings of high fluid intake and urinary volume have been reported in children with sickle cell anemia (57). Experience in Ghana (58) demonstrated that exposing the patient with sickle cell anemia to cold weather or a cold environment (which is known to help bring on crisis) induces a diuresis that may aggravate the existing polyuria. Thus, one should be aware of the need to protect patients with sickle cell disease from dehydration under stressful circumstances, usually characterized by extrarenal losses of body fluids.

Enuresis appears to be more frequent in children with sickle cell anemia than in normal children of similar age and fluid intake (59,60). Although the exact mechanism of enuresis is unknown in these as well as in other children without hemoglobinopathies, the hyposthenuria and altered circadian rhythm of urine excretion present in sickle cell anemia are undoubtedly important contributory factors.

Hematuria

Hematuria represents the most dramatic of the renal abnormalities of sickle cell conditions. It can be massive (9,61), or associated with a sickle cell crisis, or only manifest itself as a microscopic finding. It can cause significant morbidity (9,61-63) and although it is usually self-limited, it may be persistent and even life-threatening. Hematuria has been reported in most sickle cell disorders. In the review of Lucas and Bullock (62) of 64 patients with hematuria, 62% had HbAS, 27% had HbSC, and 11% had HbSS genotypes; the hematuria originated in the left kidney in 80% of the cases and arose from both kidneys in only 11%. The typical patient was a young man with painless gross hematuria, usually associated with trauma to the renal area. Others (63), however, have not substantiated this predilection of the hematuria for the left side.

The exact frequency of hematuria in relation to the abnormal hemoglobin present and/or the side of bleeding is not known with certainty. As pointed out by Serjeant (2), despite the fact that hematuria appears to be more frequent in patients with HbAS or HbSC than with HbSS, it cannot be concluded that patients carrying these genotypes are more prone to develop hematuria, since differences in age, selection relative to symptoms, and particularly frequencies of these genotypes in the general population preclude direct comparisons. For example, it should be remembered that the infrequency (63) of hematuria in patients with HbSS is more apparent than real, since the inheritance of the HbAS genotype is approximately 40 times more common than HbSS.

Likewise, the reason for the possible predominancy of bleeding from the left side is not clear but must be related to the different distribution of the venous return in each kidney. It has been suggested (63) that the fact that on the left side, the spermatic, inferior phrenic, and adrenal veins enter the left renal vein, while on the right side these veins usually enter the inferior vena cava directly explains the higher incidence on the left.

The presence of painless recurrent hematuria in patients with sickle cell disease or trait requires a complete urologic evaluation to avoid missing the diagnosis of a malignancy (64). Conversely, in patients with painless hematuria and absence of urologic abnormalities, a hematologic assessment to exclude the presence of a hemoglobinopathy should always be performed, even in patients of apparent nonblack origin.

Of interest is the demonstration of coagulation abnormalities in patients with sickle cell trait and significant hematuria. Brody et al. (65) reported on the presence of von Willebrand syndrome in five patients with HbAS and bleeding limited to the genitourinary tract. These authors concluded that the von Willebrand syndrome should be a major diagnostic consideration in these patients and, if documented, treatment with cryoprecipitate is indicated and effective. Whether the presence of two genetically determined abnormalities explains the apparent higher incidence of hematuria in sickle cell trait remains entirely speculative (65).

The pathogenesis of hematuria in sickle cell disorders is not clearly established, but it is thought to relate to the vascular abnormalities described in the juxtamedullary area (66), with congestion of vessels and hemorrhage into the mucosa of the renal pelvis (10). The bleeding arises just beneath the pelvic mucosa, where masses of sickled red blood cells engorge and rupture venules. The combination of selective ischemia of the inner medullary vasculature with increased cortical blood flow may create a situation favoring hematuria. Studies in animals (67) have shown that the nutrient vessels for the pelvic mucosa come from divisions of the efferent vessels of juxtamedullary glomeruli (which also give rise to the vasa recta and peritubular capillaries). It is conceivable that if resistance to the flow of blood is increased in the vasa recta because of selective ischemia associated with sickling and/or vascular damage or obliteration (10,67), more blood will be shunted to the peritubular and pelvic mucosal capillaries, thereby explaining the anatomic renal pelvic findings (10).

The fact that alkali, distilled water, and diuretics may be of help in persistent severe hematuria, as reported by Knochel (68), supports the above explanation. This author has suggested that these agents act by minimizing sickling in the vasa recta by reducing medullary hyperosmolality (water or loop diuretics) or medullary acidity (alkali therapy) and reducing the overperfusion of peritubular and renal pelvic capillaries, thus ameliorating the hematuria (4). Of the many other therapies proposed for persistent and severe gross hematuria in sickle cell disease or trait the administration of the urokinase inhibitor epsilon aminocaproic acid has received recent attention (63,69). This medication inhibits the activation of fibrinolysin by urokinase and thus favors clotting. When given in the lowest effective dose (to avoid possible thrombotic complications) and reserved for patients with severe and persistent bleeding, it appears to be both effective and safe (2,69).

Papillary Necrosis

Occasionally renal papillary necrosis is found in kidneys removed for the treatment of persistent hematuria (10,70). Rarely, papillary necrosis may be diagnosed radiologically (40). The most common form of renal papillary necrosis observed in sickle cell disease or trait is the more limited medullary variety (71), with a lesser occurrence of the papillary type (40). These lesions are the result of the repeated sickling episodes with consequent vascular dilatation, occlusion, hemorrhage, and focal scarring.

SELECTED FUNCTIONAL ABNORMALITIES

Renal acidification

The observations that in vitro acidosis enhances the sickling of erythrocytes from patients with sickle cell disease (72) and that experimentally induced metabolic acidosis of long duration may result in sickle-cell crisis (73), along with the data of Barreras and Diggs (74) showing that some patients with sickle-cell disease in painful crisis have metabolic acidosis and an increase in the perçent of sickled cells, raised the possibility that metabolic acidosis might be a precipitating factor. These findings resulted in the recommendation of alkali therapy for the prevention and treatment of sickle cell crisis (73,74).

Acid-base status. Investigators in the West Indies (75), Nigeria (76), and the United States (77) have found no evidence of metabolic acidosis during the steady state (no sickle cell crisis) or during crisis (75), but have found changes consistent with a mild chronic respiratory alkalosis. Oster and co-workers (78) found normal blood gas values in sickle-cell trait volunteers.

The available data suggest therefore that under most circumstances metabolic acidosis does not play a major role in the precipitation of sickle cell crises. This observation (75) raises serious doubts about the rationale of using alkali therapy for this complication of sickle cell disease. Indeed, two controlled studies have shown the failure of alkali therapy for the treatment or prevention of crisis. In a double-blind study of children, the rapid infusion of sodium bicarbonate did not relieve the symptoms of painful sickle cell crisis when compared with infusion of comparable quantities of saline (79). In a crossover study (80), bicarbonate was given orally to children with HbSS for 12 months of a 2-year period in doses adjusted to maintain the urine either neutral or alkaline. There was no significant reduction in crisis frequency during bicarbonate therapy. In addition, we have demonstrated the absence of adverse effects with short-duration (5 to 8 hr) acid loading with NH_4Cl in sickle cell patients (77). Furthermore, in our laboratory, Oster et al (77,78) demonstrated no sickling or increase in percent of sickled cells and no changes in oxygen pressure or in red blood cell 2, 3-diphosphoglycerate following mild, acutely induced, short-duration metabolic acidosis in HbSS or HbAS subjects.

Incomplete syndrome of renal tubular acidosis. In response to a short-duration acid load, 79% of the patients with HbSS studied by Ho

Ping Kong and Alleyne (81), 100% of those studied by Goossens et al. (82), and 29% of those studied by ourselves (77) were unable to decrease urine pH below 5.30. Since none of the patients studied by these investigators was acidemic or hyperchloremic before acid loading, and a generalized proximal tubular reabsortive defect was excluded by the absence of glucosuria, phosphaturia, or bicarbonate wasting, the observed acidification defect is consistent with the incomplete syndrome of distal renal tubular acidosis (83). The reduction in acid excretion in the HbSS patients resulted mainly from decreased titratable acid, since ammonium excretion was not decreased (Table 2) and was appropriate for the urine pH in most cases (77,81,82). The distal tubules of the HbSS patients apparently require a greater than normal stimulus to generate a normal urine to blood hydrogen ion (H+) gradient, since each of the HbSS subjects with an abnormal response to NH_4Cl loading showed enhanced urinary acidification (lowering pH below 5.30) after either dietary sodium restriction with concomitant mineralocorticoid administration or infusion of sodium sulfate (77,81)--two maneuvers known to stimulate distal tubular H+ secretion. Neutral sodium phosphate infusion did not correct the acidification defect in the HbSS patients (81), but there was a significant increase in titratable acid excretion, suggesting that the distal tubular H+ secretory mechanism was probably intact. There was no definite evidence of an abnormality of bicarbonate reabsorption in HbSS patients (81). Similar results were obtained in patients with HbSC (82). In contrast, subjects with HbAS exhibited a normal response to acid loading (78,81,82) despite clearly abnormal renal concentrating

TABLE 4. Maximum Renal Response to Acid Loading

	HbAA (N=9)	HbAS (N=9)	HbSS (N=20)
Urine pH	4.88 ± 0.07 (4.70 - 5.30)	4.81 ± 0.07 (4.45 - 5.01)	5.19 ± 0.06[b] (4.82 - 5.70)
Titratable acid (μEq/min)	29 ± 3	26 ± 3	21 ± 2[c]
Ammonium (μEq/min)	52 ± 4	51 ± 5	44 ± 4
Net acid (μEq/min)	79 ± 4	74 ± 6	60 ± 5[d]
$\frac{U_{NH_4}V \times 100}{U_{TA}V + U_{NH_4}V}$[a] (%)	68 ± 3	67 ± 3	70 ± 2

Adapted from Oster et al. (Ref.77). Values are mean ± SE; ranges are in parentheses.
a At the time of maximal net acid excretion.
b P<.001 in comparison with HbAA. c P<.01 in comparison with HbAA.
d P<.05 in comparison with HbAA.

ability. The response to oral bicarbonate loading was also studied in our laboratory (77). Of 13 HbSS patients, 10 did not show increased urinary Pco_2 above 2 SD below the mean of the controls (<31 mmHg). Of 7 patients with normal responses to NH_4Cl (minimal urine pH<5.3), 5 had low urinary Pco_2. However, since the urine HCO_3 concentrations of the HbSS patients were significantly lower than those of the controls, we cannot be certain that the low urine Pco_2 levels were the result of an acidification defect. The majority of subjects with HbAS had normal urinary CO_2 tension.

The precise pathophysiologic mechanisms underlying the acidification defect in patients with sickle cell anemia, particularly the elucidation of enhanced H+ back diffusion versus decreased H+ secretion, remain incompletely defined, as in most types of renal tubular acidosis. However, the response to sulfate and phosphate infusions suggests that enhanced back diffusion of H+ might be the mechanism involved in the genesis of the syndrome of incomplete renal tubular acidosis in sickle cell disease.

We (77) as well as others (81,82) have not had the opportunity to study a patient with sickle cell disease whose glomerular filtration rate was not lowered and had renal tubular acidosis when first seen. Hyperkalemic hyperchloremic distal renal tubular acidosis has been reported recently in patients with sickle cell disorders (84), suggesting the possibility of selective hypoaldosteronism (85) or an impairment of distal tubular sodium transport which prevents generation of a favorable electrical gradient for potassium and hydrogen (84).

Uric acid metabolism

Since overproduction of uric acid is an expected consequence of the increased red blood cell turnover observed in chronic hemolytic disorders, abnormalities of urate homeostasis are to be expected in patients with sickle cell disease. Although the metabolic abnormalities of sickle cell disease appear in early childhood and urate overproduction must begin early in life, hyperuricemia is rare in children (86). Evidence for an enhanced production of uric acid is supported by the fact that the mean urinary uric acid excretion exceeds the normal values in more than half the adults with this disorder who are on a purine-free diet (87). Reports of secondary gout are notably rare (86,88-92), considering the sixfold to eightfold increase in red blood cell turnover that occurs in sickle cell anemia.

Several factors may influence the low incidence of gout in sickle cell disease. First, the clinical recognition of gout depends on the duration and magnitude of hyperuricemia. Although increased levels of serum uric acid have been reported in 37% of 104 patients with HbSS disease and in 22% of 37 patients with HbSC disease (86,88-92), in most cases the values were not elevated above 8 mg/100 ml for prolonged periods. Furthermore, in only a handful of patients with clinically apparent gout (88,91) were the serum uric acid levels elevated above 10 mg/100 ml for any extended period of time. These findings may be important in determining the risk of gouty arthritis as well as the possibility of developing asymptomatic renal disease.

Second, the shortened life span of patients with severe sickle cell disease may preclude the appearance of the laboratory or clinical manifestations associated with secondary gout, which in part are related to the duration of hyperuricemia. Thus the possibility exists that with survival of more patients with sickle cell disease into advanced decades of life, gouty arthritis and tophaceous disease may become a more frequent complication.

Third, the usual musculoskeletal manifestations of sickle cell disease (episodes of aching pains in bones and joints) may mask true gouty arthritis. In a recent survey, Espinoza et al. (89) found that 46% of 70 patients with sickle cell disease showed signs involving the joints. Thus, in addition to its relatively low frequency, the joint manifestations, when present, might be attributed to sickle cell crisis rather than to gout. More than half the patients reported as having clinical gout were women; and the disease was usually diagnosed at a relatively young age, a situation that should suggest secondary gout rather than the primary idiopathic form.

Finally, the kidney in young patients with sickle cell disorders may show an adaptive response that helps to maintain normal urate homeostasis. It is reasonable to assume that the loss of this compensatory renal response coupled with the persistent enhanced production of uric acid may be responsible for the appearance of marked hyperuricemia and secondary gout in some of these patients. Diamond et al. (92) have reported studies of seven young normouricemic HbSS adults with uric acid overproduction. Urate clearance was higher in these patients than in normal subjects or in patients with primary hyperuricemia due to uric acid overproduction. The higher clearance was not the result of increased filtered load of urate or a direct result of urate overproduction (Table 5). Furthermore, this elevated urate clearance persisted when the urate load was decreased by the administration of allopurinol or increased by the feeding of yeast RNA. The greater clearance of urate in HbSS patients was entirely attributable to a greater pyrazinamide-suppressible clearance of urate, representing either enhanced urate secretion or diminished reabsorption of secreted urate (93). These data suggest increased tubular secretion of urate rather than decreased reabsorption of secreted urate. The mechanism for the compensatory renal increase in urate excretion is not apparent.

TABLE 5. Uric Acid Homeostasis in Patients with Sickle Cell Anemia

	Sickle Cell Anemia	Subjects with Primary Gout with Uric Acid Overproduction	Normal Subjects
Number of subjects	7	10	10
Serum uric acid (mg/100 ml)	4.9 ± 0.4	8.7 ± 0.6	5.3 ± 0.3
Urine uric acid[a] (mg/24 hr)	824 ± 77	843 ± 70	406 ± 42
GFR (ml/min)	130 ± 15	113 ± 8	110 ± 5
Urate clearance/GFR x 100(%)	12.1 ± 1.4	7.3 ± 0.6	7.5 ± 0.5

Adapted from Diamond et al. (ref.92). Values are mean ± SE

[a] Uric acid overproduction is defined as a daily urinary excretion greater than 590 mg in patients on a purine-free diet for five days.

On the other hand, Walker and Alexander (90) have suggested that uric acid excretion might be reduced in some patients with HbSS and hyperuricemia. Of eight patients with HbSS, four had a persistent hyperuricemia and decreased urate clearances. This study has shown that the sickle cell disease patients with hyperuricemia were those with the lowest creatinine clearances. It is apparent that because of urate overproduction in these patients, the decrease in renal function need not be great to result in a "normalization," or a "relative" decrease of urate clearance.

With one exception (89), patients with sickle cell trait have been reported to exhibit normal values for both serum uric acid (90,94) and urate excretion (90).

Renal potassium handling

Since potassium excretion primarily reflects secretion in the distal nephron and surgical papillectomy markedly suppresses the increase in potassium excretion following potassium chloride (KCl) loading (95), and because of the predominance of lesions of the renal medulla and papilla in sickle cell diseases, De Fronzo and coworkers (96) have examined renal potassium handling in patients with sickle cell anemia. In response to an intravenously administered KCl load, HbSS patients excreted significantly less potassium than control subjects. The administration of sodium sulfate and furosemide also resulted in a subnormal increase in potassium excretion. The defect in potassium excretion could not be explained by hypoaldosteronism, by abnormalities in baseline insulin levels, by decreased delivery of sodium to the distal exchange site, or by enhanced fecal losses of potassium (96). Despite the impairment in renal potassium excretion, hyperkalemia did not develop during acute KCl loading, suggesting the presence of an extrarenal mechanism for potassium adaptation in these patients (96).

We have retrospectively evaluated (97) the urinary potassium excretion in HbSS and HbAS subjects and in HbAA volunteers from data obtained in our laboratory during several renal function studies that included ammonium chloride and sodium bicarbonate but not KCl loading (77,78). There were no significant differences among the serum potassium levels of the three groups. In the HbSS subjects there was a significantly smaller augmentation of renal potassium excretion by $NaHCO_3$ loading compared with controls; the response of the HbAS group was intermediate. This difference in potassium excretion between sickle cell disease and control subjects was not apparent during daily urinary collections, hydropenia, or after acid loading with NH_4Cl. We have also compared responses to oral KCl loading of control and sickle cell trait subjects (98). Both before and after KCl loading there were no differences between groups in serum potassium concentrations or in percent urinary excretion of administered potassium.

It should be emphasized that hyperkalemia was not observed by De Fronzo et al. (96) or by us in our retrospective analysis (96) and that in the absence of decreased renal function (84), it has not been reported in patients with sickle cell disorders (77,78,99,100). Thus, although impairment in potassium excretion in patients with sickle cell anemia does not present a clinical problem, it is conceivable that progressive renal (predominantly medullary and papillary) damage may ultimately predispose these patients to hyperkalemia.

REFERENCES

1. Herrick JB: Peculiar elongated and sickle-shaped red blood corpuscles in a case of severe anemia. Arch Intern Med 6:517,1910.
2. Serjeant GR: The Clinical Features of Sickle Cell Disease. New York, North-Holland/American Elsevier, 1974.
3. Friedman EA, Sreepada TK, Sprung CL, et al: Uremia in sickle-cell anemia treated by maintenance hemodialysis. N Engl J Med 291:431,1974
4. Buckalew VM Jr, Someren A: Renal manifestations of sickle cell disease. Arch Intern Med 133:660, 1974.
5. Alleyne GAO, Statius van Eps LW, Addae SK, et al: The kidney in sickle anemia. Kidney Int 7:371, 1975.
6. Vaamonde CA, Oster JR, Strauss J: The Kidney in Sickle Cell Disease in Suki WN, Eknoyan G (Eds): The Kidney in Systemic Disease, 2nd Ed., New York, Wiley Biomedical, 1981, p. 159.
7. Sydenstricked VP, Mulherin WA, Houseal RW: Sickle cell anemia: report of two cases in children, with necropsy in one case. Am J Dis Child 26:132, 1923.
8. Diggs LW, Ching RE: Pathology of sickle cell anemia. South Med J 27:839, 1934.
9. Goodwin WE, Alston EF, Semans JH: Hematuria and sickle cell disease: unexplained gross unilateral renal hematuria in Negroes, coincident with the blood sickling trait. J Urol 63:79, 1950.
10. Mostofi KF, Vorder Bruegge CF, Diggs LW: Lesions of kidneys removed for unilateral hematuria in sickle cell disease. Arch Pathol Lab Med 63:336, 1957.
11. Bernstein J, Whitten CF: A histologic appraisal of the kidney in sickle cell anemia. Arch Pathol 70:407, 1960.
12. Miller RE, Hartley MW, Clark EC, et al: Sickle cell nephropathy. Ala J Med Sci 1:233, 1964.
13. McCoy RC: Ultrastructural alterations in the kidney of patients with sickle cell disease and the nephrotic syndrome. Lab Invest 21:85, 1969.
14. Pitcock JA, Muirhead EE, Hatch FE, et al: Early renal changes in sickle cell anemia. Arch Pathol 90:403, 1970.
15. Antonovych TT: Ultrastructural changes in glomeruli of patients with sickle cell disease and the nephrotic syndrome. Abs Am Soc Nephrol 5:3, 1972.
16. Strauss J, Pardo V, Koss MN, et al: Nephropathy associated with sickle cell anemia: an autologous immune complex nephritis: I. Studies on nature of the glomerular-bound antibody and antigen identification in a patient with sickle cell disease and immune deposit glomerulonephritis. Am J Med 58:382, 1975.
17. Pardo V, Strauss J, Kramer H, et al: Nephropathy associated with sickle cell anemia: an autologous immune complex nephritis: II. Clinicopathologic study of seven patients. Am J Med 59:650, 1975.
18. Elfenbein IB, Patchefsky A, Schwartz W et al: Pathology of the glomerulus in sickle cell anemia with and without nephrotic syndrome. Am J Pathol 77:357, 1974.
19. Ozawa T, Mass MF, Guggenheim S, et al: Autologous immune complex nephritis associated with sickle cell trait: diagnosis of the haemoglobinopathy after structural and immunological studies. Br Med J 1;369, 1976.
20. Welt LG, Lyle CB Jr: The kidney in sickle cell anemia: in Strauss MB, Welt LG (eds): Diseases of the Kidney, ed 2. Boston, Little Brown &

Co, 1971, p 1207.

20a. Strom T, Muehrcke RC, Smith RD: Sickle cell anemia with the nephrotic syndrome and renal vein obstruction. Arch Intern Med 129: 104, 1972.
21. Kimmelstiel P: Vascular occlusion and ischemic infarction in sickle cell disease. Am J Med Sci 216:11, 1948.
22. Walker BR, Alexander F, Birdsall TR, et al: Glomerular lesions in sickle cell nephropathy. JAMA 215:437, 1971.
23. Arakawa M, Kimmelstiel P: Circumferential mesangial interposition. Lab Invest 21:276, 1969.
24. Margolies MP: Sickle cell anemia: a composite study and survey. Medicine 30:357, 1951.
25. Henderson AB: Sickle cell anemia: clinical study of fifty-four cases. Am J Med 9:757, 1950.
26. Halankar A, Frumkin E, Dunn I, et al: Renal findings in sickle cell anemia, in Hercules JI, Schechter AN, Eaton WA, et al (eds): Proceedings First National Symposium on Sickle Cell Disease, Washington, DC, June 1974. Department of Health, Education and Welfare, Publication No. 75-723, 1974, p 311.
27. Berman LB, Schreiner GE: Clinical and histologic spectrum of the nephrotic syndrome. Am J Med 24:249, 1958.
28. Evans PV, Symmes AT: Bone marrow infarction with fat embolism and nephrosis in sickle cell disease. J Indiana State Med Assoc 50: 1101, 1957.
29. Sweeney MJ, Dobbins WT, Ettledorf JN: Renal disease with elements of the nephrotic syndrome associated with sickle cell anemia. J Pediatr 60:42, 1962.
30. Barnett HL, Bernstein J: Clinical pathological conference. J Pediatr 73:936, 1968.
31. Berman LB, Tublin I: The nephropathies of sickle-cell disease. Arch Intern Med 103:602, 1959.
32. Arruda JAL, Verbicario LPDS, Ruch TEA, et al: Elementos de sidrome nefrotica associados a anemia falciforme. O hospital 79:107, 1971.
33. Addae SK: The kidney in sickle cell disease: V. Clinical manifestations. Ghana Med J 12:352, 1973.
34. Susmano S, Lewy JE: Sickle cell disease and acute glomerulonephritis. Am J Dis Child 118:615, 1969.
35. Nicholson GD: Post-streptococcal glomerulonephritis in adult Jamaicans with and without sickle cell anemia. West Indian Med J 26:78, 1977.
36. Roy S, III, Murphy WM, Pitcock JA, et al: Sickle-cell disease and poststreptococcal acute glomerulonephritis. Am J Clin Pathol 66:986, 1976.
37. Alleyne GAO: Personal communication, 1979.
38. Manis T, Friedman EA: Sickle hemoglobinopathy and the kidney. Contrib Nephrol 7:211, 1977.
39. Avram MM: Survival in uremia due to systemic diseases. Kidney Int 13 Suppl 8:S55, 1978.
40. Harrow, BR, Sloane JA, Liebman NC: Roentgenologic demonstration of renal papillary necrosis in sickle-cell trait. N Engl J Med 268:969, 1963.
41. Whalley PG, Pritchard JA, Richards JR Jr: Sickle cell trait and pregnancy. JAMA 186:1132, 1963.
42. Barrett-Connor E: Bacterial infection and sickle cell anemia. An

analysis of 250 infections in 166 patients and a review of the literature. Medicine 50:97, 1971.
43. Tellem M, Rubenstone AI, Frumin AM: Renal failure and other unusual manifestations of sickle-cell trait. Arch Pathol 63:508, 1957.
44. Morgan AG: Renal function in sickle cell patients over 40 years old. Kidney Int 16:934, 1979.
45. Frascino JA, Grabstald H: Acute renal failure in sickle cell trait. Urology 6:219, 1975.
46. Koppes GM, Daly JJ, Coltman CA Jr, et al: Exertion-induced rhabdomyolysis with acute renal failure and disseminated intravascular coagulation in sickle cell trait. Am J Med 63:313, 1977.
47. Pote HH Jr, Capaldo R, Lyons H, et al: Hemodialysis in sickle cell disease: 24 months experience. Trans Am Soc Artif Intern Organs 4:51, 1975.
48. Friedman EA, Rao TKS, Sprung CL, et al: Hemodialysis and transfusion for uremic patients with sickle-cell disease. N Engl J Med 291: 1361, 1974.
49. Elberg AJ, Baker R, Koch K, et al: Transfusion requirement in patients with sickle cell disease on hemodialysis. N Engl J Med 294:444, 1976.
50. Drueke T, Zingraff J, Sari R, et al: Dialysis for renal failure in patients with sickle-cell disease. N Engl J Med 293:1153, 1975.
51. Rao TKS: Hemodialysis and transplantation in systemic diseases: the facts, in Friedman EA, (ed): Strategy in Renal Failure. New York: John Wiley & Sons, 1978, p 321.
52. Smith AJ, Tefera M, Kim HS: Hemodialysis (HD) induced sickle crisis, abstracted. Am Soc Nephrol 11:52A, 1978.
53. Chatterjee SN, Lundburg G, Berne TV: Sickle cell trait: an additional cause of renal allograft failure. Clin Res 24:125A, 1976.
54. Spector D, Zachary JB, Sterioff S, et al: Painful crises following renal transplantation in sickle cell anemia. Am J Med 64:835, 1978.
55. Chatterjee SN: National study of natural history of renal allografts in sickle cell disease and trait. Nephron 25:199, 1980.
56. Hatch FE, Diggs LW: Fluid balance in sickle-cell disease. Arch Intern Med 116:10, 1965.
57. Saxena UH, Scott RB, Ferguson AD: Studies in sickle cell anemia: XXV. Observations on fluid intake and output. J Pediatr 69:220, 1966.
58. Addae S, Addae F: Effect of acute heat stress on some renal functions in the sickle cell patient. Ghana Med J 10:14, 1971.
59. Noll JB, Newman AJ, Gross S: Enuresis and nocturia in sickle cell disease. J Pediatr 70:965, 1967.
60. Suster G, Oski FA: Enuresis in sickle cell anemia. Am J Dis Child 113:311, 1967.
61. Abel MS, Brown CR: Sickle cell disease with severe hematuria simulating renal neoplasm. JAMA 136:624, 1948.
62. Lucas WM, Bullock WH: Hematuria in sickle cell disease. J Urol 83:733, 1960.
63. Allen TD: Sickle cell disease and hematuria: a report of 29 cases. J Urol 91:177, 1964.
64. Carrion H, Machiz S, Politano VA: Sickle cell disease and transitional cell carcinoma of the renal pelvis: a case report. J Urol 109:569, 1973.
65. Brody JI, Levison SP, Jung C: Sickle cell trait and hematuria associated with von Willebrand syndromes. Ann Intern Med 86:529, 1977.

66. Statius van Eps LW, Pinedo-Veels C, de Vries GH, et al: Nature of concentrating defect in sickle-cell nephropathy: microradioangiographic studies. Lancet 1:450, 1970.
67. Moffat DB, Fourman J: The vascular pattern of the rat kidney. J Anat 97:543, 1963.
68. Knochel JP: Hematuria in sickle cell trait: the effect of intravenous administration of distilled water, urinary alkalinization, and diuresis. Arch Intern Med 123:160, 1969.
69. Black WD, Hatch FE, Acchiardo S: Aminocaproic acid in prolonged hematuria of patients with sicklemia. Arch Intern Med 136:678, 1976.
70. Akinkugbe OO: Renal papillary necrosis in sickle-cell haemoglobinopathy. Br Med J 3:283, 1967.
71. Margulies SI, Minkin SD: Sickle cell disease: the roentgenologic manifestations of urinary tract abnormalities in adults. Am J Roentgenol 107:702, 1969.
72. Greenberg MS, Kass EH, Castle WB: Studies on the destruction of red blood cells: XII. Factors influencing the role of S hemoglobin in the pathologic physiology of sickle-cell anemia J Clin Invest 36:833, 1957.
73. Greenberg MS, Kass EH: Studies on the destruction of red blood cells. XIII. Observations on the role of pH in the pathogenesis and treatment of painful crisis in sickle-cell disease. Arch Intern Med 101:355, 1958.
74. Barreras L, Diggs LW: Bicarbonates, pH and percentage of sickled cells in venous blood of patients in sickle cell crisis. Am J Med Sci 247:710, 1964.
75. Ho Ping Kong H, Alleyne GAO: Acid-base status of adults with sickle-cell anemia. Br Med J 3:271, 1969.
76. Oduntan SA: Blood gas studies in some abnormal hemoglobin syndromes. Br J Haematol 17:535, 1969.
77. Oster JR, Lespier LE, Lee SM, Pellegrini EL, Vaamonde CA: Renal acidification in sickle-cell disease. J Lab Clin Med 88:389, 1976.
78. Oster JR, Lee SM, Lespier LE, Pellegrini EL, Vaamonde CA: Renal acidification in sickle cell trait. Arch Intern Med 136:30, 1976.
79. Schwartz E, McElfresh AE: Treatment of painful crises of sickle cell disease: a double blind study. J Pediatr 64:132, 1964.
80. Mann JR, Stuart J: Sodium bicarbonate prophylaxis of sickle cell crisis. Pediatrics 53:414, 1974.
81. Ho Ping Kong H, Alleyne GAO: Studies on acid excretion in adults with sickle-cell anemia. Clin Sci 41:505, 1971.
82. Goossens JP, Statius van Eps LW, Schouten H, et al: Incomplete renal tubular acidosis in sickle cell disease. Clin Chim Acta 41:149, 1972.
83. Buckalew VM Jr, McCurdy DK, Ludwig GD et al: Incomplete renal tubular acidosis: physiologic studies in three patients with a defect in lowering urine pH. Am J Med 45:32, 1968.
84. Battle DC, Itsarayoungyen K, Arruda JAL, Kurtzman NA: Hyperkalemic hyperchloremic metabolic acidosis (MA) in patients with sickle cell hemoglobin. Kidney Int 18:12A, 1980.
85. Vaamonde CA, Perez GO, Oster JR: Syndrome of aldosterone deficiency, in Arruda JAL, Kurtzman NA (eds): Symposium on disorders of tubular transport. Mineral Electrolyte Metab 5:121, 1981.
86. Diamond H, Meisel A, Holden D, et al: Hyperuricemia in sickle cell disease, in Hercules JI, Schechter AN, Eaton WA, et al (eds):

Proceedings First National Symposium on Sickle Cell Disease, Washington, DC, June 1974. US Department of Health, Education and Welfare, Publication No. 75-723, 1974, p 371.
87. Diamond H, Sharon E, Holden D, et al: Renal handling of uric acid in sickle cell anemia. Adv Exp Med Biol 41:759, 1974.
88. Gold MS, Williams JC, Spivak M, et al: Sickle cell anemia and hyperuricemia. JAMA 206:1572, 1968.
89. Espinoza LR, Spilberg I, Osterland CK: Joint manifestations of sickle cell disease. Medicine 53:295, 1974.
90. Walker BR, Alexander F: Uric acid excretion in sickle cell anemia. JAMA 215:255, 1971.
91. Ball GV, Sorensen LB: The pathogenesis of hyperuricemia and gout in sickle cell anemia. Arthritis Rheum 13:846, 1970.
92. Diamond HS, Meisel A, Sharon E, et al: Hyperuricosuria and increased tubular secretion of urate in sickle cell anemia. Am J Med 59:796, 1975.
93. Diamond HS, Paolino JS: Evidence for a post-secretory reabsorptive site for uric acid in man. J Clin Invest 52:1491, 1973.
94. Vaamonde CA, Oster JR: Unpublished observations.
95. Finkelstein FO, Hayslett JP: Role of medullary structures in the functional adaptation of renal insufficiency. Kidney Int 6:419, 1974.
96. DeFronzo RA, August P, Black H et al: Impaired renal tubular K secretion in sickle cell disease. Ann Intern Med 90:310, 1979.
97. Vaamonde CA, Oster JR: Urinary potassium excretion in sickle-cell disorders. Mineral Electrolyte Metab 2:142, 1979.
98. Oster JR, Lanier DC Jr, Vaamonde CA: Renal response to potassium loading in sickle cell trait. Arch Intern Med 140:534, 1980.
99. Kuranstin-Mills, J, Kudo M, Addae SK: Cation content and transport characteristics of the sickle-cell erythrocyte and their relationship with structural changes in the membrane. Clin Sci Mol Med 46:679, 1974.
100. Statius van Eps LW, Schouten H, Slooff PAM, et al: Sodium, potassium and calcium in erythrocytes in sickle cell anemia. Clin Chim Acta 33:475, 1971.

Acknowledgement.

The original research discussed in this chapter was supported by the National Institutes of Health, Grant HL-15999, and by designated Veterans Administration research funds (VA-8943-07) and Training Grant in Nephrology (TP-139).

HYPONATREMIA - AN APPROACH TO THE AFFECTED CHILD

Alan B. Gruskin, M.D., H. Jorge Baluarte, M.D., James W. Prebis, M.D., Martin S. Polinsky, M.D. and Howard W. Rosenblum, M.D.

Hyponatremia is amongst the more common disorders of electrolyte imbalance observed in children. Failure to recognize its presence may lead to catastrophic problems. Moreover, appropriate therapy which in certain cases may be life saving, depends initially upon the proper diagnosis being made. Nine combinations define the relationship between serum sodium concentration and total body water, one normal and eight abnormal (Figure 1).

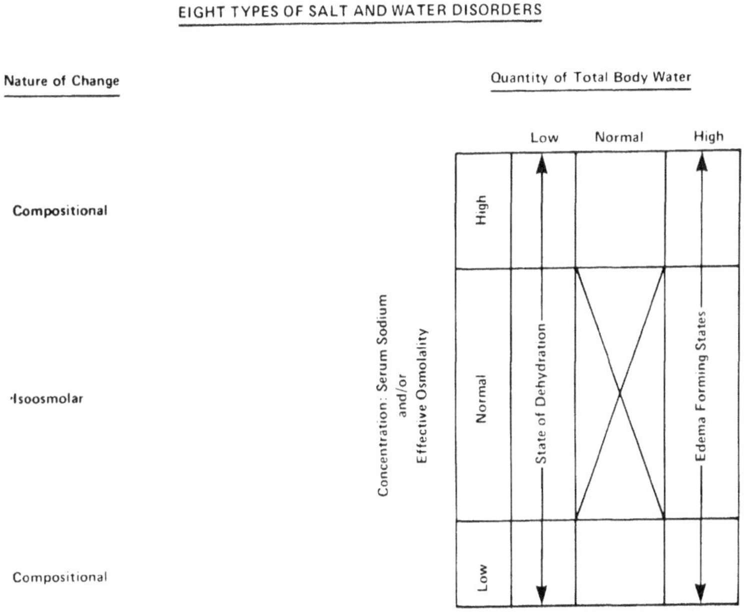

Figure 1

Hyponatremia occurs in association with diminished, normal, and increased amounts of total body water. Hyponatremia in most patients develops as a result of the retention of water in excess of sodium or the replacement of sodium losses by hypoosmotic solution. This review will consider disorders of fluid-electrolyte-homeostasis associated with hyponatremia and will focus primarily on issues related to clinical aspects of hyponatremia. It will deal with fou aspects of the problem - definitions, pathogenesis, clinical features and diagnosis. Treatment will not be considered.

DEFINITIONS

Clinical hyponatremia may be viewed as being present when the serum sodi concentration is less than 130 mEq/L. Although sodium is present in serum water its concentration in blood is usually expressed in terms of serum volum i.e. mEq/L, millequivalents per liter of serum (1). Noteworthy is the fact that a liter of serum contains 6-8 percent solid particles with the remaining 92-94% of serum being water.

The term hyponatremia refers to a reduction in the number of milliequiva lents of sodium per liter of serum water. This term should not be confused with the term sodium deficiency which is used to define a reduction in the total number of sodium particles within the body. Sodium deficiency may or m not be associated with hyponatremia. Depending upon what has happened to the quantity of water within the body and its distribution between extracellular and intracellular compartments, total body sodium deficiencies or excesses may be associated with isonatremia, hyponatremia and or hypernatremia.

Hypo-osmolality, while usually associated with hyponatremia should be viewed as being different from hyponatremia. Osmolality or milliosmolality (mosm) is a colligative property and is a measure of the number of particles p kilogram of water, i.e. per 1000 gm of water, and must be viewed differently from the usual measurements of serum concentrations of electrolytes which are expressed in milliequivalents per liter of serum.

Because sodium and its accompanying anions are the most abundent extra-cellular ions, the serum concentrations of sodium generally parallel the seru concentrations of osmotically active particles. The serum osmolality, althou easily measured, may be estimated using the following formula (2):

$$\text{Posm} = \text{twice the sodium concentration in mEq/L} + \frac{\text{urea (mg\%)}}{2.8} + \frac{\text{glucose (mg}}{18}$$

In most clinical situations, measurements of serum osmolality, when done by freezing point determination, usually agree within 10 mosm of the calculated osmolality.

Serum osmolality also differs from "effective osmolality" which is the term used to describe the concentration of osmotically active particles which do not cross the imaginary semipermeable membrane between extracellular and intracellular compartments. Solutes such as urea, ethanol, methanol, and eth lene glycol being highly permeable exert little influence on "effective osmo-lality" because they easily cross the semipermeable membrane; solutes such as sodium chloride, glucose, mannitol, fructose and glycerol exert a major in-fluence on "effective osmolality" because they do not readily penetrate the intracellular compartment. It is the difference in "effective" solute con-centration between extra and intracellular compartments which determines the fractional distribution of the total body water between these two compartment

PATHOGENESIS

The occurrence of hyponatremia may be viewed as a two step process-factors leading to hyponatremia and factors which enable hyponatremia to persist. Extrarenal and/or intrarenal mechanisms may be operative in hyponatremic patients (1,2).

Extrarenal mechanisms leading to hyponatremia include the ingestion and/or administration of hypotonic solutions in patients with low or absent rates of glomerular filtration. The net extrarenal loss of sodium in excess of water often accompanied by the ingestion and/or replacement of deficits with hypotonic solutions may participate in either the generation and/or persistence phases of clinical hyponatremia.

Many different intrarenal mechanisms may participate in enabling hyponatremia to develop and persist. These mechanisms determine the kidney's ability to dilute urine. Normally, the ingestion of hypotonic fluids leading to hyponatremia results in the excretion of a maximally hypo-osmotic or dilute urine and a return to normal of extracellular osmolality and serum sodium concentration. The ability to appropriately and maximally dilute glomerular filtrate depends upon four factors (2).

1. The quantity of isotonic glomerular filtrate delivered from the proximal tubule to sites within the nephron where hypotonic urine may be formed determines the amount of hypotonic urine excreted

2. The active reabsorption of chloride within the water impermeable diluting segment of the ascending loop of Henle. This process reduces the solute content of the solution entering the ascending loop and forms a hypotonic solution

3. The continued reabsorption of sodium within the distal convoluted tubule further reducing urinary osmolality, i.e. urinary solute concentration

4. A water impermeable collecting duct which is operating in the absence of antidiuretic hormones, thereby permitting the excretion of a maximally dilute urine.

The failure and/or excess activity during the course of a disease of one or any combination of the above four factors to operate normally may generate hyponatremia and/or enable hyponatremia to persist.

CLINICAL FEATURES

The clinical manifestations of hyponatremia range from vague to life threatening complaints. They are not specific for hyponatremia per se and primarily reflect alterations in three organ systems-cardiovascular, central nervous system and gastrointestinal. The signs and symptoms which may be associated with hyponatremia are tabulated in Table I.

Table I: Hyponatremia: Associated Signs and Symptoms

Signs	Symptoms
Apathy	Altered consciousness
Agitation	Coma
Anorexia	Cheyne-Stokes respirations
Diarrhea	Circulator insufficiency-shock-dea
Disorientation	CNS - death
Muscle cramps	Depressed deep tendon reflexes
Nausea	Disordered thinking
Polyuria	Hypotension
Vomiting	Pathologic reflexes
	Pseudobulbar palsy
	Seizures
	Weakness

The severity of the clinical manifestations reflect five factors (1-4):

1. The nadir of the serum sodium concentration. In general, the lower the serum sodium concentration, the more severe the clinical manifestations

2. The rate at which hyponatremia develops; the faster the fall, the greater the morbidity and mortality. When hyponatremia occurs gradually over a number of days to weeks, the patient often remains asymptomatic

3. The quantity of extracellular water. Since sodium is the principle cation controlling the distribution of water between extra and intracellular compartments, the lowering of the serum sodium concentration causes a redistribution of water between these two compartments. The less the quantity of extracellular water, the more severe the signs and symptoms of circulatory insufficiency for a given degree of hyponatremia. The larger the quantity of extracellular water, the greater the degree of intracellular water accumulation for a given degree of hyponatremia

4. The level of serum albumin. The level of serum albumin determines the plasma oncotic pressure and, in part, the distribution of water between intravascular and interstitial compartments. Consequently, any dimunition in the intravascular segment of the extracellular compartment because of hyponatremia will be further modified by the simultaneous occurrence of hypoalbuminemia

5. The age of the patient. Young children and senior citizens are more likely to become symptomatic when hyponatremia develops.

The pathogenesis of the cardiovascular symptomatology reflects primarily the distribution of water between extra and intracellular fluid compartments in response to the development of osmotic gradients between these compartments. The signs and symptoms indicating involvement of the central nervous system and gastrointestinal tract can be explained by the cell swelling which accompanies hyponatremia. Because the skull functions as a nonexpandable structure, its rigid structure limits cell swelling within the central nervous system. It is this limitation in cell swelling which is one of the major factors determining central nervous system symptomatology.

Differences in signs and symptoms due to the rate of drop of serum sodium concentration in acute vs chronic hyponatremia can be explained by the intrinsic ability of the brain to simultaneously lower its content of sodium, potassium and perhaps amino acids (5,6). These differences reflect the formation and/or removal of "idiogenic" osmols, i.e. the addition of and/or removal of previously unavailable solutes from the "effective" pool of particles in the central nervous system. These osmols are part of large molecular weight compounds and do not exist as individual ions. The degree to which these solutes remain a segment of such compounds is related to the osmolality of the solution surrounding these compounds.

DIAGNOSIS OF HYPONATREMIC DISORDERS

The recognition of clinical disorders associated with hyponatremia may be approached by seeking the answers to five questions (Figure 2).

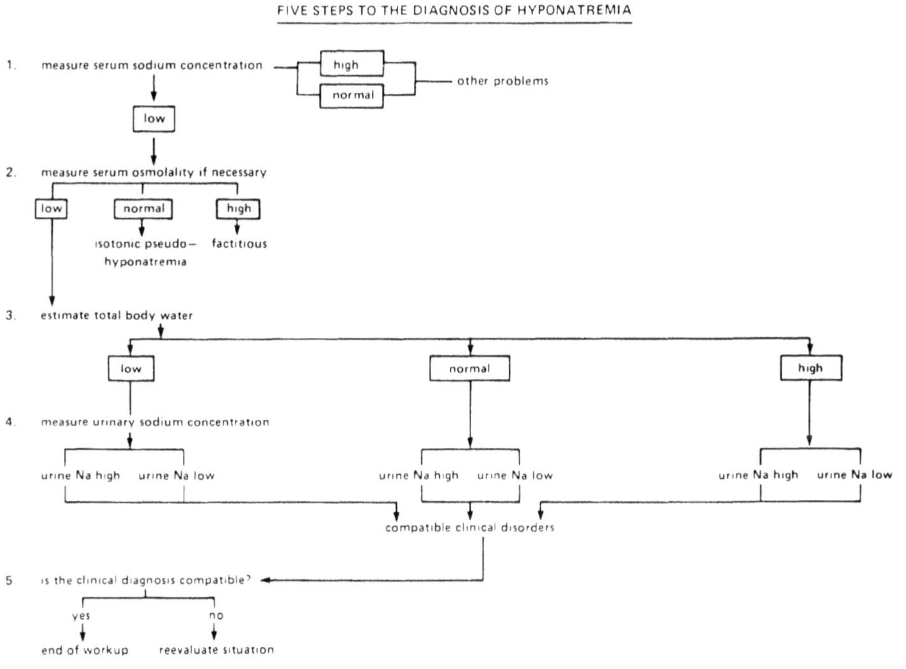

Figure 2

1. Is the serum sodium concentration truly low, or does the presence of pseudohyponatremia or factitious hyponatremia account for the finding of hyponatremia?

2. Is the serum osmolality low, normal or high?

3. Is total body water low, normal or high?

4. Is the urinary sodium concentration less than 10 mEq/L or greater than 20-30 mEq/L?

5. Is the clinical diagnosis compatible with the laboratory findings?

When hyponatremia is found, it must be decided whether the low serum sodium is real or is due to the occurrence of pseudo or factitious hyponatremia. If these differences cannot be resolved on the basis of available data obtained by history, physical examination and routine laboratory studies then the measurement of serum osmolality and serum lipids and/or proteins is indicated.

Serum osmolality may be low, normal or high in patients with hyponatremia (Table II).

Table II: Differential Diagnosis of Serum Osmolality

A) Low

1) True hyponatremia
   a) multiple diseases
   b) may have small increases in sugar, lipids, proteins and/or urea

B) Normal

1) Pseudohyponatremia
   a) hyperlipidemia
   b) hyperproteinemia
2) True hyponatremia plus additional osmotic particles
   a) glucose
   b) urea
   c) isotonic mannitol

C) High

1) Factitious hyponatremia
   a) hyperglycemia
   b) hypoglycemia
   c) galactosemia
   d) fructosemia
   e) hypotonic mannitol
2) True hyponatremia in conjunction with
   a) hyperglycemia
   b) other sugars
   c) urea-renal failure
   d) glycerol

The finding of hypo-osmolality in conjunction with hyponatremia is confirmatory of the diagnosis of hyponatremia in most clinical situations. Iso-osmolality in association with hyponatremia is usually due to the presence of pseudohyponatremia, i.e. the replacement of serum water by serum lipids and/o proteins (1,2). When plasma water is replaced by lipids, the concentration of sodium per liter of serum which will include lipid will be low, yet the osmolality, i.e. the number of particles per 1000 gm of water, will be very close to normal. The amount of water which will be replaced by lipid and/or protein can be estimated by the formula H_2O/100 ml serum = 99.1 -(1.03 x total lipids gm/dl) -(0.73 x total protein gm/dl) (7).

Factitious hyponatremia may be operationally defined as a clinical situation in which dilutional hyponatremia occurs because of the shift of water from intracellular to extracellular compartments because of the addition to the extracellular space of nonpermeant solutes, either real or functional (1,2). The serum sodium concentration should decrease by approximately 1.6 mEq/L for each increase of 100 mg/dl in blood glucose above the normal of 100 mg/dl because of the addition to the extracellular compartment of water from the intracellular compartment. The serum sodium concentration is usually low and serum osmolality increased when factitious hyponatremia has occurred. In certain unusual circumstances, serum osmolality may be normal when hyponatremia exists. Such a situation could exist because of the addition to serum of the precise number of particles such as glucose, galactose, mannitol, etc. to balance the reduction in serum osmolality due to the hyponatremia. More often, when nonpermeant particles are added to the extracellular compartment during the course of a disease process and/or therapeutic intervention, the serum osmolality will be elevated and the sodium depressed due to the osmotic effect of these solutes on transcompartmental water movement.

An estimate of total body water is essential in evaluating patients with hyponatremia because the pathogenesis as well as the etiology of hyponatremia is different in patients when total body water varies from low to high. An initial indication of the directional changes in total body water can be estimated by data obtained as part of a history. A history of acute weight loss, or rapid weight gain, vomiting, diarrhea, rapid respirations, excessive sweating, ingestion of drugs known to alter water balance such as alcohol or chlorpropamide, abdominal swelling, changes in urinary frequency and/or volume, edema, etc. is suggestive of an alteration in total body water. Changes in vital signs in the direction of shock as well as clinical findings of dehydration such as diminished turgor, dry mouth, sunken eyeballs, etc. indicate the presence of a decrease in total body water. Increases in total body water are suggested by the findings of edema, ascites, pulmonary edema, congestive heart failure, etc.

The urinary sodium concentration may be used as an indicator of the magnitude of the tubular reabsorption of filtered sodium. Avid sodium reabsorption is suggested when the urinary sodium concentration is less than 10-15 mEq/L. Conversely, the finding of urinary sodium concentration greater than 20-25 mEq/L suggests the failure of the kidney to maximally reabsorb sodium. In hyponatremic states associated with extracellular volume contraction, the finding of a low urinary sodium concentration suggests an extrarenal etiology of the sodium loss. A low urinary sodium concentration in an obviously volume expanded patient suggests the presence of a disorder known to be associated with an edema forming state. The finding in a hyponatremic patient of a urinary sodium concentration greater than 20-25 mEq/L suggests the presence of a disorder associated with an excessive loss of sodium by the kidney (Table III).

Extracellular Volume	Urinary Sodium Concentration <10-15 mEq/L	Urinary Sodium Concentration >20 mEq/L
Contracted	Gastrointestinal losses diarrhea fistula post-op tube drainage vomiting Third space losses burn muscle trauma pancreatitis peritonitis	Diuretic excess Metabolic alkalosis with bicarbnaturia Mineralocorticoid exesss Osmotic diuresis glucose, glycerol, mannitol,urea Post-obstructive diuresis Renal tubular acidosis with bicarbonaturia Sodium losing nephropathies
Expanded (edematous)	Cardiac failure Cirrhosis Hepatic failure, acute Nephrotic syndrome	Acute renal failure, acute tubular necrosis Chronic renal failure, slowly progressive
Euvolemic to mildly expanded but non-edematous	Iatrogenic water loading? Psychogenic water loading? Syndrome ADH excess with patient ingesting low sodium diet	Antidiuretic hormone excess, drugs, emotion, pain, syndrome ADH excess Glucocorticoid deficiency Hypothyroidism

Table III: Relationship of Urinary Sodium Concentration to Various Diseases

A large number of clinical disorders may be associated with hyponatremia (Table IV). The delineation of the specific clinical features of these disorders is not the purpose of this review. Unless the history, physical examination and laboratory findings are compatible with one of the more common disorders known to be associated with hyponatremia it is our practice to consult a list tabulating the various diagnoses and to proceed in the above mentioned sequence to evaluate the patient initially for disorders compatible with the history, physical and available laboratory studies and, finally, to consider the remaining diagnostic possibilities.

Table IV: Etiology of Hyponatremia - Adapted from Cooke, R.E., Parenteral Fluid Therapy. In Nelson, W.E., Textbook of Pediatrics, Seventh Edition, W.B. Saunders, Co., Phila. 1959, p.191 and References 1,2 and 18.

I. Diminished extracellular volume
- A. Excessive loss (often with water replacement)
  - 1) Gastrointestinal: diarrhea, vomiting, fistula, tube drainage, salivary losses
  - 2) Renal: glomerular and interstitial disorders, ATN (recovery phase), post obstructive diuresis, transport defects (adrenal-insufficiency, RTA, mineralocorticoid excess) diuretics, SIADH?, cerebral salt wasting?
  - 3) Skin: excessive normal sweat, abnormal sweat (cystic fibrosis, adrenal insufficiency)
  - 4) Third space: burn, muscle trauma, pancreatitis, peritonitis, emphysema, thoracentesis, parencentesis
- B. Inadequate intake (may occur simultaneously with disorder of excessive loss)
  - 1) Low sodium diet
  - 2) Parenteral therapy (low sodium content)
  - 3) Resin therapy which may bind sodium
- C. Redistribution
  - 1) Acid base disorders
  - 2) Malnutrition, chronic severe
  - 3) Potassium deficiency
  - 4) Trauma

II. Euvolemic to mildly expanded extracellular volume (May be accompanied by decreased output)
  - 1) Factitious hyponatremia
  - 2) Glucocorticoid deficiency
  - 3) Hypothyroidism
  - 4) Iatrogenic water loading (parenteral) therapy, mist tent, tap water enema
  - 5) Oral intake (with diminished ouput)
  - 6) Pseudohyponatremia
  - 7) Psychogenic water drinker
  - 8) Reset osmostat
    - a) Cerebrovascular accident
    - b) Infection, tuberculosis
    - c) Malnutrition
  - 9) Syndromes with excessive levels of antidiuretic hormone (SIADH)

Table IV continued

III. Hyperexpanded extracellular volume (may be associated with diminished output)
1) Edema forming disorders - cardiac failure, cirrhosis, malnutrition, nephrotic syndrome, acute hepatic failure, renal failure, acute or chronic
2) Excessive intake - oral, ↑environmental humidity i.e. incubators, mist tent, parenteral therapy, (excessive input of all types prevalent in preterm infant)

Relatively few reports designed to evaluate the incidence of various disorders associated with hyponatremia in children and neonates are available (8) In our patient population, hyponatremia occurs most frequently as a consequenc of gastroenteritis, renal failure, and excessive antidiuretic hormone release. The remaining disorders are observed less often.

ASPECTS OF HYPONATREMIC DISORDERS IN RELATION TO TOTAL BODY WATER

Hyponatremia Associated with a Diminished Volume of Extracellular Fluid(1,2)

Diminished extracellular volume leads to the reabsorption of a greater fraction of the glomerular filtrate as well as an increase in the secretion oi antidiuretic hormone (ADH). The control of extracellular volume by the body supercedes the control of concentration of sodium. Consequently, when hyponatremia develops in a fluid deprived individual, additional ADH is also beinc released, and maximal quantities of water will be retained. This sequence of events may worsen the degree of hyponatremia.

In children with gastroenteritis, hyponatremia occurs becuase of the los: from the body via the gastrointestinal tract of sodium in excess of water and/ or the replacement of gastrointestinal losses with hypo-osmotic solutions. Th ingestion and/or intravenous administration of hypo-osmotic solutions in patients experiencing sodium loss through sweating, especially children with cystic fibrosis, or movement of iso-osmotic fluid into potential spaces such as peritoneal and pleural cavities or intracellular spaces (traumatically injured muscle) may also lead to hyponatremia.

If renal function is normal, the occurrence of the above disorders will usually be associated with a low urinary sodium concentration (usually less than 10 mEq/L), a low urine output, and a urine of high specific gravity. Exceptions to these urinary findings would be expected if advanced renal failure with an associated defect in sodium transport and renal concentrating capacity were present. The persistence of the hyponatremic state in these dis orders is due to the influence of hyponatremia on renal function: increased proximal absorption of glomerular filtrate with a low sodium concentration, diminished delivery of filtrate to the cortical diluting segment, and increase secretion of ADH resulting in the maximal conservation of water by the collecting ducts.

The generation of hyponatremia in the remaining hyponatremic disorders associated with a diminished extracellular volume is due to the excessive los: of sodium by the kidney, often accompanied by the continued ingestion of intra venous administration of hypotonic solutions or the failure of the extracellular compartment to receive sufficient amounts of sodium and water to replace losses. The urinary sodium concentration in these patients usually exceeds 20 mEq/L.

The use of diuretics may result in hyponatremia. The generation of hyponatremia occurs as a consequence of the failure of sodium reabsorption within the nephron leading to extracellular volume contraction and increased ADH release. Simultaneously, the inability of the nephron to lower the sodium concentration of the tubular fluid because of the pharmacologic action of diuretics on active transport sites decreases the ability of the kidney to excrete free water. The persistence of hyponatremia reflects the ongoing influence of these alterations on renal function. The loss of potassium may also result in the exchange of extracellular sodium for intracellular potassium and a reset osmostat.

Hyponatremia and extracellular volume contraction occur commonly in children with advanced renal insufficiency. The level of GFR determines the filtered load of sodium and sets by this mechanism the maximum quantity of sodium which can be excreted. Because of intrinsic changes occurring in nephron function as GFR falls, especially when the GFR falls to levels of less than 25-35 ml/min/1.73m^2, the renal excretion of sodium cannot be reduced when sodium intake decreases. Consequently, hyponatremia does not frequently occur in patients whose level of renal function exceeds this rate unless oral intake ceases and the renal losses of sodium are replaced with hypotonic solutions. Hyponatremia occurs when the GFR is less than 10-15 ml/min/1.73m^2 and a normal diet including the drinking of hypo-osmotic solutions is ingested. The occurrence of volume contraction, hyponatremia, and a high urinary sodium concentration in an otherwise well child associated with chronic renal insufficiency and a GFR exceeding 25-35 ml/min/1.73m^2 suggests the presence of a tubulo-interstitial disorder and/or some form of cystic disease.

Hyponatremia in Association with an Expanded Extracellular Fluid Volume (1,2)

Hyponatremia in association with an expanded extracellular volume occurs in two general clinical settings: 1) renal failure in which the urinary concentration of sodium exceeds 20 mEq/L and 2) edema forming disorders - cirrhosis, heart failure, and nephrosis in which the urinary concentration of sodium is generally less than 10 mEq/L.

The generation phase of hyponatremia associated with advanced renal failure is due to the limitation imposed on the renal excretion of solute free water by a low GFR and not a limitation in the renal diluting mechanism. The persistence of hyponatremia reflects a combination of the continued ingestion of hypotonic solutions sufficiently large to maintain an expanded extracellular volume and the limited ability of the kidney to excrete free water.

The majority of patients with generalized edema occurring in response to the development of cirrhosis, heart failure or the nephrotic syndrome will have normal serum levels of sodium. The development of hyponatremia in a few of these patients probably occurs as a consequence of changes in each of these clinical syndromes (9,10,11) leading to an associated increased release of ADH perhaps reflecting changes in baroreceptor response. Another mechanism which may be operative in children with advanced heart and/or liver failure is an enhanced reabsorption of glomerular filtrate in the proximal tubule and diminished delivery of filtrate to the diluting sites.

Hyponatremia Associated with Clinical Apparent Euvolemia (1,2)

The primary mechanism leading to the generation of hyponatremia associate with clinical apparent euvolemia is excessive secretion of ADH. The disorders associated with excessive serum levels of ADH do lead to a small increase in extracellular volume but the quantity is of an amount which does not lead to clinically apparent edema. A weight gain of 7-9% of body weight is needed before edema will be clinically apparent. Because the kidneys of these patients respond as if there were an increase in "effective" extracellular volume, urinary sodium excretion reflects sodium intake. When sodium restriction is imposed in such patients, the urinary sodium excretion will decrease to levels less than 10 mEq/L; otherwise, urinary sodium excretion exceeds 20 mEq/L.

In our experience, one of the more common problems in children leading to hyponatremia has been the syndrome of inappropriate antidiuretic hormone release. The term inappropriate is perhaps a misnomer,for in truth the ADH release is often quite proper for the given physiologic set. The word inappropriate is perhaps best appreciated if it is viewed as reflecting too much ADH for a given serum sodium concentration. The criteria which ought to be demonstrated prior to making a diagnosis of excessive ADH activity include the following (12,13):

1. normal renal, adrenal and pituitary function
2. extracellular fluid hypo-osmolality
3. persistent urinary excretion of sodium despite hyponatremia
4. the excretion of a urine whose concentration, i.e. osmolality is inappropriately high for the level of serum sodium. The urinary osmolality is always greater than that of a maximally dilute urine and may either be less and/or greater than the corresponding serum osmolality. In our experience, the urinary osmolality has often been less than the simultaneously determined serum osmolality.
5. severe water restriction corrects hyponatremia

Many disorders may be associated with the excessive secretion of ADH, the abnormal production of ADH and/or the failure of normal ADH metabolism to occur (Table V). Additionally, a number of drugs are known to alter ADH metabolism (2,14). Emotional stress (15) and physical pain may also alter ADH metabolism.

Table V: Etiology of the Syndrome of ADH Excess (Relative and Absolute)

1. CNS: infection, tumor, injury, vascular accidents, Guillain-Barre syndrome
2. Drug related:

Drug related:	Acetaminophen (Tylenol)	Morphine
	Barbiturates	Navane
	Carbamazepine (Tegretol)	Nicotine
	Chlorpropamide	Phenformin
	Clofibrate	Polymyxin B
	Cyclophosphamide	Thiazides
	Elavil	Tolbutamide
	Indomethacin	Vincristine
	Isoproterenol	

3. Endocrine: myxedema, cortisol deficiency, pituitary stalk section
4. Heart: Congestive heart failure, left atrial stretching

Table V continued

5. Infections: acute childhood infectious disorders, especially viral
6. Liver: hepatic failure, elevated portal vein pressure
7. Metabolic: acute intermittent porphyria
8. Pulmonary: infections, fibrosis, tumors, ventilation (CPAP)
9. Renal: changes in sodium handling by the kidney related to volume contraction and/or diuretics, hypoalbuminemia
10. Surgery related: anesthesia or premedication, peritoneal reflexes, intracranial manipulation, post-op pain

The precise nature by which hyponatremia occurs in patients with thyroid (16) and glucocorticoid deficiency (17) has been only partially defined. Glucocorticoid deficiency may be associated with elevated levels of ADH occurring as a consequence of an alteration in myocardial function while thyroid deficiency may lead to alterations in GFR and thereby decrease distal delivery o glomerular filtrate. Although it has been suggested that thyroid deficiency may be associated with increased ADH activity, confirmation of such a relation ship is still needed.

Reset Osmostat

Hyponatremia can occur because of the readjustment of those mechanisms normally controlling the serum sodium concentration. There have been a few reports of chronically ill and/or malnourished patients whose serum osmolality has fluctuated around a reduced level of serum sodium (18). In these patients the osmotic control of ADH around the lower level of serum sodium was apparent ly normal. Such patients are very unusual and such a diagnosis should be considered only after all other diagnoses have been systematically eliminated.

REFERENCES

1. Humes, H.D., Narins, R.G. and Brenner, B.M.: Disorders of Water Balance. The Kidney in Health and Disease: IX Hospital Practice, March, 1979, p.133.
2. Berl, T. and Schrier, R.W.: Water Metabolism and the Hypo-Osmolar Syndrome In Sodium and Water Homeostasis, ed. Brenner, B. and Stein, J.H., Cont. Issues In Nephrology I, Churchill-Livingstone, New York, Edinburgh and London, 1978, p.1.
3. Arieff, A.I. and Guisado, R.: Effects on the central nervous system of hypernatremic and hyponatremic states. Kidney International 10:104, 1976.
4. Arieff, A.I., Liach, F. and Massry, S.G.: Neurological manifestations and morbidity of hyponatremia: Correlation with brain water and electrolytes. Medicine 55:121, 1976.
5. Covey, C.M. and Arieff, A.I.: Disorders of Sodium and Water Metabolism and Their Effects on the Central Nervous System. In Sodium and Water Homeostasis. ed. Brenner, B. and Stein, J.H., Cont.Issues In Nephrology I, Churchill-Livingstone, New York, Edinburgh and London, 1978, p.212.
6. Thurston, H.J., Hauhart, R.E., Jones, E.M. and Ater, J.L.: Effects of salt and water loading on carbohydrate and energy metabolism and levels of selected amino acids in the brains of young mice. J.of Neurochemistry 24: 953, 1975.
7. Waugh, W.H.: Utility of expressing serum sodium per unit of water in assessing hyponatremia. Metabolism 18:706, 1969.

8. Varavithya, W. and Hellerstein, S.: Acute symptomatic hyponatremia. Medical Progress. J. Pediatr. 71:269, 1967.
9. Humes, H.D., Gottlieb, M.N.and Brenner, B.M.: The Kidney in Congestive Heart Failure With Emphasis on the Role of the Renal Microcirculation in the Pathogenesis of Sodium Retention. In Sodium and Water Homeostasis. ed. Brenner, B.M. and Stein, J.H., Cont.Issues in Nephrology I, Churchill Livingstone, New York, Edinburgh and London, 1978, p.51.
10. Levy, M.: The Kidney in Liver Disease. In Sodium and Water Homeostasis. ed. Brenner, B.M. and Stein, J.H., Cont.Issues in Nephrology I, Churchill-Livingstone, New York, Edinburgh and London, 1978, p.73.
11. Coggins, C.H.: Nephrotic and Nephritic Edema. In Sodium and Water Homeostasis. ed. Brenner, B.M. and Stein, J.H., Cont. Issues in Nephrology I, Churchill-Livingstone, New York, Edinburgh and London, 1978, p.117.
12. Bartter, F.C. and Schwartz, W.B.: The syndrome of inappropriate secretion of antidiuretic hormone. Am.J.Med. 42:790, 1967.
13. Schwartz, W.B., Bennett, W., Curelop, S. et al: Syndrome of renal sodium loss and hyponatremia probably resulting from inappropriate secretion of antidiuretic hormone. Amer.J.Med. 23:529, 1957.
14. Moses, A.M. and Miller, M.: Drug-induced dilutional hyponatremia. New Eng. J.Med. 291:1234, 1974.
15. Linshaw, M.A., Hipp, T.J. and Gruskin, A.B.: Infantile psychogenic water drinking. J.Pediatr. 85:520, 1974.
16. Michael, U.F., Kelley, J., Alpert, H. and Vaamonde, C.A.: The role of dista delivery filtrate in the impairedrenal dilution of the hypothyroid rat. Am.J.Physiol. 230:699, 1976.
17. Boykin, J., McCool, A., McDonald, K. Robertson, G. and Schrier, R.: Mechanism of effect of glucocorticoid deficiency on renal water excretion in the conscious dog. Clin.Res. 24:269A, 1976.
18. Taclob, L.T. and Needle, M.A.: Hyponatremic syndromes. Med.Clin.N. Am. 57: 1425, 1973.
19. Supported in part by NIH Clinical Research Center Grant No.RR-75, HL23501, and the Hoechst Roussel Pharmaceutical Co.

RENAL HANDLING OF POTASSIUM IN CHRONIC RENAL INSUFFICIENCY

Jacques J. Bourgoignie, M.D.

PATHOPHYSIOLOGY

The regulation of extracellular fluid (ECF) potassium concentration and potassium balance is complex because only 1 to 2 percent of total body potassium is extracellular. Moreover, the excretion of potassium is not exclusively renal.[1-3]

Extrarenal adaptations

Several factors influence the distribution of potassium between the intra-and extracellular compartments (Table I). Alkalosis, an increased level of ECF potassium and the hormones aldosterone, insulin and epinephrine facilitate cellular uptake.[-8] Conversely, sudden increases in ECF osmolality tend to redistribute potassium outside cell membranes leading to hyperkalemia.[1-3] Little is known about the influences of these factors in chronic renal disease. A decreased intracellular potassium content associated with a decreased transmembrane potential difference has been described in patients with chronic renal disease.[9] This might facilitate the entry of potassium intracellularly and, thereby, buffer and minimize increases in ECF potassium. However, a decreased extrarenal uptake of potassium has been claimed to occur in uremic patients and rats.[10,11] Except for the colon, extrarenal potassium adaptation has not been demonstrated in chronic renal failure.

Table 1. Factors Affecting Potassium Distribution

1. Acid-Base Status
2. Insulin
3. Aldosterone
4. Epinephrine (B-adrenergic system)
5. Hyperosmolar Status

The colon secretes potassium, but its contribution to balance (about 10 percent of intake) is negligible in health. When glomerular filtration rate (GFR) decreases, secretion of potassium by the colon increases. Nevertheless, this mechanism cannot replace the kidneys and remains of little significance in patients with a creatinine clearance in excess of 10 ml/min or in dogs and rats with a GFR 25 to 40 percent of normal.[12-14] In contrast, stool potassium increases markedly and averages 35 percent of intake in patients with end-stage renal failure and a creatinine clearance below 5 ml/min.[15] Fecal potassium excretion is independent of sodium intake, and proportional to stool wet weight and potassium intake. The mechanism responsible for increased stool potassium in chronic uremia is aldosterone-dependent, and has been associated with an increase in colonic mucosal Na-K ATPase.[10] The changes are limited to the colon and do not occur in the jejunum.[16] Patients with hyperaldosteronism also exhibit increases in fecal potassium that disappear after correction of the hyperaldosteronism.[17] An increase in Na-K ATPase in the colon also occurs in normal animals given a high dietary potassium;[18,19] this response is also abolished by adrenalectomy.

Renal adaptations

The same adaptations occur in individual nephrons. Thus, patients with chronic renal failure, on an average potassium intake, typically exhibit normal fasting concentrations of serum potassium and maintain potassium balance on a 24-hour basis.[12] This implies an increased ability of the remaining nephrons to excrete potassium. Markedly increased rates of potassium excretion per nephron have been demonstrated in chronic renal insufficiency. In fact, the amount of potassium excreted may exceed the amount of potassium filtered. Since the amount of potassium remaining in the early distal tubule averages less than 10 percent of the filtered load in superficial nephrons from intact and remnant kidneys, the kaliuresis results predominantly from an increase in potassium secretion by distal nephron segments.[14,20] Adaptive mechanisms for tubular secretion of potassium have been demonstrated by micropuncture in the late distal and collecting tubules of normal rats exposed to a high potassium intake, as well as in rats with a decreased renal mass.

The adaptive mechanisms that facilitate excretion after an acute potassium challenge, have not been fully characterized (Table II). Potassium adaptation and homeostasis in chronic uremia can be dissociated from the dictates for sodium, hydrogen and phosphorus balance.[21] The adaptation occurs after GFR reduction by renal artery construction, showing no direct role for the filtered load of potassium. Insulin, glucagon and aldosterone have been proposed as effectors of potassium excretion. Studies in dogs with chronic renal insufficiency show no regulatory role for insulin or glucagon.[22] In the dog, transient hyperkalemia develops after induction of an 80 percent reduction in nephron mass, and potassium excretion per nephron increases. Within one week, however, fasting serum potassium returns to control values and 24 hr balance is restored. The same adaptation occurs in adrenalectomized dogs with a remnant kidney provided with a low, fixed dose of mineralocorticoid hormone, as well as in animals given supramaximal doses of mineralocorticoids.[13] These observations mitigate against any regulatory role for aldosterone. Nevertheless, the hormone appears important in its permissive action. Indeed, the rate of potassium secretion is blunted in the absence of normal plasma levels of aldosterone. Moreover, in patients with moderate renal insufficiency and hypoaldosteronism, hyperkalemia is common and can be corrected by administration of exogenous mineralocorticoids. Finally, spironolactone, a tubular aldosterone antagonist, decreases urinary potassium excretion and increases circulating potassium concentration.[23-25]

Table 2. Factors Affecting Potassium Secretion

1. Aldosterone
2. Dietary Potassium
3. Acid-Base Status
4. Tubular Flow Rate
5. Serum Potassium
6. Nephron Mass

Urinary potassium excretion is also influenced by sodium delivery and/or tubular fluid flow rate in the distal tubule and by uptake of potassium at the peritubular membrane.[2,26] Changes in serum potassium rapidly modify active peritubular uptake, leading to proportional changes in both intracellular potassium and rates of potassium secretion from cell to tubular lumen. The ability of acute acid-base disturbances to alter potassium secretion probably reflects changes in peritubular uptake of potassium, alkalosis enhancing and acidosis decreasing it. Chronic (but not acute) administration of aldosterone restores distal tubular intracellular potassium content in adrenalectomized rats, presumably by increasing renal Na-K ATPase in the baso-lateral membrane and, thereby, facilitating potassium uptake. All these factors undergo changes in chronic uremia.

In-vitro experiments utilizing the isolated perfused kidney or the isolated cortical collecting tubule have conclusively shown that the adaptation for potassium secretion was intrinsic to the nephrons.[27-29] Fine et al have shown that both transepithelial potential difference and aldosterone contribute to the adaptation in cortical collecting tubule of uremic rabbits;[29] but neither factor accounts for the phenomenon entirely. Transepithelial potential difference across the isolated cortical collecting tubule and aldosterone levels were greater in uremic than in normal rabbits fed a high-potassium diet. However, both factors were quantitatively similar in normal and in uremic rabbits fed a normal potassium diet, despite the fact that potassium secretion was significantly increased in the latter. Fine et al also found that intracellular potassium content per unit tubule length was increased in uremic rabbit because of an increased size of cortical collecting tubules.[29] Nevertheless, the same intracellular potassium concentration was found in equally hypertrophied tubules of uremic rabbits adapted from a normal to a high potassium diet. Although, in intact animals fed a high potassium diet and in chronically uremic animals, enhancement of potassium secretion has generally been attributed to an increase in Na-K ATPase activity of the outer medullary tissue, increases in Na-K ATPase activity were not associated with higher rates of potassium secretion in these studies. Therefore, uncertainty remains regarding the mechanisms underlying the adaptive increase in potassium secretion. In the isolated kidney, kaliuresis varies directly with changes in potassium concentration of the perfusing solution.[27,28] It appears that aldosterone and other factors set the sensitivity level of the peritubular membrane to acute changes in serum potassium concentration by modifying Na-K ATPase activity.

Response to an acute potassium load

Data in the literature suggest that the failing kidney responds with the same kaliuresis as the normal kidney to an acute potassium challenge.[13] Recent observations from our laboratories indicate otherwise, and point to an impaired ability of the remnant kidney to excrete a potassium load.[22] We compared the dynamics of potassium excretion after an oral load in normal and in chronically uremic dogs with a remnant kidney and a GFR about 30 percent of normal. Irrespective of previous dietary intake, varying from 15 to 100 mEq of potassium per day, fasting serum potassium and daily urinary potassium excretion were similar in normal and remnant dogs. However, after orogastric administration of 50 mEq potassium chloride, serum potassium rose significantly more (Fig. 1) and kaliuresis significantly less in remnant than in normal dogs. In 5 hours, the normal animals excreted 61 to 67 percent of the potassium load, but the remnant dogs excreted only 30 to 39 percent.

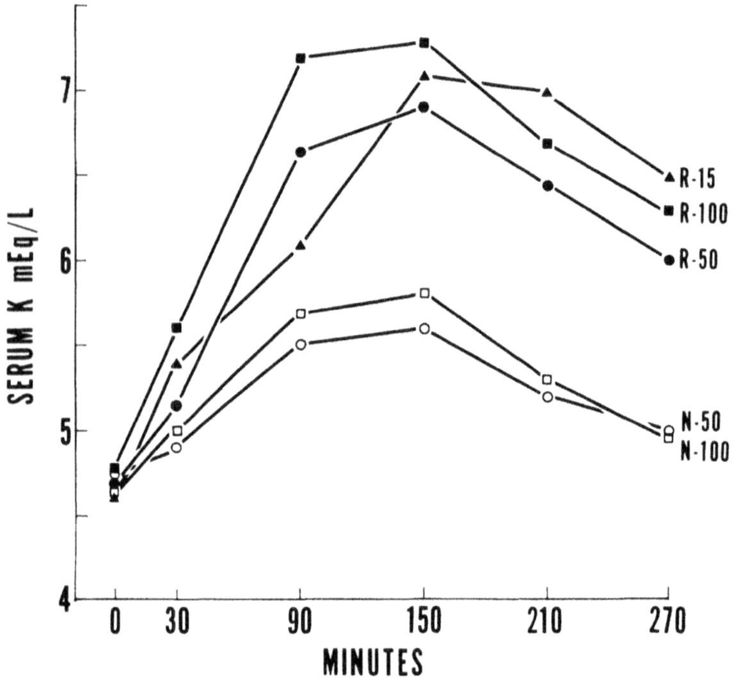

FIGURE 1. Changes in serum potassium in normal (N) dogs and in dogs with chronic renal insufficiency (R) after orogastric administration of 50 meq KCl at time 0. Fasting serum potassium before the challenge varied from 4.6 to 4.8 meq/L in all groups. N-50, N-100 and R-15, R-50 and R-100 refer to normal and uremic animals respectively maintained on 15, 50 or 100 meq potassium diets. There were 6 animals in each group.

Although the kaliuresis correlated directly with the concentration of serum potassium in all groups, this relationship was markedly attenuated in the remnant animals, and independent of previous dietary potassium intake (Fig. 2). The same change in circulating potassium induced a smaller kaliuresis in remnant than in normal animals.

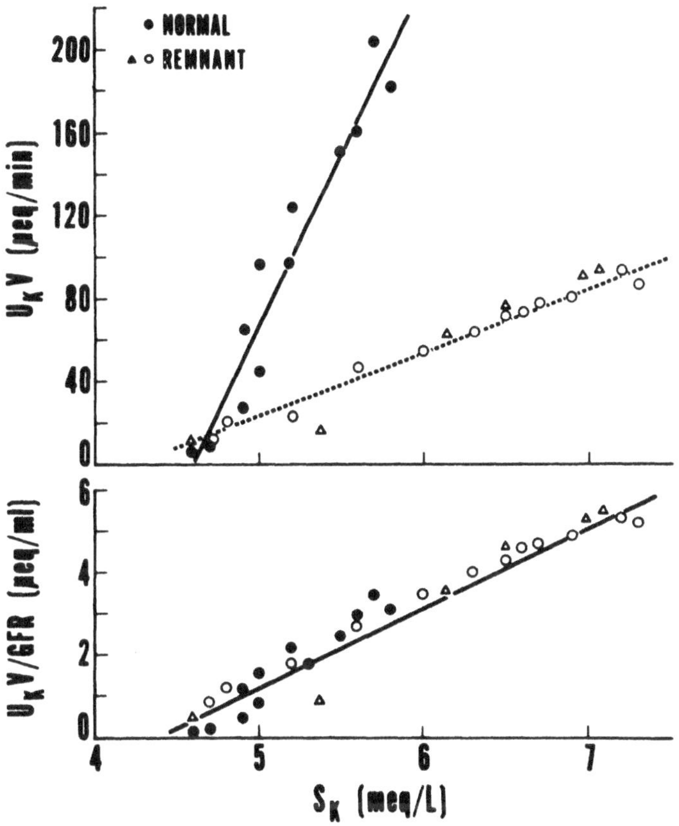

FIGURE 2. Mean absolute (UKV) and per ml GFR (U_kV/GFR) urinary potassium excretion rates for the groups of normal and uremic dogs depicted in Fig. 1. Circles indicate animals on 50 or 100 meq potassium diets; Δ, animals on 15 meq. (Reprinted with permission from Kidney International [22]).

The fasting levels of circulating aldosterone were identical in normal and remnant dogs; and like serum potassium, aldosterone increased more and remained elevated longer in remnant than in normal dogs (Fig. 3).

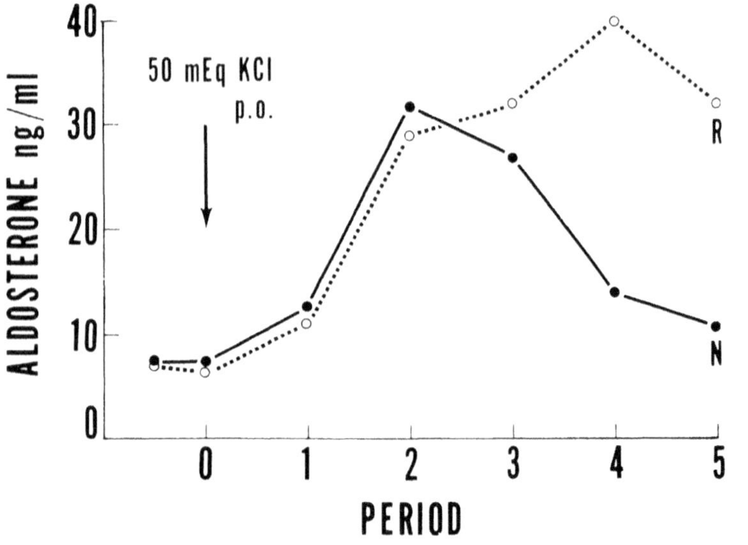

FIGURE 3. Effects of KCl on circulating aldosterone in normal (N) and remnant (R) dogs. (With permission from Kidney International [22]).

Thus, the blunted kaliuresis of remnant dogs occured despite a prolonged hyperkalemia and hyperaldosteronism. Plasma insulin and glucagon levels and the acid-base status of the animals did not change during the acute potassium challenge.[22] The data also indicated a greater extrarenal buffering of potassium in the chronically uremic dog than in the normal animals.[22] These experiments clearly demonstrate that the aggregate of surviving nephrons in the remnant kidney is limited in its ability to excrete potassium. After a potassium challenge, potassium retention occurs. As a result, an augmented and prolonged hyperkalemia and stimulation of aldosterone ensue. The diseased kidney, however, cannot respond normally, and excretion of the load is prolonged. When balance is re-established, usually within 24 hours, fasting serum potassium and aldosterone levels and urinary potassium excretion rates return to normal.

These observations agree with the enhanced hyperkalemia observed in patients with chronic renal insufficiency given a potassium challenge.[30] In agreement with data in the isolated perfused kidney, the results, also suggest that changes in serum potassium may directly effect an end-organ response. In this context, the adaptations in potassium excretion, although imperfect, can be viewed as an attempt to shorten the time over which balance is restored after administration of a potassium load.

CLINICAL REMARKS

The clinical consequences of these observations are important for the care of patients with chronic renal insufficiency. First, there is little need to restrict potassium intake in the average patient with chronic renal insufficiency under steady state condition until end-stage renal failure occurs. However, under conditions of intercurrent illness with increased catabolism and metabolic acidosis, K intake should be reduced. Second, if hyperkalemia develops in a patient with chronic renal failure and a plasma creatinine below 10 mg/dl, causes other than renal insufficiency may be implicated including metabolic acidosis, increased catabolism, dietary indiscretion, administration of blood, or drugs that either contain potassium (penicillin) or prevent cellular entry of potassium (beta-adrenergic antagonists); drugs that inhibit angiotensin activity directly (converting enzyme inhibitors) or indirectly (prostaglandin synthetase inhibitors) may lead to hyperkalemia by blunting the stimulation of aldosterone secretion, particularly in states of volume depletion. Third, the danger of severe life-threatening hyperkalemia contraindicates the use of potassium-sparing diuresis in patients with chronic renal impairment, in patients simultaneously receiving oral potassium supplements, or in insulinopenic diabetic patients, even those with normal renal function, who may be prone to develop hyperkalemia in relation to hypoaldosteronism or complicating events of acidosis or hyperglycemia. Fourth, due to release of potassium from muscle during cell depolarization, depolarizing muscle relaxants such as succinylcholine may result in hyperkalemia. Patients with renal insufficiency and a decreased excretory ability are particularly susceptible to the effects of these agents.[31] Fifth, oliguric patients are prone to develop hyperkalemia because of the influence of distal tubular fluid flow rate on potassium secretion. Severe hyperkalemia may develop in patients with chronic renal insufficiency experiencing acute episodes of dehydration or oliguria from urinary retention or acute decreases in GFR.[1] Sixth, in end-stage renal disease, constipation induced by phosphate-binding gels, or otherwise, should be avoided as it can lead to hyperkalemia by preventing the contribution of the colon to potassium excretion. Seventh, since potassium excretion both in the colon and in the nephron is mediated by Na-K ATPase, inhibition of this enzyme by digitalis glycosides would be associated with a reduction in cellular uptake of potassium. Hyperkalemia has been described with digitalis intoxication.

Acknowledgments

The secretarial assistance of Ms. Rosa Alvarez is deeply appreciated. This work was supported by U.S. Public Health Service Grant AM 19822.

REFERENCES

1. Schultze, RG, Nissenson AR: Potassium: physiology and pathophysiology: in Maxwell MH, Kleeman CR(eds): Clinical disorders of fluid and electrolyte metabolism. McGraw-Hill Book Co, 1980, pp 113-145.

2. Gabow PA, Peterson LN: Disorders of potassium metabolism: in Schrier RW(ed): Renal and electrolyte disorders. Little, Brown and Co, Boston, 1980, pp 183-223.

3. Kliger AS, Hayslett JP: Disorders of potassium balance: in Brenner BM, Stein JH(eds): Contemporary issues in Nephrology. Vol. 2. Acid-Base and Potassium Homeostasis. Churchill Livingstone

Publishers, New York, 1978, pp 168-204.

4. Alexander EA, Levinsky HG: An extrarenal mechanism of potassium adaptation. J Clin Invest 47:740-748, 1968.

5. Santeusanio F, Falooma GR, Knochel JP, et al: Evidence for a role of endogenous insulin and glucagon in the regulation of potassium homeostasis. J Lab Clin Med 81:809-817, 1973.

6. Cox M, Sterns RH, Singer I: The defense against hyperkalemia. The roles of insulin and aldosterone. New Engl J Med 299:525-532, 1977.

7. DeFronzo RA, Sherwin RS, Dillingham M, et al: Influence of basal insulin and glucagon secretion on potassium and sodium metabolism: Studies with somatostatin in normal dogs and in normal and diabetic human beings. J Clin Invest 61:472-479, 1978.

8. Rosa RM, Silva P, Young JB, et al: Adrenergic modulation of extrarenal potassium disposal. New Engl J Med 302:432-434, 1980.

9. Bilbrey GL, Carter NW, White MG, et al: Potassium deficiency in chronic renal failure. Kidney Intern 4:423-430, 1973.

10. Schon DA, Silva P, Hayslett JP: Mechanisms of potassium excretion in renal insufficiency. Am J Physiol 227:1323-1330, 1974.

11. Kahn T, Kaji DM, Nicolis G, et al: Factors related to potassium transport in chronic stable renal disease in man. Clin Sci Mol Med 54:661-666, 1978.

12. Van Ypersele de Strihou C: Potassium homeostasis in renal failure. Kidney Int 11:491-504, 1977.

13. Schultze RG, Taggart DD, Shapiro JP, et al: On the adaptation in potassium secretion associated with nephron reduction in the dog. J Clin Invest 50:1061-1068, 1971.

14. Bank N, Aynedjian HA: A micropuncture study of potassium excretion by the remnant kidney. J Clin Invest 52:1480-1490, 1973.

15. Haynes CP, McLeod ME, Robinson RR: An extrarenal mechanism for the maintenance of potassium balance in severe chronic renal failure. Trans Assoc Am Physicians 80:207-217, 1967.

16. Bastl C, Hayslett JP, Binder HJ: Increased large intestinal secretion of potassium in renal insufficiency. Kidney Int 12:9-16, 1977.

17. Edmonds CJ, Godfrey RC: Measurement of electrical potentials of the human rectum and pelvic colon in normal and aldosterone-treated patients. Gut 11:330-337, 1970.

18. Silva P, Charney AN, Epstein FH: Potassium adaptation and Na-K ATPase activity in mucosa of colon. Amer J Physiol 229:1576-1579, 1975.

19. Hayslett JP, Myketey N, Binder HJ, et al: Mechanism of increased potassium secretion in potassium loading and sodium deprivation. Amer J Physiol 239:F378-F382, 1980.

20. Giebisch G: Renal potassium excretion: in Rouiller C, Muller AF(eds): The kidney: Morphology, biochemistry, physiology Vol. 3. Academic Press, New York, 1971, pp 329-401.

21. Espinel CH: Effect of proportional reduction of sodium intake in the adaptive increase in glomerular filtration of nephron and potassium and phosphate excretion in chronic renal failure in the rat. Clin Sci Mol Med 49:193-200, 1975.

22. Bourgoignie JJ, Kaplan M, Gavellas G, et al: Renal handling of potassium in dogs with chronic renal insufficiency. Kidney Int In Press

23. Perez G, Siegel L, Schreiner GE: Selective hypoaldosteronism with hyperkalemia. Ann Intern Med 76:757-763, 1972.

24. Oh MS, Carroll HH, Clemmons JE, et al: A mechanism for hyporeninemic hypoaldosteronism in chronic renal disease. Metabolism 23: 1157-1166, 1974.

25. Schamberlan M, Sebastian A, Biglieri EG: Prevalence, pathogenesis, and functional significance of aldosterone deficiency in hyperkalemic patients with chronic renal insufficiency. Kidney Int 17: 89-101, 1980.

26. O'Connor G, Kunau RT: Renal transport of hydrogen and potassium: in Brenner BM, Stein JH(eds): Contemporary issues in nephrology, Vol 2. Acid-base and potassium homeostasis. Churchill Livingstone, New York, 1978, pp 1-30.

27. Silva P, Ross BD, Charney AN, et al: Potassium transport by the isolated perfused kidney. J Clin Invest 56:862-869, 1975.

28. Silva P, Brown RS, Epstein RH: Adaptation to potassium. Kidney Int 11:466-475, 1977.

29. Fine LG, Yanagawa N, Schultze RG, et al: Functional profile of the isolated uremic nephron. Potassium adaptation in the rabbit cortical collecting tubule. J Clin Invest 64:1033-1044, 1979.

30. Gonick HC, Kleeman CR, Rubini ME, et al: Functional impairment in chronic renal disease. III. Studies of potassium excretion. Am J Med Sci 261:281-290, 1971.

31. Kunau RT, Stein JH: Disorders of hypo- and hyperkalemia. Clin Nephrology 7:173-190, 1977.

HIGHLIGHTS: CYSTINOSIS

Ronald J. Kallen, M.D.

Cystinosis in children is a rare, heritable inborn error of metabolism leading to extensive accumulation of cystine in many organs and tissues with consequent organ dysfunction, most notably the kidneys (nephropathic cystinosis). This condition has no relationship to cystinuria. Patients with cystinosis do not have cystine urolithiasis. Cystinosis is inherited as an autosomal recessive. Both parents are asymptomatic carriers without detectable stigmata of disease. Each pregnancy carries a 25% risk of an affected child and a 50% risk of an asymptomatic carrier child. Means are available for antenatal diagnosis. The clinical features of nephropathic cystinosis may be described as follows:

1. Apparently-well infants during the first 6 months of life
2. Profound failure-to-thrive in later infancy with marked growth retardation
3. Blondness
4. Photophobia
5. Recurrent dehydration and acidosis with minor flu-like illness
6. Salt and fluid craving
7. Profound polyuria
8. Rickets
9. Fanconi syndrome with renal tubular acidosis (proximal type)
10. Normal intelligence
11. Insidious hypothyroidism
12. Characteristic opacities of the lens on slit-lamp examination
13. Widespread deposition of cystine in many organs
14. Cystine crystals in bone marrow
15. Progressive renal failure

Cystinosis with renal involvement may not appear until the second decade (juvenile form). The usual clinical presentations are failure-to-thrive with rickets, incidental findings of glycosuria and tubular proteinuria, and delayed onset of nocturnal bladder control. The exact metabolic defect is not known. There are no known enzyme deficiencies. The defect appears analogous to other "storage" diseases, with sequestration of cystine in lysosomes rendering it unavailable for cell metabolism.

Current therapy includes use of vitamin D, phosphate supplementation, sodium and potassium citrate, and thyroid hormone replacement as thyroid "reserve" declines (rising TSH).

Cysteamine is being studied in a multicenter collaborative trial (National Institutes of Health, University of California at San Diego, and University of Michigan) and elsewhere as means of depleting cells of cystine. Preliminary results in terms of preservation of renal function, are encouraging. In one recent report (New Eng. J. Med. 304:41, 1981), creatinine clearance improved in two out of five children; however, Fanconi syndrome and growth retardation persisted.

DISCUSSION

José Strauss, M.D., Moderator

MODERATOR: Regarding sickle cell nephropathy, in terms of the hypothesis of the ischemia being the pathophysiologic event that starts the sequence, as we have proposed, really it's all conjectural. We don't have the necessary information. There is no experimental animal. We tried to develop an experimental model while Rawle McIntosh was still alive, but did not really succeed. We don't have proof that that happens. The other phenomenon that we interpreted as supporting the concept of hypoxia being responsible or at least involved is the fact that when we took piglets and allowed them to breathe 10% oxygen, there was a natriuresis which Finberg and his group have reported to occur in sickle cell crisis. I don't know whether you have any comments on the hypoxia, the natriuresis and the hyponatremia which subsequently developed.

RESPONSE: As you have said, there are no animal models for sickle cell disease. We looked at this, obviously, because there is a limit as to what we can do in patients. We came up with the deer in the Florida Keys. There are only a few hundred of them left - a small deer which is so peculiar that it's just the opposite of the patients. It sickles at 100% oxygen. It's really not a model for what we see in sickle cell disease. Regarding the theory of hypoxia, nobody has evaluated it as far as I know, but there is suggestive data. For instance, the available data like the beautiful micro-angiographic studies of the Dutch workers and the worsening of the renal problem with age. The fact that once the patient has a concentration defect he will always have it, only proves that there is no more hypertonicity in the medulla. In a young child you expect that he will concentrate his urine under conditions of hydropenia up to > 1000 mOsm/kg but in this disease they lose this capacity very early in life. Therefore, I think that you will have to study people who are very young to be able to prove this. The blood transfusions show in a sense that if you eliminate the S hemoglobin there is presumably no more hypoxia. Of course, it could be just an ischemic effect. There is a lot of data against the old theory that the transport of sodium chloride is affected in the ascending limb of the Loop of Henle in these patients; for instance, the lack of salt wasting. As such, it does not exclude the Loop of Henle hypothesis because it may be that there is a selective reabsorption of sodium recaptured downstream.

MODERATOR: The natriuresis and hyponatremia, by the way, as proposed by Finger and collaborators would occur during the sickle cell crisis; if that were the case, they may not be present in the periods between crises. Am I correct?

RESPONSE: I have to confess I'm not familiar with this study, but I am with other studies from the West Indies. There they have looked at renal function during sickle cell crises. What happened there is that sodium excretion went down. I don't know of anybody who has shown enhanced sodium excretion under conditions of a crisis. Since there is no animal model, we are stuck with the hypothesis.

QUESTION: Am I not correct that there's been a recent report of trying to maintain patients with chronic hyponatremia in an attempt to avoid crises with some success?

RESPONSE: You are correct. I am familiar with the abstract which was published some time last year.

MODERATOR: The entire paper is out now.

COMMENT: This again follows the old thoughts where to a high intake of water of about 3.8 to 4 liters a day is added a relatively low sodium intake. These patients drop their serum sodium to 124-125 mEq/L and they have a significantly decreased number of crises. I think the patients have something like seven or eight crises in six or eight months as a baseline of the study with normal serum sodium. Then, with this treatment in a period of actual practice, the number of crises was zero within a period of a few months. When the patients somehow didn't follow this regimen carefully, the crises reappeared within a relatively short period of time. To me what these data show is that hyposmolality may dilute the concentration of the S hemoglobin.

QUESTION: Do they show data on sodium excretion?

MODERATOR: I don't recall. But, to me, the main claim was that the oxygen dissociation curve with hyponatremia was "improved" with the oxygen carrying capacity being increased. As the cell swells up, the curve is actually shifted to the left. The question which remains to be answered is whether or not tissue oxygenation improves.

COMMENT: I thought they showed that dilution of S hemoglobin did the trick. It's obvious. You could do the same thing by blood transfusion early in the game. I don't remember how old these patients were. There were only two patients in the abstract.

MODERATOR: There are more patients in the final paper and as I recall, the emphasis was on the size of the red cell. Even though there were not enough patients and the difference in the number of crises may not be definitive, it is suggested that they are doing something desirable. The question is, what should we improve? Should we improve the oxygen carrying capacity at the expense of the oxygen releasing ability or should we do the reverse? That's a question that in oxygen transport circles has never been settled. The only way this question will be settled is by measuring tissue oxygen and then see if, with one or the other of the available tools, tissue oxygenation is indeed improved. Increasing the oxygen carrying capacity does not necessarily mean that one is doing what the tissues actually need. Satisfying the tissue needs (whatever that means) should be the final goal.

COMMENT: It would be interesting to discuss the pathogenesis of RTA in sickle cell disease because the fact is, you have found a defect in urine pH and a normal ammonium production, which is an incomplete form of RTA. Then, there are patients in a more evolved state with high potassium and hypoaldosteronism-hyporeninism, more fitting in type four RTA. But most patients have normal potassium. Then, which type of RTA could it be, which pathogenesis could be involved? The fact that potassium secretion is also impaired is very similar to the situation of the "short circuit effect".

For that you should speculate that there is a defect in sodium reabsorption with an abolished negative transtubular potential because sodium is not reabsorbed. But, you have mentioned that the sodium transport is completely normal. My question is, there are studies done looking at the pCO_2 in the urine that have been able to assess the distal secretion of hydrogen ion and the possibility to correct this transtubular electrical gradient by means of sulfate or other substances that increase the electronegativity in the lumen.

RESPONSE: We have done that. I think they have a distal type, an incomplete syndrome of distal RTA. I think 40% of the patients studied showed this. We could not show salt wasting. These patients on a low salt diet conserved sodium normally. In the literature I know of two patients. One in the Dutch group. In one of their patients they mention this but don't show any data. They have studied a number of patients. The other one is included in a recent report. We and the group in the West Indies have shown that they conserve sodium normally. That's in response to DOCA or when you put them on a low sodium diet. We have indeed given them sodium sulfate. When you do that, you can sometimes improve in some of them but this is not a complete reversal; as we have shown in cirrhotic patients, they all reverse to normal; that is, their capacity to generate a steep gradient after giving them sodium sulfate. Perhaps this means that there is in these patients,back diffusion of hydrogen or a low electronegativity of the lumen, and that the so-called "electrical component" was the culprit.

We also measured Δ pCO_2. After a bloody fight in the nephrology acid-base field, finally it appears that urine minus blood pCO_2 is an acceptable way of looking in vivo in an animal or a human at distal hydrogen secretion, most likely collecting duct secretion. This you do simply by giving orally or by infusing IV sodium bicarbonate, thus increasing the bicarbonate in the urine and the generation of CO_2. This CO_2 is subtracted from blood pCO_2 and this difference relates to distal hydrogen secretion for reasons that I will not go into detail to explain. The trait patients we studied all have normal ΔpCO_2's. The patients with sickle cell disease were split in between and they were split almost half and half. They all had low urine-blood CO_2 difference but half of them had inability to generate a normal pH less than 5.3 and the other half reached normal pH's. Another group has shown that the volume status of the individual has a tremendous importance in ΔpCO_2. Volume contraction will tend to increase the difference and volume expansion will make for a nice correlation between ΔpCO_2 and urine bicarbonate concentration.

QUESTION: In your patients with sickle cell, was there a correlation between the level of ΔpCO_2 and the actual concentration of the urine? Was it a low CO_2?

RESPONSE: You mean the bicarbonate? Unfortunately we didn't measure the bicarbonate in the urine because this work is five-six years old. At the time we didn't realize the importance of bicarbonate excretion. We were measuring pCO_2 with the blood gas analyzer.

QUESTION: But it is a concentration defect; it's a low concentration of bicarbonate.

RESPONSE: Well, now it's volume that's an important factor. We will have to look into it. For us it looked like in some maybe back diffusion of hydrogen was important. But, we were not sure because there was enough sodium available in the urine. These people are not like cirrhotic patients who have low sodium in their urine. These people have sodium in their urine and, under those conditions, the syndrome of incomplete RTA that has been described in view of the findings in cirrhotics may or may not apply. It was easy to understand why it was thought to be due to the low electrical potential.

QUESTION: I know of only one report of a few cases of sickle cell disease patients with what looked like proximal RTA. In your patients studied with bicarbonate infusion - Did you rule out proximal RTA?

RESPONSE: I think we did. First of all, we didn't do a lot of bicarbonate infusions in these patients except in the ΔpCO_2 studies in which we weren't measuring bicarbonate. We were just measuring ΔpCO_2 concentration and pH. Although we could recalculate the data for bicarbonate, we have moved to other fields. Under base line conditions the bicarbonaturia we have shown is negligible; this is typical of incomplete RTA. Therefore, it is very difficult to believe that they would have significant proximal RTA if the bicarbonaturia is negligible under normal bicarbonate concentration. But workers in Jamaica have done these studies and shown that the bicarbonate Tm and bicarbonate proximal tubular reabsorption are normal.

QUESTION: I was asking this question because the work I referred to remains the isolated one to have found a proximal RTA.

RESPONSE: I'm not familiar with that work.

MODERATOR: What would you guess would happen if the patients with sickle cell disease were studied with the methodology presented earlier in this Seminar-- volume expansion.

RESPONSE: I think it would be normal. I think that all the data presented here showed that free water clearance is normal under the condition of hypertonic saline. It's very clear in the data presented that with the technique of fractional clearances there would be no abnormality. And that is quite curious because when you study free water clearance, it is not only Henle's Loop that is involved. The whole distal diluting segment should participate in the formation of free water.

Most of the free water is formed in the thick ascending loop but it is quite unexpected to find a normal free water formation with the enormous lesions shown us in the medulla. It's fantastic. I cannot understand it.

COMMENT: Well, I'm not sure. I think the theory of selective hypoxia may explain it. During water diuresis, or sodium diuresis, or mannitol diuresis, the urine flow is increased. Blood flow to the medulla, even if it is increased, will dilute the hemoglobin there, sickling may decrease and the concentration will decrease. You may change the pH. You are doing all the things that favor the patient. That's why some years ago it was said that one desirable approach to the hematuria of these patients, a frequent problem, is to minimize sickling. You minimize sickling by giving water, by giving bicarbonate, maybe mannitol, or diuretics. All these approaches will improve circulation and if you give enough oxygen, the active transport mechanisms should be normal. The fractional excretion of sodium is normal under conditions of solute diuresis. If there is a difficulty of salt wasting, it is only under the conditions of ischemia. It is hard to prove. Finally, many of the findings in the blood of these patients could be due to ADH release as a result of pain, hypertonicity, etc.

MODERATOR: I want to emphasize before we leave the subject, that what was just said is crucial in terms of providing a good perfusion of the tissues. The treatment that some people have advocated of giving packed red cells really could be a dangerous maneuver if it is not coupled with what is probably the most important part, the providing of circulating volume. In terms of the inducement of hyponatremia, really there is no clear proof yet that it does work and in some patients, it may be dangerous if done without controls of urinary excretion of sodium since, as we were saying before, it has been proposed that in some of these patients there is increased sodium loss. Therefore, ideally, these patients should be individualized,carefully monitored, and treated according to the findings.

COMMENT: I'd like to comment about transplantation in sickle cell anemia. We've had some experience with a couple of patients. First, one of the children that we transplanted eventually died because she refused to let us remove her gall bladder and developed gall stones. Evidently, gall bladder disease has been a problem in some of the patients who have had transplants with sickle cell disease. In fact,some people have suggested that if you have SS disease, you ought to remove the gall bladder before you transplant. The second problem is speculation. What do you do after a transplant as the sickle hemoglobin starts to rise? What a number of people have been doing is keeping them chronically transfused which presents a number of mechanical problems and raises the question of what's going to happen over the long haul with the chronic transfusion in terms of their transplanted kidney. I'm not aware of, and I gather from the survey that there has not been any recurrence of disease in the transplanted kidney. At least it hasn't been reported yet.

COMMENT: You are absolutely right. All that was in the report, which was briefly presented to you today, is just a one year follow-up. Of course, here in Miami if you could have a successful renal transplant you would be able to physiologically do a number of studies in these patients. If you could it would be a fantastic model because presumably even if the kidney had had Acute Tubular Necrosis and recovered, it would offer the opportunity to unravel what sickling may do to these patients in a variety of functions very early in the game. This is hard to do with a little child subjected to a number of studies. To my knowledge, it has not been done.

QUESTION: A question about this survey you reported that I missed, you mentioned 30 transplants that had been done; nine had SS disease and 21 were traits. So that the number of patients with SS disease that have been transplanted is indeed very small.

QUESTION: Were your two cases among these nine?

RESPONSE: No. Our two were not and I can't remember what our patients had. One had SS; the other SC or SS, I'm not sure.

COMMENT: This brings a very important question. Why trait patients with end-stage renal disease? Unfortunately, this review could not answer this because there was no histopathological description.

COMMENT: There are some reports of people with trait having hematuria.

RESPONSE: Not only some reports. If you take hematuria, the majority of hemoglobinopathy patients with hematuria have AS hemoglobin (trait). The second largest group is the one with SC disease, and the third is the one with SS disease. Unfortunately a statement that sickle cell disease has less hematuria than the other forms has crept up in the literature. That's wrong. It follows the distribution of the genes. There are many more AS patients; eighty percent of the black population, compared with SS which is 2% or less. If anything, you should see more because the anatomical abnormalities are more extense in the SS patients.

MODERATOR: We reported (in the paper you quoted from the group of the late Rawle McIntosh and I) a case of trait (AS) with the complete form of the nephropathy, the renal tubular epithelial antigen in the circulation and glomeruli, and the membranoproliferative nephritis (MPGN). We may have failed to tell you to include in that group a patient who just now is getting ready to start hemodialysis who was picked up as part of the International Study, a membranoproliferative glomerulonephritis who has sickle cell trait. She was treated with the drug therapy under comparison for MPGN. We finally had to take her out of that group. We did not know whether she accidentally had the trait and the association was not related in a cause and effect fashion but with the progression that she had, the course resembles more the patients with the sickle cell nephropathy than patients with membranoproliferative. We don't have but one patient with idiopathic MPGN (Type I); she is doing quite well. So, there is no question that the trait seems to be able to produce the nephropathy. Maybe we can switch now to other areas. Any other questions or comments?

QUESTION: I would like to ask a question. In the chronic renal failure model with one kidney, there was a decrease in potassium excretion. Does that apply also to nonglomerular entities?

RESPONSE: The decrease in potassium excretion does apply irrespectively of what the etiology of the renal disease is in each patient-- whether it was glomerular or tubular, they react similarly. Although they sometimes have minimally decreased GFR, I grant you that there are specific diseases where you may see more frequently hyperkalemia. One thing I could comment on is the differences in the literature between various studies and ours.

We followed essentially the same protocol. It seems that it is all due to the fact that their animals were fed at the time of the potassium challenge. If you give food with potassium, there will be sequestration of potassium in the GI tract, much slower reabsorption; you will miss the peak because by 5 hours not enough potassium had been reabsorbed. But you will see it--to answer your question--in most types of diseases.

MODERATOR: I may have missed this in your presentation of the experimental preparation with which you have worked so extensively. Does the GFR return to normal at the same time within those seven or eight days?

RESPONSE: The GFR does not change. In the remnant it will increase slightly but from a very low value. Let's say it was 8-9 ml/min before you did the nephrectomy. That's the period of time you are talking about, I think. It may go up to 12 or 13 ml/min. We have dogs now that have been staying for two years with a GFR of 14 or 15 ml/min. They will regenerate or hypertrophy a little bit immediately after nephrectomy but then they remain stable.

MODERATOR: And never goes back to the combined GFR that you had prior to the nephrectomy?

RESPONSE: No. The combined GFR is the normal GFR essentially because they have one intact kidney and one diseased kidney. It's a slightly decreased GFR but not much. But, if you take the intake kidney out, the GFR is going to fall off and remain low.

COMMENT: We had one child with the hemolytic uremic syndrome who was anuric for a period of time and then developed essentially a total infarction of his colon. He had to have a colectomy up to his ileum. His GFR gradually started to improve and we had a terrible time trying to control his potassium by diet. I'm aware that a fair amount of potassium adaptation in chronic renal disease occurs because of increased potassium secretion in the gut. I wonder whether you've done any animal studies with your model, removing part of the gut and looking at what happens with the potassium level. Do you think it would be worth doing?

RESPONSE: Yes. There is very little known about potassium-- the contribution of the colon to potassium balance. The only studies I know are those in vivo --in patients. The authors don't mention the actual diet in the paper. All the numbers are in percent of intake, so one doesn't know exactly what levels they are speaking of. But in animals, in rats at least, the colon seems to contribute to potassium but we have not done any such studies.

QUESTION: Looking at your data, there is an extrarenal component of the response to potassium loading --it's increased in your patients. That obviously must be a compensatory mechanism. That increase in serum potassium is less than what really happened, simply because now there is more potassium in the cell.

COMMENT: That's correct. The only thing we wanted to show here was that there was at least no defect in uptake. But if one assumes there was no uptake in extrarenal tissues, these animals at the end of 5 hours should have a serum potassium of about 13 mEq/L. At least those given the potassium intravenously. So it could not be compared. Obviously, the extrarenal tissue is important. Whether it's an adaptation or a regulation,I am not sure , or whether it is not simply a function of the gradient that exists between extracellular potassium and intracellular potassium.

QUESTION: Regarding Bartter Syndrome, is there anything to the proposed special structures or any organic explanation for some of the changes? Specifically, we had a patient with the syndrome whom we biopsied and the pathologist observed what seemed a short-cut circuit, as I recall, connecting the proximal with the distal tubule. We never reported that. We thought that it may be an artifact. Is there anything to that?

RESPONSE: Well, there was a publication in 1969 about some glomerular-distal tubular shunts in patients with Bartter Syndrome. In this work by electron microscopy they found these funny shunts between Bowmans capsule and the distal tubular cells. I think your observation could be in this line of thinking. It doesn't explain very well the distal defect. If you get a proximal defect, if the filtrate goes directly to the distal part and escapes the proximal tubular reabsorption, it doesn't fit very well with the functional data. This thing is always quoted in all reviews on Bartter syndrome. Nobody seems to put much attention to it. I think the observation has been previously published.

QUESTION: In your list I think you said that gentamycin could produce a potassium depletion. Have you seen this clinically? I am familiar with some dog work where this was found recently. We have looked extensively in over a hundred rats treated with gentamycin with various protocols and we have not seen that.

COMMENT: I put it in the list because there are observations of hypokalemia after gentamycin administration. That's the only thing I can tell.

QUESTION: What is the mechanism?

RESPONSE: I don't know because we know that gentamycin makes specifically a proximal tubulopathy and that all studies done on the distal part of the nephron are intact. It's hard to understand why hypokalemia should follow. Gentamycin administration is a drug that specifically acts on the proximal tubule. I am aware of a case of a distal RTA, not very well documented. I asked a famous American professor--he was visiting us--and he said "Oh, that's very well known". But really I think that all distal effects of gentamycin toxicity should be very carefully questioned.

QUESTION: On this topic, was the hypokalemia associated with loss of potassium in the urine or redistribution of potassium? Could it be secondary to hypomagnesemia?

RESPONSE: The report I quoted was a paper on drug induced hypokalemia. It was interesting because most of these cases are patients with malignancies. They have some infection during the course of leukemia and it was very frequently quoted, the situation that a basic disease precipitated this hypokalemic state. I don't recall now all the details but they were infectious on top of some leukemic disorder.

QUESTION: Were these gentamycin toxicity or were they because of some of the other antibiotics.

RESPONSE: They reported that gentamycin induced hypokalemia.

COMMENT: Some other synthetic penicillins? Carbenicillin will increase the distal transtubular gradient.

COMMENT: The other report is on carbenicillin and also is of hypokalemia associated with antibiotic treatment and associated with malignant neoplasms.

COMMENT: That's different.

QUESTION: Is it not possible theoretically if you have a proximal tubular defect with gentamycin that sooner or later you would encounter a patient that had a big enough defect, delivered enough sodium distally, that he might get hypokalemic on that basis although that's not a distal defect?

RESPONSE: These are clinical observations. They are not worked up as far as the pathogenesis of hypokalemia. It was just a report of the association of the treatment and the biochemical abnormalities without any physiopathological studies. Hypomagnesemia has been described after gentamycin.

COMMENT: Along the same point as the malignancies, I thought there was some relationship to lysozumuria in malignancies with high load of potassium and destruction of the cells with the hypokalemia and increased kaliuresis. Then, it would be a secondary hypokalemia. Isn't that so?

COMMENT: Our rats with gentamycin toxicity excrete tons of lysozyme in the urine. They don't have hypokalemia or wasting of potassium.

COMMENT: Then, it's something else.

QUESTION: To go back to the sickle cell discussion, I come from the Middle East and the problem there is rather different from what we have been discussing. At least we can identify two groups of SS patients. One, people coming from the African society where for the severe SS disease they develop crises and fail to grow and have all the problems. The other group of patients with proven SS disease are those who are usually Arabian people who have less severe disease. Many of them are found by accident. Usually they live quite normal lives. My question is, first of all, do you see these varieties in your population? If you do, or don't, how would you explain the variations in response to various modalities of treatment. I know there are so many variables you are discussing but is it all degree of renal disease or could it be the hemoglobinopathy itself or the type of it that is maybe affecting response to the treatment? You say 40% responded to one treatment and so on. Is it a different spectrum of one disease or are we having one type of disease or more than one?

RESPONSE: You probably are correct. I'm not a hematologist. We would need a geneticist to answer you properly. There are a number of factors that influence results. The percent of F hemoglobin a patient may have is important. It has been shown that the disease is less severe, including renal manifestations, if they have a high F content. I think there are variations dependent upon where the patient comes from. This is absolutely right. For a long time in this country they neglected the black population that grew older. Everybody thought they weren't reaching this age because they died before that and it is not true. Therefore, there must be a difference between one group and another. There are patients who reach over sixty; people from the West Indies wrote a beautiful book on sickle cell four or five years ago and they insisted on this point. There is a sub-group of people with sickle cell disease who grow to be sixty and some who have no renal function, obviously-- 2/3 of them in one group studied. So you probably are right. Do these factors have an impact on the pathology? The answer is yes. I don't know what treatment you were referring to.

RESPONSE: Only noting what you explained, that only 40% of them respond. Have you been screening your patients for different hemoglobins or just saying that they have hemoglobin SS and then screening their renal functions?

RESPONSE: We did this study in cooperation with the hematologists who have a sickle cell disease center here. All our patients were seen by the people in the sickle cell center-- a rather good screen. Most of them were known to the hematologists.

QUESTION: About cystinosis. As you said, this must be a very rare disease, but maybe we are missing it. I am wondering, we see so many young patients who come with rickets. We say this is renal tubular acidosis. What I am asking is, what is the most useful diagnostic test looking at your data, for a clinician who is not aware of the situation may easily miss it unless he uses certain laboratory tests or clinical approaches. Are you suggesting a muscle biopsy or a bone marrow biopsy or a test that will prove it or biochemical information to determine the diagnosis?

RESPONSE: Probably, the easiest thing to do is the slit lamp examination by an opthalmologist. The findings are so characteristic that that would confirm the presence of the disease. The question really is, since the Fanconi Syndrome can be seen with rickets or nutritional rickets, are you missing this more rare condition in your particular population, are you seeing individuals with rickets and Fanconi Syndrome who are going on to chronic renal failure? That would be the natural history of unrecognized cystinosis. In terms of a ready diagnosis, the slit lamp is probably the quickest way to make that diagnosis.

COMMENT: We have two brothers who started cystinosis very early in life, the first year of life. Now they are 10 and 9 years old and they don't have any renal insufficiency. Their tubular disorder was treated and now everybody is surprised. The years go by and they have maintained a rather normal GFR. Unfortunately, we don't have cystine content.

Are you aware of any case of adolescent cystinosis starting early in life? I believe there is a possibility that these patients had adolescent cystinosis of early onset. Since this was an adult type of cystinosis diagnosed in 16 and 11 year old girls, I don't see why the adolescent type could not be present in infancy. Are they different diseases or the same disease with different degrees of severity? I am surprised. I was expecting to get cystine contents; if they have very high levels I will be obliged to make the diagnosis of nephropathic cystinosis, but I'm puzzled because we gave such a bad prognosis to the parents and the children are doing all right, growing quite well.

QUESTION: They are growing well, then they don't have the full expression?

RESPONSE: They have a full blown Fanconi Syndrome.

QUESTION: Fanconi Syndrome per se, but they are not azotemic.

COMMENT: They are very interesting.

COMMENT: I think that's possible. I don't recall whether the intermediate or juvenile form of Fanconi Syndrome manifests early in life or not but it's possible that these may evolve into renal failure later and become examples of the intermediate form.

MODERATOR: Thank you everybody.

III

HYPERTENSION

THE HYPERTENSION PROBLEM IN CHILDREN

Mary Jane Jesse, M.D.

Prior to 1970 the problem of hypertension in children revolved around renal disease, central nervous system disease, coarctation of the aorta, and rare endocrine or collagen disease.

The pediatric community began in 1970 to study blood pressure levels in children, and ten years later there are now available data which allow the pediatrician to identify children whose blood pressure levels are persistently at the highest levels for age and sex.

Numerous studies have been completed to determine whether blood pressure level at a given age is predictive of a level at a later age.

Programs have been developed to aid the pediatrician in managing the child with elevated blood pressure. The programs advise methods of diagnosis as well as therapy.

As in so many cases, however, there are some dangers if the pediatrician overreacts to a statistically determined definition of hypertension.

These and other aspects of identification, and management of elevated blood pressure in children must be understood in any discussion of hypertension.

STANDARDS FOR CHILDREN'S BLOOD PRESSURE

In May of 1977, the report of the Task Force of Blood Pressure Control in Children (1) was published by Pediatrics as a supplement. The data regarding blood pressure of children included in this Task Force report, are the result of recording of blood pressures by specific protocol at the University of Iowa and the Mayo Clinic, in 11,309 children from the age of 5 through 18, and children between 2 and 5 years of age totaling 306 children.

From these data blood pressure charts which presented the various percentiles for age were published, and are now available for inclusion in the chart of each child which the pediatrician sees (1).

The study of these children revealed some surprises. For example, in boys at age 13, the 95th percentile for blood pressure was 140/95 mm of mercury. In 18-year old boys, blood pressures of 145/90 represented the 90th percentile. In females, the 95th percentile at age 14 had reached 140/90 mm of mercury, and at age 18 that blood pressure reading was the equivalent of the 90th percentile. Since those levels are commonly used as a measure of mild hypertension in adults, it was a surprise to find that "mild hypertension" was identified in children from 13 to 18 in at least 5% of the population.

PERCENTILES OF BLOOD PRESSURE MEASUREMENT

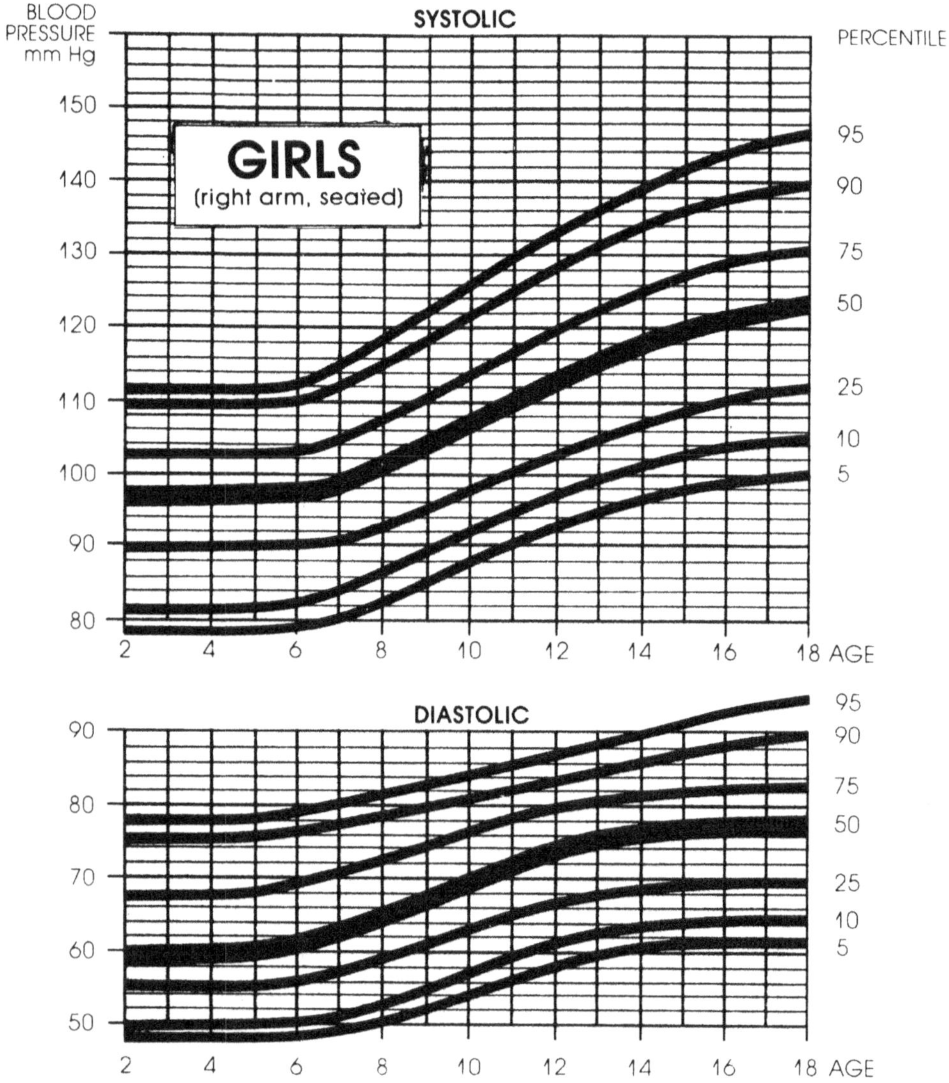

Blood pressure measurement percentiles prepared by the National Heart, Lung, and Blood Institute's Task Force on Blood Pressure Control in Children, (Supplement) Vol. 59, No. 5 Part 2, May, 1977.

"Because it does not follow that a single high pressure is an abnormal finding, the charts are not intended for use in assessment of an individual child's blood pressure at a single point in time but rather for the plotting of pressures during growth and maturation . . . a single elevated measurement (i.e., greater than the 95th percentile) in an apparently healthy child does not necessarily reflect disease; it is necessary to repeat these measurements over time to obtain a trend."

PERCENTILES OF BLOOD PRESSURE MEASUREMENT

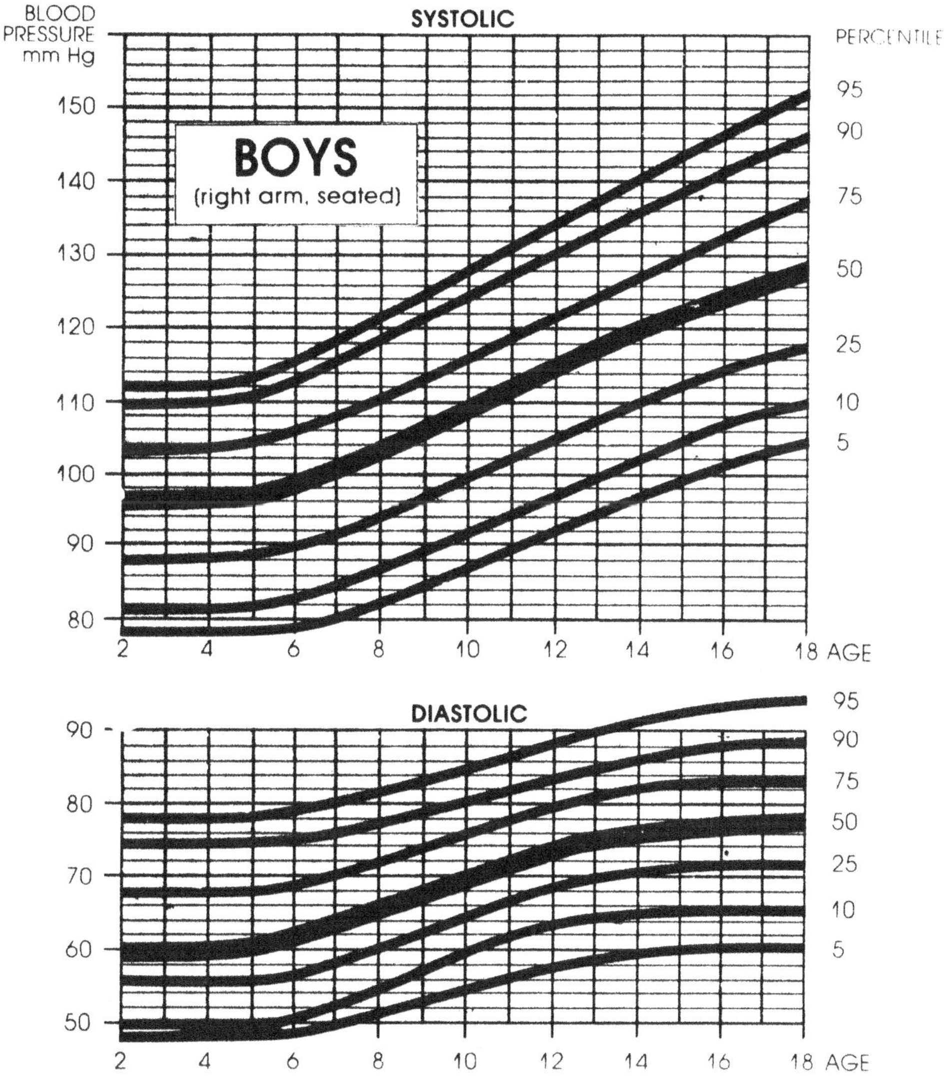

Blood pressure measurement percentiles prepared by the National Heart, Lung, and Blood Institute's Task Force on Blood Pressure Control in Children, (Supplement) Vol. 59, No. 5 Part 2, May, 1977.

"Because it does not follow that a single high pressure is an abnormal finding, the charts are not intended for use in assessment of an individual child's blood pressure at a single point in time but rather for the plotting of pressures during growth and maturation . . . a single elevated measurement (i.e., greater than the 95th percentile) in an apparently healthy child does not necessarily reflect disease; it is necessary to repeat these measurements over time to obtain a trend."

The charts which allow sequential recording of blood pressure levels in children, become a valuable adjunct in the health care program of children who are followed either by their own physicians, or by school physicians and Public Health medical personnel.

It became apparent from follow-up studies, that it was extremely important to repeat blood pressure levels in children and to identify children with high "normal" blood pressures only after having repeated the blood pressure at 3 separate visits to the health care provider.

This resulted from the finding of several investigators, which indicated that on the 2nd and 3rd measurement of blood pressure in children, less than 2% of children found to be in the 95th percentile would have blood pressure levels remaining in that percentile, and would commonly be found to have much lower pressures at the 2nd and 3rd examination (2).

PREDICTABILITY OF BLOOD PRESSURE IN CHILDHOOD

A number of studies have been completed to determine whether the blood pressure level at a given age is predictive of a level at a later age.

In adults 35 to 70 years of age, tracking correlations for systolic blood pressure equal 0.6, and 0.5 for diastolic pressure reported over a 4-year follow-up interval.

In adults who were followed for over 2-year periods the correlation coefficient for systolic and diastolic blood pressure rose to about 0.7 (3).

In a 4-year follow-up interval for children in the Boston area, Zinner et al.(4) reported correlations of 0.25 for systolic pressure and 0.14 for diastolic pressure. This finding, among a group of children age 2 to 14 years of age at entry, was of statistical significance, but of very small biological significance. It would predict that over a 4-year period in children age 2 to 14 years of age, the chances of predicting what the blood pressure might be 4 years later is only of the order of 6%. For diastolic pressure, the chances of making a significant prediction are of the order of 2%.

In a study of 820 children studied repeatedly over a 6-year period, the group at the University of Iowa (2) reported correlation coefficients of 0.3 for casual systolic blood pressure and 0.18 for diastolic blood pressure. The chances of predicting blood pressure over a 6-year period then are of about the same order as the previous study.

The group in Iowa reported on the correlation coefficients over a 2 year period at age 15. The correlation coefficients for systolic blood pressure over a 2 year period in the 15-year old group was .42 and for diastolic blood pressure the coefficient was .39. At age 16, a group was followed over a 2-year period, and the coefficient for the systolic blood pressure had risen to .57 and for diastolic pressure to .28.

It would thus appear that the chances of predicting a blood pressure over a 2, 4 or 6 year period are not very high. It is also apparent that the correlation coefficients do not begin to approach those found in adults until after the age of 16 years.

Thus, the relatively low orders of magnitude for the tracking correlations reported during childhood provide no evidence that hypertensive adults may be identified with any degree of certainty solely on the basis of casual blood pressure determinations during infancy or early childhood.

This finding serves to emphasize the need for practicing physicians to remain aware of several assumptions which underly the decision to intervene on blood pressure levels in infancy or childhood. First, it must be proven that it is feasible to lower blood pressure levels in infants and young children for extended periods of time. It must also be determined that lowering blood pressure in childhood is more beneficial than lowering the elevated pressure in adulthood. Third, and probably most important, is the consideration that the anticipated benefits of the therapy will exceed the risks.

There also appears to be some confusion as to what should be done about elevated systolic blood pressures in childhood and/or adolescence. Since the data are not clear as to how to approach the problem of systolic hypertension in the adult population, it is apparent that treating of systolic blood pressure elevations in childhood is even more tenuous.

It was, therefore, the opinion of the Task Force on Blood Pressure Control in Children that the level of diastolic blood pressure should be the guide as regards consideration of the institution of therapy.

EVALUATION OF CHILDREN AND INFANTS WITH ELEVATED BLOOD PRESSURE

The accepted program (1) for evaluation of blood pressure in children has been designed as a result of the data presented above. The child whose initial blood pressure measurement is found to be less than the 95th percentile should be referred to his usual continuing health care program which should include repeated measurements of his blood pressure. If on the initial examination the diastolic blood pressure is greater than the 95th percentile, the blood pressure measurement should be repeated at another visit. If at that visit the blood pressure is less than the 95th percentile that child would be referred to his continuing health care regimen and, of course, blood pressure should be repeated at each visit. If the diastolic pressure on the 3rd visit continues to be greater than the 95th percentile, investigation may be indicated. The medical history should be repeated, the physical examination should be repeated, and a urinalysis should be performed. If the patient is obese or a cause is identified for hypertension, a BUN or creatinine may not be indicated. Otherwise, measurement of the blood urea nitrogen and creatinine would be appropriate.

If the diastolic pressure is less than 90 mm of mercury at ages 3 through 12 and less than 100 mm of mercury at ages 13 through 18, the individual should be counseled regarding weight loss if obesity is present, an exercise program, and a diminution of salt intake. If, on the other hand, the diastolic pressure is greater than 90 in children ages to 12 and greater than 100 in ages 13 to 18, that child should be referred on for further investigation.

MANAGEMENT OF ELEVATED BLOOD PRESSURE LEVELS IN CHILDHOOD

If the blood pressure measurements correspond to those described above, and all the usual causes, that is coarctation of the aorta, renal disease, adrenal disease, etc. have been ruled out, a stepped care program for lowering the blood pressure is outlined in detail in the Task Force on Blood Pressure Control in Children. This program in essence suggests the use of Thiazide as the first step in treatment in the group age 7 to 12 years of age, and that individualized therapy in the group 13 to 18 should be considered. In this age group drug therapy is not always required. Weight control, avoidance of salt abuse, and systematic follow-up may accomplish the purpose of lowering the diastolic blood pressure.

If either of these steps do not accomplish a lowering of the diastolic blood pressure in either of the age groups, the use of beta blockers of Methyldopa may be the appropriate next step. If these steps fail, the use of a vasodilator may be considered. The drugs which affect blood pressure as vasodilators constitute something of a problem in children since Clonidine, as an example, has not yet been evaluated in children, and since Guanethidine has a number of side effects which may not be desirable. The best advice for the practicing pediatrician may be to consult with a specialist in hypertension when one runs into a patient who requires a vasodilator, or a patient who is refractory to the outlined methodology. Children with diastolic pressures greater than 100 mm of mercury should probably be hospitalized for their work-up.

CONCLUSION

The data as reviewed present a great deal of information to the practicing pediatrician as to how to manage elevated blood pressure in children. There are clearly pitfalls along the way, if a systematic approach is not taken to the identification, evaluation, and management of elevated blood pressure levels in childhood. Based on the data as currently recognized, there is little evidence to support drug intervention on systolic blood pressure elevation. Based on the low correlation coefficients for blood pressure levels in children for a 2, 4 or 6-year period, it appears that careful and systematic follow-up of blood pressure levels in children is very important in terms of establishing a therapeutic regimen. If all other causes of hypertension have been ruled out, and the elevation of diastolic blood pressure is persistent, great care must be taken in terms of drug intervention, in order to guard against risks of therapy being greater than benefit to the patient.

There is no question that the emphasis on blood pressure levels in childhood has had a salutary effect on the raising of consciousness in the pediatric practice community, as well as in the population of parents and patients.

The tremendous amount of effort which has been expended in collecting the data reported here, will have been justified if the practicing physician, particularly those who look after children, make the taking of blood pressure in their patients as systematic a part of the physical examination as examining the ears or the throat.

It is hoped as the years progress, that the scientist who is examining the etiology of elevated blood pressures will make major contributions in our understanding of the population data observations which have been produced, and in our management of children who are proven to be persistently hypertensive.

REFERENCES

1. Blumenthal, Sidney, M.D. et al.: Report of Task Force on Blood Pressure Control in Children. Pediatrics 59:5, Part 2, 1977.

2. Clarke, William R., PhD et al.: Tracking of Blood Lipids and Blood Pressures in School Age Children: The Muscatine Study. Circulation 58:4, 1978.
3. Feinleib, M. M.D. et al.: Relationship between blood pressure and age. Read before the 97th annual meeting of the American Public Health Association, Philadelphia, November 1969.
4. Zinner, S.H., M.D. et al.: A longitudinal study of Blood Pressure in Childhood. American Journal of Epidemiology 100:437, 1975.

THE EVALUATION OF THE CHILD WITH HYPERTENSION

Donald E. Potter, M.D.

The evaluation of the child with hypertension has two goals. One is to determine the effect of hypertension on the body. This is accomplished by examination of the ocular fundi and heart, chest x-ray and electrocardiogram. The second, and more important, is to determine the cause of the hypertension.

It has often been stated that hypertension in children, especially prepubertal children, almost always has a cause that can be identified.[1,2] It has therefore been recommended that all prepubertal hypertensive children have an extensive evaluation or work-up to determine the cause of their hypertension, and that a diagnosis of primary or essential hypertension can be made only after a negative work-up has been completed.

This viewpoint concerning the nature of hypertension in children largely reflects studies of severe hypertension in selected children published prior to 1970.[1,3] During the last decade, information derived from studies of blood pressure in larger populations of asymptomatic children[4-7] has resulted in modification of this viewpoint and changes in the recommendations for evaluation of hypertensive children. In this paper the information on which previous and more recent recommendations for the evaluation of hypertension in children are based will be reviewed, the causes of hypertension will be outlined, and a sequence for the evaluation of hypertension will be discussed.

STUDIES OF HYPERTENSION IN CHILDREN

The results of three studies in which the causes of hypertension were evaluated in children are summarized in Table 1. In the study from London, all children admitted to a children's hospital over a 10-year period with a sustained diastolic blood pressure greater than 120mm were evaluated. An etiology of the hypertension was determined in 52 of 55 children and was attributed to renal disease, including renal artery stenosis, in 37. The hypertension associated with polyarteritis nodosa probably also had a renal mechanism as well.

In Muscatine, Iowa, the blood pressure of 6,622 asymptomatic school children was screened and hypertension was defined as a blood pressure either greater than the 95th percentile for normal children of the same age and sex or greater than 140/90, on four different occasions. Of the 41 children who were identified as hypertensive only 29% were in the prepubertal age range. Twenty-three were obese and a cause of hypertension other than obesity was identified in only 5.

TABLE 1. Studies of Hypertension in Children

	London [3]	Muscatine [7]	St. Louis [4]
Number of children	55	41	74
Age, years	-	6-12(12) 13-18(29)	3-12(69) 13-16 (5)
Number obese	-	23	39
Number with cause	52	5	5
Pyelonephritis	18		2
Other renal disease ± pyelo	13	1	3
Glomerulonephritis	6		
Renal artery stenosis	5	1	
Coarctation of aorta	6	2	
Pheochromocytoma	1		
Cushing syndrome	1		
Polyarteritis nodosa	1		
Contraceptive pills		1	

In Saint Louis, 74 children in a pediatrician's practice were identified as hypertensive and 69 were in the prepubertal age range. Hypertension was defined as a blood pressure greater than the 90th percentile for normal children, repeatedly, or greater than the 95th percentile for normal children, occasionally, for one year. Only one child had a diastolic blood pressure greater than 90mm. Forty-five children had systolic hypertension only, 39 were obese, and a probable cause of hypertension other than obesity was identified in only 5, all associated with the kidney.

The results of the London study indicate that in children with severe hypertension, a cause of the hypertension can almost always be identified and is most often due to kidney disease. Although the Saint Louis study can be criticized because the definition of hypertension included children with blood pressure lower than the 95th percentile, the results of that study and the Muscatine study indicate that in most children with mild hypertension, no cause of the hypertension can be found. An extensive evaluation of children with mild hypertension is therefore unwarranted.

CAUSES OF HYPERTENSION

As stated by Rance and associates,[8] "The list of common causes (of hypertension) is short and the list of rare causes long." The list of causes in Table 2 is not complete but covers the major categories of organ system pathology causing hypertension. Most of the causes not listed are either very rare or are acute clinical conditions with which hypertension is sometimes associated. The former include porphyria, familial dysautonomia and mercury poisoning and the latter, burns, poliomyelitis, orthopedic traction and Guillian-Barre syndrome. The list in Table 2 can be simplified into categories of obesity, ingestions, the brain, thyroid, aorta, adrenal gland, endocrine tumors and the kidney. Renal artery stenosis needs to be considered separately from the other renal causes of hypertension because the diagnostic approach is different.

EVALUATION OF HYPERTENSION

The American Academy of Pediatrics Task Force on Hypertension has formulated guidelines for the evaluation of hypertension in children.[9] These guidelines reflect information derived from the studies of hypertensive children noted above and take into account the more common causes of hypertension listed in the table. The guidelines will be reviewed and provide the background for the more extensive evaluation of severe hypertension described in this paper.

Hypertension is defined as a blood pressure greater than the 95th percentile for normal children on three or more occasions. The initial evaluation of children who meet this criterion is a complete history, including family history, a physical examination, urinalysis and urine culture, hemoglobin and hematocrit, serum electrolytes, and BUN and creatinine. If this work-up is negative and the diastolic blood pressure is less than 90mm in a child 3-12 years of age or less than 100mm in a child 13-18 years of age, no further work-up is recommended, but the child should have periodic surveillance of blood pressure, yearly reevaluation, and counseling regarding such factors as salt intake, physical activity, and weight control. Although not specified in the guidelines a child with severe hypertension should also have a chest x-ray and EKG to look for evidence of target organ damage.

TABLE 2. Causes of Hypertension

Obesity	Adrenogenital syndrome
Drugs	Cushing syndrome
Contraceptives	Primary aldosteronism
Steroids	Pheochromocytoma
Amphetamines	Neuroblastoma, ganglioneuroma
Lead	Wilms tumor
Increased intracranial pressure	Renal parenchymal disease
Thyrotoxicosis	Hydronephrosis
Coarctation of the aorta	Renal artery stenosis

This preliminary work-up should provide clues to most of the causes of hypertension. The history should establish the diagnosis of drug ingestion and should elicit the well-known symptoms of hyperthyroidism. Children with pheochromocytoma usually have headaches and sweating and, sometimes, palpitations. Abdominal pain may be the first clue to the presence of neuroblastoma or Wilms tumor although both of these tumors usually present as abdominal masses. A history of urinary tract infections suggests chronic pyelonephritis, the commonest cause of severe hypertension in children, but a negative history does not rule out this condition, which is frequently silent. A previous history of hematuria or acute nephritis strongly implies chronic glomerulonephritis as the cause of hypertension.

The physical examination will identify many of the causes of hypertension and will provide clues to the diagnosis of others. Obesity is an obvious example of the former, although the association of obesity and hypertension may be fortuitous and does not prove a cause and effect relationship. Increased intracranial pressure severe enough to cause hypertension should be recognized by the clinical setting and a careful neurological exam. Thyrotoxicosis causes systolic hypertension only and is identified by the classic signs. Coarctation of the aorta is recognized by differential pulses and blood pressure in the arms and legs.

The physical signs of Cushing syndrome - growth failure, the characteristic pattern of obesity, and plethora - are obvious in most children but more mild cases can be missed. The form of adrenogenital syndrome resulting from 11β-hydroxylase deficiency is recognized by virilization of both sexes whereas the form resulting from 17-hydroxylase deficiency causes feminization of males but no signs in prepubertal females.

Of the hormone secreting tumors, neuroblastoma, which secretes catecholamines, and Wilms tumor, some of which secrete renin, are usually large enough to be detected by abdominal palpation. Pheochromocytoma and ganglioneuroma, on the other hand, are usually too small to be detected. The presence of neurofibromas or cafe-au-lait spots should be sought since neurofibromatosis is associated with an increased incidence of both pheochromocytoma and renal artery stenosis, the latter being more common in children.[10]

Abdominal palpation should also detect infantile polycystic kidneys, which almost always present as flank masses, and may detect the unusual case of hydronephrosis causing hypertension. An abdominal bruit suggests the presence of renal artery stenosis.

The urinalysis should suggest the presence of acute or chronic glomerulonephritis or interstitial nephritis, which are invariably accompanied by hematuria, proteinuria, or both. Hematuria also occurs in 30% of children with Wilms tumor.[11] Pyelonephritis may or may not be accompanied by pyuria, and hydronephrosis sometimes, but not always, is associated with proteinuria. A positive urine culture strongly implicates pyelonephritis in the causation of hypertension but a negative culture does not exclude it.

The measurement of hemoglobin and hematocrit, in the author's opinion, has little value in detecting causes of hypertension and need not be performed. Serum electrolytes are seldom useful but the rare case of primary aldosteronism may be suggested by the presence of hypokalemic alkalosis. Hypokalemic alkalosis may also be present in children with renal artery stenosis and secondary aldosteronism, but frequently is not.

The BUN and serum creatinine are important screening tests for renal disease severe enough to cause impaired function. Elevated levels may occasionally be the first clue to a congenital nephropathy, obstructive uropathy, or chronic pyelonephritis associated with normal urinalysis but are more commonly confirmatory evidence of an already suspected renal disease.

It is apparent that most of the secondary causes of hypertension in children should be identified, or strongly suspected, as a result of this evaluation. These include obesity; drug ingestion; CNS causes; thyrotoxicosis; coarctation of the aorta; most cases of Cushing syndrome, adrenogenital syndrome, neuroblastoma, Wilms tumor, hydronephrosis, and renal parenchymal disease; and some cases of pheochromocytoma. This evaluation is of less help in identifying primary aldosteronism, ganglioneuroma, and renal artery stenosis.

EXTENDED EVALUATION

If the basic work-up has directed suspicion to one of the primary causes of hypertension, the appropriate diagnostic tests for that condition should be performed. If the work-up is negative, the decision to proceed to more extensive evaluation is based on the severity of hypertension. Evidence of hypertensive changes in the ocular fundi or on cardiac evaluation would also influence the decision, but these changes rarely occur in the absence of severe hypertension. The criteria for further evaluation formulated by the Task Force, a diastolic pressure greater than 90mm in children 3-12 and greater than 100mm in children 13-18, are generally appropriate but may need to be modified for the individual child. For example, diastolic pressures consistently between 95 and 100mm in a 13-year old, prepubertal girl are an indication for further evaluation.

The studies which are usually included in an extended evaluation, and the conditions they are designed to detect, are listed in Table 3.

TABLE 3. Extended Evaluation of Hypertension

IVP (rapid sequence)	Plasma aldosterone
Pyelonephritis	Primary aldosteronism
Hydronephrosis	Renal artery stenosis
Polycystic kidneys	
Wilms tumor	Plasma renin
Neuroblastoma	Primary aldosteronism
Renal artery stenosis	Renal artery stenosis
Plasma DOC	Urinary catecholamines
Adrenogenital syndrome	Pheochromocytoma
	Neuroblastoma, ganglioneuroma
Urinary free cortisol	
Cushing syndrome	Renal arteriography and renal vein renin
	Renal artery stenosis

On occasion, other studies of the kidney, such as ultrasound and biopsy, may also be indicated. The rationale for these studies and their interpretation will be discussed. Other reviews of the subject are recommended.[12,13]

The rapid sequence intravenous pyelogram is the most important study and perhaps should be part of the basic evaluation of all children with hypertension. The presence of segmental scars establishes the diagnosis of chronic pyelonephritis. The pyelogram also establishes the diagnosis of hydronephrosis, confirms the suspected diagnosis of polycystic kidneys and is the most useful study for distinguishing between the masses of neuroblastoma and Wilms tumor. With renal artery stenosis there may be delayed uptake of the dye by the affected kidney at one and two minutes, followed by hyperconcentration and delayed excretion on later films. These signs, however, were absent in 46% of children with confirmed stenotic lesions of the main renal artery or segmental arteries in one series.[14] The affected kidney is sometimes smaller than the normal kidney. Notching of the pelvis or upper ureter by collateral vessels which have developed in response to renal artery stenosis is seen occasionally and is a clue to the diagnosis.

The urinary free cortisol level is used as a screening test for Cushing syndrome. Since Cushing syndrome is a rare cause of hypertension and is almost always associated with clinical findings, the yield from this test in asymptomatic children will be very low. Similar considerations apply to the measurement of desoxycorticosterone (DOC) as a test for adrenogenital syndrome, which is almost always suspected on clinical grounds. Measurement of urinary 17-ketosteroids and 17-hydroxysteroids, which are elevated in 11β-hydroxylase deficiency and decreased in 17-hydroxylase deficiency, can also be used to detect adrenogenital syndrome and will distinguish between the two forms.

Twenty-four hour urinary catecholamines (epinephrine and norepinephrine) are the most reliable tests for pheochromocytoma whereas urinary metanephrines and vanyilylmandelic acid are used for the diagnosis of neuroblastoma and ganglioneuroma. Neuroblastoma usually presents on physical or radiologic examination, however, and is rarely first suspected from the measurement of catecholamine metabolites.

The measurement of plasma renin activity may be helpful in the diagnosis of primary aldosteronism, where it is usually low, and renal artery stenosis, where it is usually high. However, because renin secretion is influenced by such factors as age, posture, diet, and time of day, as well as by many of the antihypertensive drugs, interpretation of results can be difficult. Also, one-third of patients with significant renal artery stenosis had normal values in one adult series[15] and there are false negative results with primary aldosteronism as well. Thus a normal level is of little value but a high level, in a sample appropriately drawn and interpreted, strongly suggests renal artery stenosis (or rarely, a renin secreting tumor) and virtually excludes primary aldosteronism.

The measurement of plasma aldosterone is used for the diagnosis of primary aldosteronism, caused by adrenal hyperplasia or an adenoma, and secondary aldosteronism resulting from renal artery stenosis. Many children with renal artery stenosis have normal levels, however. Plasma aldosterone concentration is affected by time of day, position, and sodium intake, similarly to renin, and levels can be difficult to interpret.

Renal arteriography and catheterization of the renal veins for renin measurements are necessary for the evaluation of renal artery stenosis. Although demonstration of a stenotic lesion on the arteriogram is essential to the diagnosis, the presence of a lesion does not prove that it has functional significance or that its removal will result in correction of the hypertension. Studies in adults have shown that when the renal vein concentration of renin on the side of the stenosis is >1.5 times the concentration on the unaffected side, the chances that surgical repair or nephrectomy will relieve the hypertension are greater than 80%.[15,16] Evidence that renin release is suppressed in the contralateral kidney - a renin concentration in the contralateral renal vein < 1.3 times the concentration in the vena cava distal to the kidneys - increases the chances of a favorable result from surgery even further.[15] Although the value of these studies in children has been questioned,[17] in one center the 15 children who benefited from surgery all had renal vein renin ratios >1.5 and 13 had contralateral renal vein to vena cava ratios < 1.3.[18] In children with segmental arterial lesions renin data obtained from catheterization of segmental veins may be required to establish the significance of the lesions. Although it is customary to perform venous catheterization immediately prior to arteriography, demonstration of a segmental lesion by arteriography necessitates segmental vein catheterization at the end of the procedure. A recent study[19] indicates that venous studies can be performed with equal validity before or after arteriography.

All of the studies of this evaluation, with the exception of renal arteriography and renal venous studies can be performed on an outpatient basis, at least in older children, although it is easier to control variables of diet, medication, and time of blood sampling if the child is in the hospital. Because they are the most invasive procedures, arteriography and renal vein catheterization are usually performed at the end of the evaluation, after all other studies are negative. Since the measurements of hormone levels often take several weeks to perform, these results will not be available prior to the performance of arteriography if the evaluation is undertaken during a single hospital admission.

The decision to perform renal arteriography and vein catheterization in an asymptomatic child in whom the preceding evaluation has been negative may be difficult. The ^{131}I-hippurate scan has been advocated as a screening test to identify the children who have renal artery stenosis and will require arteriography. As usually performed, however, this test is relatively insensitive,[20] and although a computer technique to improve sensitivity has been developed,[21] it is not available for general use. It is the author's contention that arteriography and vein catheterization should be performed in any prepubertal child with severe, unexplained hypertension. The following case illustrates this viewpoint:

A 12-year old boy had had intermittent, unilateral, morning headaches for several years but was otherwise in good health. During a hospital admission for hernia repair his blood pressure was 130/100. Blood pressure over the next 7 months varied from 120/90 to 150/130. Physical examination was negative with the exception of narrowing of the retinal arterioles. White blood cell count was 6,800, hemoglobin, 14.0 g/dl. Urine was cloudy, specific gravity was 1.020, pH 7.0, there was no protein or glucose, and sediment was loaded with amorphous phosphates.

Serum sodium was 139 mEq, potassium 4.7 mEq, chloride 103 mEq, and CO_2 27 mEq per dl. BUN was 16 mg and creatinine 0.9 mg per dl. Chest x-ray was negative. Electrocardiogram showed possible left ventricular hypertrophy. Intravenous pyelogram (not rapid sequence) was normal. Urinary catecholamine excretion was 58 mcg in 24 hours (normal 0-130). Serum aldosterone level was 65.6 ng/dl (normal 4-13). Repeat value was 16.3 mg/dl. Plasma renin level was 3.4 ng/ml/hour (normal 1.1-7.9). Femoral vein catheterization was performed; renin values were: left renal vein 2.8 ng, right renal vein 2.1 ng, left common iliac 2.6 ng/ml/hour. Renal arteriogram showed a stenosis of a segmental branch of the left superior renal artery (Figure 1). Numerous small collaterals were identified. Catheterization of left segmental renal veins was performed; renin values were 3.1 and 4.2 ng/ml/hour from two lower pole segmental veins and 13.2 ng/ml/hour from the main renal vein. It was felt that the segmental vein draining the area of the stenotic artery had not been catheterized and that the renin value of 2.8 ng/ml/hour on the first catheterization, thought to be from the left renal artery, was actually from a segmental vein.

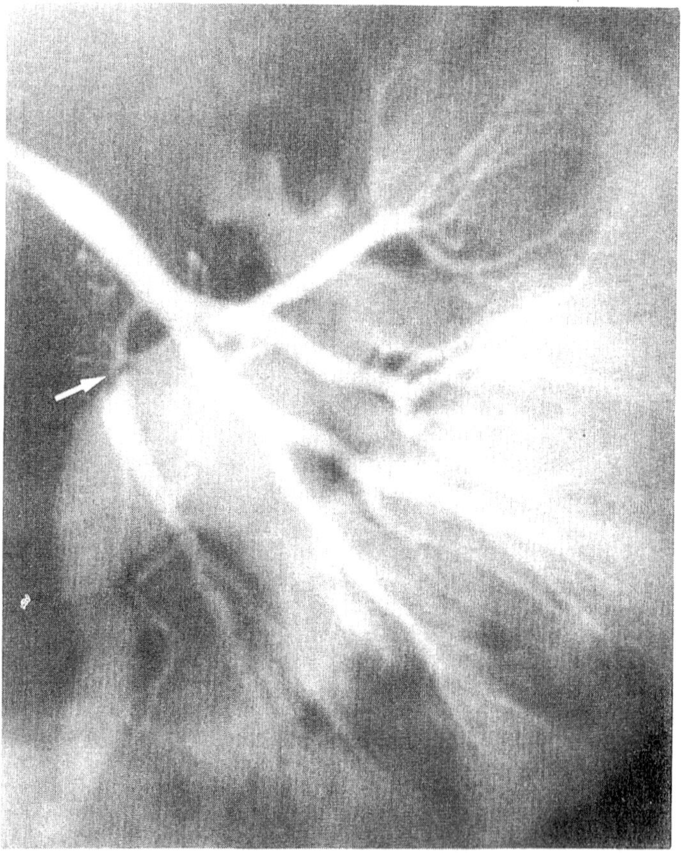

FIGURE 1. Stenosis of a branch of the upper left renal artery (arrow) with post-stenotic dilatation and the development of collateral vessels.

On the basis of the segmental stenosis identified by arteriography and the high renin value from the left renal vein obtained during the second study, a left partial nephrectomy was performed. Prior to operation the blood pressure was 150/130. The day after operation it was 140/100 and four months later it was 120/78. He was asymptomatic and taking no medication.

Comment on this case: There were no clues to the etiology of hypertension in this prepubertal boy. An outpatient work-up was negative with the exception of an elevated serum aldosterone level. A repeat level was normal. A segmental arterial stenosis was identified by arteriography but renal vein renin studies prior to arteriography were negative and a second study after arteriography was necessary before the diagnosis was confirmed. This case illustrates the value of performing a complete evaluation, including renal arteriography and venous catheterization, in children with moderately severe hypertension and the difficulty in interpreting data obtained during catheter studies. Children requiring these studies should be referred to centers with demonstrated expertise in performing them.

SUMMARY

A schema for the evaluation of hypertension has been presented which is based on the prevalence of primary hypertension and various causes of secondary hypertension in children with mild, and with severe, hypertension. Mild hypertension is usually primary or associated with obesity. A basic evaluation, consisting of history and physical examination, urine analysis and culture, and a blood chemistry panel, is indicated. Severe hypertension, at least in prepubertal children, is almost always secondary. Many of the causes will be suspected from the basic evaluation, but a more extensive evaluation is necessary to detect occult causes. Although a standard format for the evaluation can be followed, experience in the interpretation of results is helpful if diagnostic pitfalls are to be avoided.

REFERENCES

1. Loggie, J.M.H.: Hypertension in children and adolescents. 1. Causes and diagnostic studies. J Pediatr 74:331-355, 1969.
2. Rubin, M.I.: Systemic hypertension in childhood. Arch Dis Childh 42:34-39, 1967.
3. Still, J.L. and Cottom, D.: Severe hypertension in childhood. Arch Dis Childh 42:34-39, 1967.
4. Londe, S., Bourgoigne, J.J., Robson, A.M., and Goldring, D.: Hypertension in apparently normal children. J Pediatr 78:569-577, 1971.
5. Kilcoyne, M.M.: Adolescent hypertension II. Characteristics and response to treatment. Circulation 50:1014-1019, 1974.
6. Levine, L.S., Lewy, J.E., and New, M.I.: Hypertension in high school students. NY State J Med 76:40-44, 1976.
7. Rames, L.K., CLarke, W.R., Connor, W.E., Reiter, M.A., and Lauer, R.M.: Normal blood pressures and the evaluation of sustained blood pressure elevation in childhood: The Muscatine study. Pediatrics 61:245-251, 1978.

8. Rance, C.P., Arbus, G.S., Balfe, J.W., and Kooh, S.W.: Persistent systemic hypertension in infants and children. Pediat Clin North Am 21:801-824, 1974.
9. Report of the Task Force on Blood Pressure Control in Children. Pediatrics 59(Suppl): 797-820, 1977.
10. Tilford, D.L. and Kelsch, R.C.: Renal artery stenosis in childhood neurofibromatosis. Am J Dis Child 126:665-668, 1973.
11. Levitt, S.B.: Neoplasms of genitourinary tract. In Rudolph, A.M. (ed): Pediatrics, 16th Edition. New York: Appleton-Century-Crofts, 1977, Chapter 26.
12. Robson, A.M.: Special diagnostic studies for the detection of renal and renovascular forms of hypertension. Pediatr Clin North Am 25: 83-98, 1978.
13. Loggie, J.M.H., New, M.I., and Robson, A.M.: Hypertension in the pediatric patient: A reappraisal. J Pediatr 94:685-699, 1979.
14. Korobkin, M., Perloff, D.L., and Palubinskas, A.J.: Renal arteriography in the evaluation of unexplained hypertension in children and adolescents. J Pediatr 88:388-393, 1976.
15. Stockigt, J.R., Collins, R.D., Noakes, C.A., Schambelan, M., and Biglieri, E.G.: Renal-vein renin in various forms of renal hypertension. Lancet 1:1194-1197, 1972.
16. Marks, L.S. and Maxwell, M.H.: Renal vein renin. Value and limitations in the prediction of operative results. Urol Clin North Amer 2:311-325, 1975.
17. Goddard, C.: Predictive value of renal-vein renin measurements in children with various forms of renal hypertension. An international study. Helv Paediat Acta 32:49-57, 1977.
18. Dillon, M.J., Shah, V., and Barratt, T.M.: Renal vein renin measurements in children with hypertension. Br Med J 2:168-170, 1978.
19. Harrington, D.P., Whelton, P.K., MacKensie, E.J., Russell, R.P., Kaufman, S.L., Barth, K.H., White, R.I., and Walker, W.G.: Renal venous renin sampling. Prospective study of techniques and methods. Radiology 138:571-575, 1981.
20. Shames, D.M. and Korobkin, M.: A simple technique for measuring relative renal blood flow. J Nuc Med 17:876-879, 1976.
21. DeGrazia, J.A., Scheibe, P.O., Jackson, P.E., Lucas, Z.J., Fair, W.R., Vogel, J.M., and Blumin, L.J.: Clinical applications of a kinetic model of hippurate distribution and renal clearance. J Nuc Med 15:102-114, 1974.

THE RENIN ANGIOTENSIN SYSTEM IN CHILDHOOD HYPERTENSION

Alan B. Gruskin, M.D., James W. Prebis, M.D., H. Jorge Baluarte, M.D., Martin S. Polinsky, M.D., Howard Rosenblum, M.D.

Hypertension in adults is recognized as being a significant precursor of stroke, myocardial infarction, congestive heart failure and renal insufficiency. Many feel that the origins of adult hypertension occur during the childhood years and that a further understanding of normal and abnormal blood pressure regulation in children can lead to better control of abnormal (elevated) blood pressures during childhood and adulthood and perhaps prevent the long term consequences of uncontrolled hypertension.

During the past decade there has been an increased emphasis in the broad subject of childhood hypertension focusing on topics dealing with its recognition, natural history, evaluation and treatment (1-8). This review will focus on the renin angiotensin system in the hypertensive patient and consider means by which the degree of participation of the renin angiotensin system in hypertensive children may be evaluated. It is hoped that a more complete appreciation of the biochemistry and physiology of the renin angiotensin system will increase the understanding of the relationship of this system to hypertensive disorders in children and permit a more rational approach to evaluating and treating affected children.

The Renin Angiotensin System (Figure 1)

Renin is a proteolytic enzyme secreted primarily by the juxtaglomerular cells of the outer cortical glomeruli in the kidney. Its secretion into the systemic circulation is increased when the renal artery perfusion pressure is diminished, when the intratubular content of sodium, potassium and/or chloride in the region of the macula densa is reduced or when beta sympathetic activity is increased (9,10,11). Renin substrate or angiotensinogen is a globulin synthesized by the liver. Once released into the blood stream, renin functions as an enzyme which cleaves angiotensinogen into angiotensin I, a physiologically inactive decapeptide. As angiotensin I passes through the lungs it is converted by a pulmonary converting enzyme to angiotensin II, a physiologically active octapeptide.

Angiotensin II has two actions: First, it directly stimulates arteriolar vasoconstriction; secondly, it stimulates the production and release of aldosterone from the adrenal cortex (3,10,11,12). The release of aldosterone increases potassium excretion and sodium retention by the kidney. The water retention which accompanies this increase in sodium reabsorption in the distal tubule increases "effective" arterial volume, increases blood pressure and, in turn, reduces the stimulation for the renin release.

The recent development and clinical availability of two types of inibitors of the renin angiotensin system has permitted further clarification of this system (13,14,15). An oral inhibitor, Captopril, which may be given on a chronic basis, blocks the activity of the converting enzyme and, therefore, the formation of angiotensin II (15,16). There is also an intravenous preparation, Saralasin(R), which is a competitive agonist of angiotensin II and functions by competing with angiotensin II for its receptor sites located in the anterior walls (13,17)

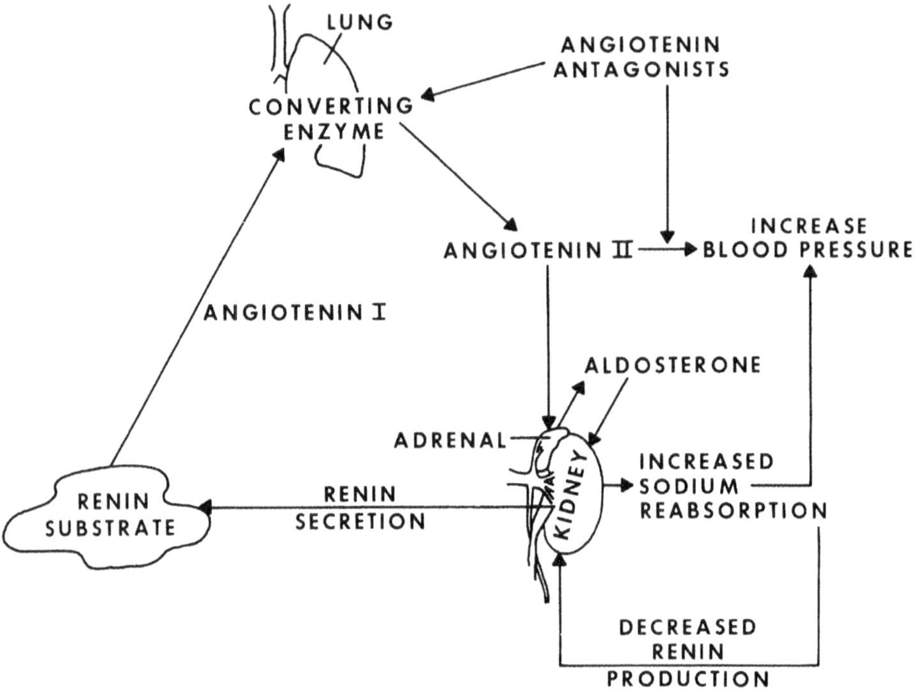

Figure 1: The renin-angiotensin-aldosterone system. Note that this system influences both the vasoconstriction and volume components of the basic blood pressure formula. Reproduced with the permission of the Publisher. Pediatr.Ann.6:373, 1977)

The Formula for Blood Pressure

Blood pressure regulation and its maintenance within normal limits is essential to life. Insufficient blood pressures reduce tissue perfusion, ultimately resulting in tissue death. When blood pressure is elevated either acutely or chronically, ischemic damage with its associated complications can occur. Consequently, it is logical to expect that the control of blood pressure is multifactorial in nature, complex in its understanding, and that the level of pressure is subject to many influences in both normal and abnormal situations. A major step in simplifying the multiple factors included in blood pressure control was the development of the volume-vasoconstriction hypothesis by Laragh and co-workers (11,18,19). We have interpreted this hypothesis using the basic pressure formula as follows (3): Pressure equals Flow times Resistance which may be physiologically interpreted to be blood pressure equals volume times vasoconstriction.

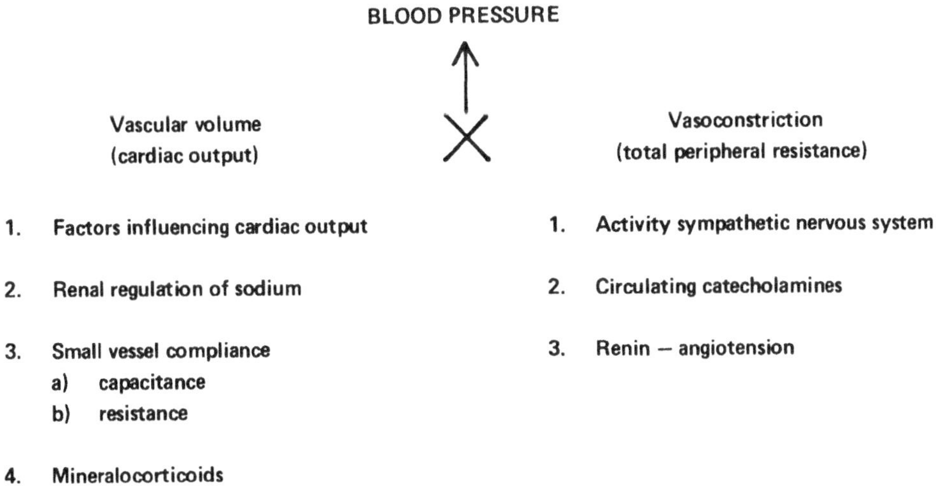

Factors influencing volume and resistance segments of the blood pressure formula.

Figure 2: Legend included as part of the figure

As indicated in Figure 2, one set of factors is known to influence the state of volume while a different set of factors influences the degree of vasoconstriction. The observed blood pressure in any patient is the resultant of the continuous interaction of each of these factors. Because the renin angiotensin aldosterone system is involved with both limbs of the blood pressure formula, careful study of the activity of this system is central to understanding blood pressure regulation in children.

Measurement of Plasma Renin Activity (PRA)

The clinical evaluation of the renin-angiotensin-aldosterone system involves measurements of PRA as well as urinary and plasma aldosterone levels. During the past few years, the measurement of PRA has become more standardized. According to Sealey, four criteria must be met if a laboratory assay for PRA is to be sensitive, reproducible and capable of detecting low values (20). These criteria include: 1) collection and handling of samples so as to inhibit the conversion of pro-renin to active renin, 2) the ability to lengthen the time of incubation of samples so as to be able to measure subnormal values, 3) adjustment of samples to a pH which prevents cryoactivation of prorenin and limits angiotensin I generation and 4) the use of angiotensinase inhibitors such as EDTA, Phenylmethylsulfonyl Fluoride and Diisopropyl Fluorosphosphate to prevent the breakdown of angiotensin. Until recently such criteria could only be met in research laboratories dealing with large numbers of specimens; however, with the advent of commercially available radioimmunoassay kits such as Renak$^{(R)}$ a sensitive, reproducible determination of PRA can be performed in most hospital laboratories.

Present methodology does not allow for the accurate measurement of angiotensin II levels; therefore, the PRA assay actually measures by radioimmunoassay the rate of generation of angiotensin I from endogenous renin substrate. Since the formation of angiotensin II is not rate limiting in vivo, the rate of generation of angiotensin I parallels the formation of angiotensin I formed per unit volume per unit time, i.e. ng/ml/hr. The length of the incubation step of the assay may be lenghtened when PRA is low until a large enough quantity of angiotensin I can be generated and its rate of activity accurately measured. Because of the many technical aspects in the assay procedure for PRA, it is worthwhile for laboratories doing many determinations to establish its own normal values from the population it serves. We have also found it helpful to assay PRA in frozen aliquots of plasma samples having known high and low values during each set of determinations as an internal check of the consistency of the radioimmunoassay. We accept as useful data assays in which the PRA for the frozen controls agree within 10-15% of the mean value of previous determinations. In our experience, approximately 5% of the assays have to be repeated because of technical problems with the assay procedure. Often samples with high levels of PRA have to be diluted and rerun because these values exceed the highest standards for the assay.

Interpretation of Levels of Plasma Renin Activity

The level of PRA in contrast to many other blood constituents such as electrolytes is not limited to a narrow range of normal values. Age, position, time of day, ingestion of drugs, and any acute and/or chronic changes in extracellular volume alters the level of PRA (9,10,12,21,22). Indeed, the failure to take into accunt the influence of these factors on PRA may account for some of the differences found by different investigators who have studied this system in normal and hypertensive individuals. The gathering of useful and more importantly reproducible data may be enhanced by rigidly controlling many of these variables, specifically the position of the patient and time of day when blood samples are drawn. Also, the evaluation of the renin-angiotensin system in hypertensive disorders is most meaningful if the patient is not receiving antihypertensives and/or diuretic agents which are known to alter PRA.

It is important that PRA in hypertensive patients be compared to PRA obtained in age related normals since PRA normally decreases with age (23-28). PRA falls during the first few weeks of life and again by 50% by the end of the first year of age. Levels of PRA fall again by 30% by four years of age and another 40-50% by 9-15 years of age. Also, PRA continues to gradually fall throughout adulthood.

The single most important clinical variable which acutely alters PRA is the volume status of the patient such that a patient with an increase in extracellular volume will have low PRA and a patient with volume depletion will have increased PRA. It has been shown that the simultaneous estimation of sodium balance and PRA permits a more meaningful interpretation of PRA than measurements of PRA alone (29). Assuming the presence of adequate renal function, the sodium excretion of an individual reflects his intake. Moreover, the higher the rate of excretion of sodium, the greater the extracellular volume of that individual and vice versa.

The process of obtaining simultaneous measurements of a 24 hour urinary sodium excretion and a PRA usually obtained in the sitting position after an individual has been upright for 4-5 hours has been given the label of renin profiling while the measurement of this relationship has been termed the renin sodium index (29). When PRA is evaluated in adults in this fashion, a nomogram describing a curvilinear relationship between PRA and sodium excretion is found (10,12); however, there are several inherent difficulties with the use of this nomogram.

Since PRA ought to be high when sodium excretion is low, it is difficult to detect an abnormally elevated PRA in association with low sodium excretion. In addition, an unusually low PRA cannot be differentiated from normal when sodium excretion is high. However, this nomogram can demonstrate an abnormally increased PRA in association with a high sodium excretion or a suppressed PRA in a patient with a low sodium excretion. In order to better identify suppressed or elevated PRA values, patients may be given diets containing high or low quantities of sodium for 3-5 days until a new steady state of sodium balance is achieved (10,11,12). Renin profiling is repeated and the degree of change in the PRA in response to the sodium diet is compared to the results found in normal subjects.

Three other means of renin profiling have been used in an attempt to reduce the need to alter diets and to reduce the length of hospital stay. The first has been to acutely reduce extracellular volume by administering potent diuretics such as Lasix, i.e. the Lasix stimulation test (21), and the second has been to give an intravenous infusion of saline (2000 ml over 2 hrs in adults)(22) to acutely increase ECF (22). In both situations, PRA is measured before and after the maneuver and the change in PRA expressed either as a percentage change, and/or absolute value compared to the response of PRA in normals similarly studied. The change in PRA is used as an indication of the degree to which the renin angiotensin system is hyperresponsive, or non responsive (Lasix stimulation) (21), suppressible or non suppressible (Saline infusion) (22). Such responses are often defined as remaining within and/or exceeding 95% confidential limits for normals. In summary,

PRA may be defined as being high, normal or low in relationship to the urinary excretion of sodium (renin sodium indexing) and as being normally responsive, hyperresponsive or nonresponsive to maneuvers designed to change extracellular volume (altered salt diets, Lasix stimulation, intravenous sodium loading).

Another technique which is helpful in evaluating the renin angiotensin system involves the administration of biochemical blockers of various segments of the system, e.g. Captopril or Saralasin (13-17). When such agents are given and a significant fall in blood pressure occurs it may be concluded that the renin angiotensin system plays a significant role in the maintenance of the elevated blood pressure.

Although the above mentioned evaluation processes of the renin angiotensin system has been extensively used to study this system in normal adults and in hypertensive adults with many forms of hypertension, similar approaches have not been extensively used in the study of childhood hypertension. There are probably less than two to three dozen studies dealing with the subject of renin profiling in children. As regards the evaluation of hypertensive children clear guidelines for determining the degree of activity of the renin angiotensin system are still in the process of being developed. The scheme which we are currently utilizing to evaluate our hypertensive children is outlined in Figure 3.

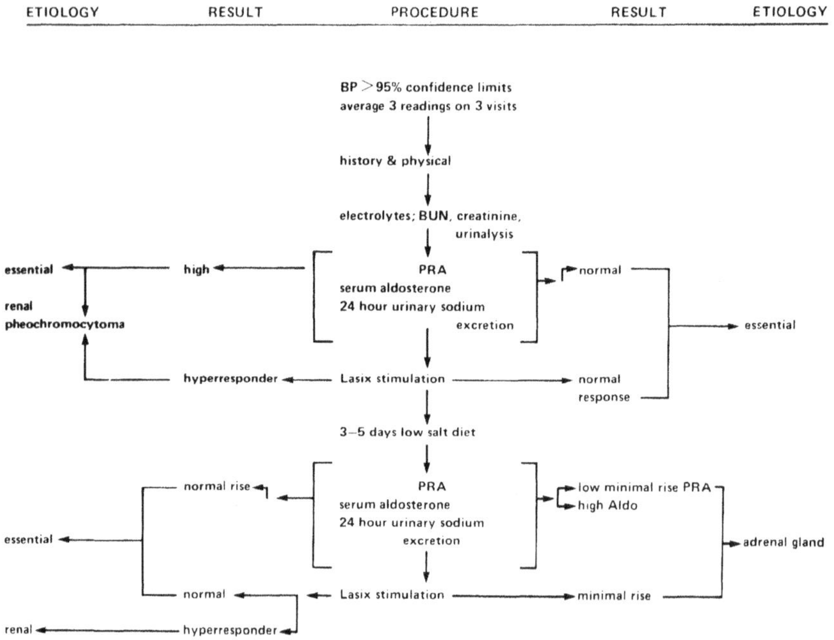

Figure 3: Stepwise evaluation of the renin-angiotensin-aldosterone system in hypertensive children.

We currently are utilizing a combination of renin profiling and the degree of change of PRA to changes in extracellular volume induced by either changes in sodium intake or by the administration of Lasix to evaluate PRA. When categorizing our patients nine combinations are possible (Figure 4). We currently determine PRA using the Renak(R) Kit made by Roche.

RENIN – SODIUM INDEX

Response of PRA to Changes in ECF	High	Normal	Low
Hyper	1	2	3
Normal	4	X	5
Minimal	6	7	8

Categories of Plasma Renin Activity

Figure 4: Multiple categories of plasma renin activity. The X indicates a normal patient.

Plasma Renin Activity in Hypertensive Disorders (Table 1)

We feel that the determination of PRA should be included amongst the initial steps in evaluating hypertensive children when the history, physical examination, routine urinalysis and determination of BUN, creatinine and electrolytes do not readily lead to a diagnosis.

Table 1: PLASMA RENIN ACTIVITY (PRA) IN HYPERTENSIVE DISORDERS

Increased PRA

Bilateral renovascular-volume contracted
Coarctation of the aorta-volume contracted
Congenital adrenal hyperplasia - salt loss
End Stage renal disease, volume contracted
Essential hypertension
Hemolytic uremic syndrome
Malignant hypertension
Post transplant
Pheochromocytoma

Solitary kidney with renal artery stenosis
Unilateral renovascular disease

Normal PRA

Bilateral renovascular-volume expanded
Coarctation of aorta-volume expanded
Corticosteroid excess-Cushing's (increased renin substrate)
End stage renal disease
Essential hypertension
Post transplant
Solitary kidney with renal artery stenosis

Decreased PRA

Anephric
Bilateral renovascular-volume expanded
Coarctation of aorta-volume expanded
Essential hypertension
11β-hydroxylase deficiency
17α-hydroxylase deficiency
Licorice ingestion (Pseudoaldosteronism)
Liddle syndrome
Mineralcorticoid excess-endogenous or exogenous
Parenchymal renal disease with volume expansion
Post streptococcal nephritis with volume expansion
Primary hyperaldosteronism adrenal tumor
bilateral hyperplasia
Solitary kidney with renal artery stenosis-volume expanded

When PRA is elevated, hyperresponsive or nonsuppressible, the kidney should be viewed as contributing to the hypertension process (10,20,30-33). Hyperactivity of the renin angiotensin system has been described in patients with unilateral renovascular and parenchymal disorders, hydronephrosis, acute renal failure, advanced chronic renal insufficiency, small vessel vascular disorders of the kidney, pheochromocytoma (34,35,36) because of catecholamine stimulation of renal renin release, malignant hypertension, Wilms tumor, cystic disorders, the juxtaglomerular cell tumor (37), and acute transplant rejection (38).

Low and/or suppressed levels of PRA suggest the presence of hypertensive disorders associated with some degree of volume expansion (10-12). The classical example of a disorder associated with low PRA is primary aldosteronism (3,39). Other disorders associated with low or suppressed PRA include a number of congenital disorders affecting the adrenal gland (40,41) Low levels of PRA may occur in children with post infectious nephritis perhaps because of acute volume expansion (42).

If renin profiling is done while the patient is ingesting a normal diet PRA is usually in the low and/or normal range in hypertensive patients with bilateral renovascular stenosis and/or coarctation of the aorta. However, hyperresponsivity of the renin angiotensin system to sodium restriction or by response to angiotensin inhibitors can be demonstrated in such patients (43,44). The reason for this is that bilateral obstruction decreases renal blood flow and alters renal function in a manner that leads to increased sodium reabsorption by the kidney, volume expansion and suppression of renin production. The removal of the influence of volume by sodium restriction permits the role of the renin angiotensin system in the hypertension process to be demonstrated. The term inappropriate elevation of PRA has been used to describe such a sequence of events.

Essential or primary hypertension occurs in association with high, normal or low levels of PRA 99-12,45). It is felt by some that the level of PRA in adults with essential hypertension has both prognostic and therapeutic implications (46). Data exist suggestiong that high levels of PRA may be associated with an increased rate of myocardial infarction, cerebral vascular accidents and an increased rate of development of vascular damage while those with low PRA are protected from such complications. Studies in hypertensive adults also suggest that the treatment of choice for patients with high levels of PRA is the use of renin inhibitors while diuretics should be used as initial therapy in patients with low levels of PRA. A similar approach may be beneficial when drug therapy is being considered for a hypertensive child. Children with essential hypertension have been shown to have high, normal and low levels of PRA (3,6,47,48), but the magnitude of the problem of essential hypertension in children including its incidence, degree and nature of the activity of the renin angiotensin system, long-term prognosis and therapy needs additional study.

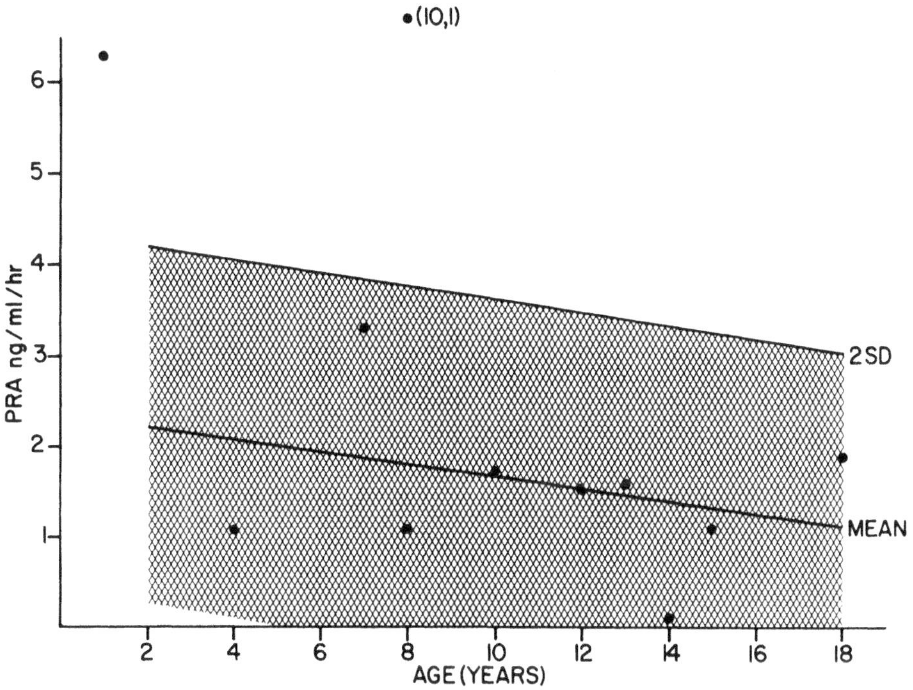

Figure 5: PRA in normals (cross-hatched area) and hypertensive children (dots)

Approximately 4 years ago we changed our renin assay to a more sensitive one which takes into account many of the newer concepts already mentioned in this article. Data we previously obtained by using a Squibb(R) kit for PRA, which is no longer available, can serve to illustrate the potential value of examining the renin angiotensin system as a means of evaluating childhood hypertension. The mean $\pm$ standard deviations of the age related urinary rates of excretion of sodium while ingesting a normal diet and the age related normal levels for PRA are shown in Figures 5 and 6. Noteworthy is the observation that sodium excretion, when corrected for body size, did not change appreciably with age while the PRA decreased with age.

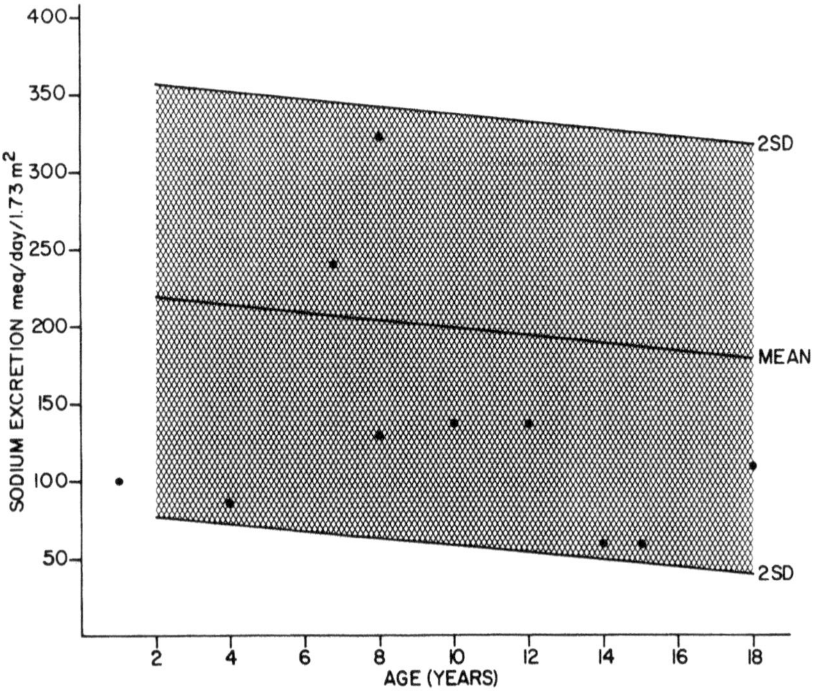

Figure 6: Twenty-four hour urinary sodium excretion in normal children (cross-hatched areas) and hypertensive children (dots).

All of the hypertensive children had rates of excretion of urinary sodium which fell within age related 95% confidence bands. PRA in two children was elevated for age and sodium excretion. One child had unilateral renal vascular disease and the other biopsy proven periarteritis. PRA in one child was low i.e. almost undetectable, and most importantly, did not increase with prolonged, severe sodium restriction. This child was shown to have low renin essential hypertension (47). All the remaining children except for one with coarctation of the aorta had essential hypertension. These data, although limited, indicate the potential value of renin profiling as a means of determining the etiology of elevated blood pressures in children.

Only a limited number of studies emphasizing renin profiling in children are available. Kilcoyne and associates have reported that their experience with renin profiling in a group of black adolescents and young adults with hypertension. They were able to identify children with essential hypertension as having low, normal and high levels of PRA (47,48). We have previously reported on the use of renin profiling to study the renin angiotensin system in children with pheochromocytoma (34) and traction relation hypertension (49).

Many of the early reports dealing with PRA and childhood hypertension have not included an indicator of extracellular volume as part of the evaluation process of the renin angiotensin system and have often failed to compare PRA to age related normals. Also, most of available studies have not addressed the issue of the responsivity of the renin angiotensin system after maneuvers designed to stimulate changes in PRA. PRA in many of the available reports has been examined in blood samples either obtained from children early in the morning or while they were supine. Such samples tend to give low values for PRA rendering the recognition of an abnormally low PRA difficult if not impossible.

Use of Renin Antagonists

Although the use of specific renin antagonists, Captopril$^{(R)}$, an oral inhibitor of the converting enzyme and Saralasin, a competitive antagonist of angiotensin II had had limited application to the study of childhood hypertension, the few studies reported in children have shown the potential value of these agents as both diagnostic and therapeutic agents (15,50). It is clear that a drop in blood pressure following the use of either agent demonstrates the participating role of the renin angiotensin system in maintaining the hypertensive process. These agents have their greatest use in recognizing hyperreninemic states and they may have value in identifying the normal reninemic hypertensive patient whose PRA is inappropriately elevated for the degree of hypertension.

The administration of Saralasin to some hypertensive adults has been associated with a seemingly paradoxical increase in blood pressure. This is due to the fact that Saralasin is a partial "agonist" of angiotensin II, and usually increases the blood pressure in patients with low renin hypertension. In contrast, Saralasin produces a slight increase or no change in blood pressure in high renin hypertensives (14). From a clinical standpoint, Saralasin would be of greatest benefit in identifying patients with high renin levels with either renovascular or essential hypertension. Saralasin testing could be used in conjunction with, but not in place of, renin profiling.

Captopril$^{(R)}$ has been used experimentally by a number of investigators including us to successfully treat children with severe, unresponsive, high renin, hypertension of various etiologies (15,50). The degree of response to therapy is felt to be correlated with the level of PRA. Because Captopril produces peripheral vasodilation with a resultant tachycardia and sodium retention, the use of a beta blocker and diuretics is often required. When Captopril is given, and consistant with the vasoconstrictor - volume hypothesis, sodium depletion may be required before the involvement of the renin angiotensin system in the hypertensive process can be demonstrated.

In conclusion, the techniques of renin profiling and the examination of the stimulated renin angiotensin system together with improved methodology has provided many new insights into the mechanism of hypertension and the issues incurred in studying clinical hypertension in adult patients. The limited number of studies in children have shown that the degree of PRA is different in children and that careful examination of the renin angiotensin system by different techniques offers the potential for a quicker and more precise noninvasive diagnosis and the promise of a better understanding of childhood hypertension and perhaps even the origins of adult hypertension.

REFERENCES

1. Gruskin, A.B.: Clinical evaluation of hypertension in children. Primary Care 1:233, 1974.
2. Katz, S.H., Hediger, M.L., Schall, J.I., Bowers, E.J., Barker, W.F., Aurand, S., Evaleth, P.B., Gruskin, A. and Parks, J.S.: Blood pressure, growth and maturation from childhood through adolescence:Result of a mixed longitudinal study from the Philadelphia blood pressure project. Hypertension 2, Supplement 1, Part II, 1980, pp.55-69.
3. Hiner, L.B. and Gruskin, A.B.: The physiology of blood pressure regulation normal and abnormal. Pediatr.Ann. 6:373, 1977.
4. Robson, A.M.: Special diagnostic studies for the detection of renal and renovascular forms of hypertension. Pediatr.Clin.North Am.25:83, 1978.
5. Londe, S.: Causes of hypertension in the young. Pediatr.Clin.North Am. 25:55, 1978.
6. Kilcoyne, M.M.: Adolescent hypertension, in New M.I., Levine, L.S. (eds.): Juvenile hypertension. New York, Raven Press, 1977,pp.25-35.
7. Loggie, J.M.H.: Prevalence of hypertension and distribution of causes, in New, M.I., Levine, L.S. (eds.): Juvenile Hypertension, New York, Raven Press, 1977, pp.1-12.
8. Kotchen, T.A., and Kotchen, J.M.: Clinical approaches to high blood pressure in the young. Cardiovascular Reviews & Reports 1(3):53,1980.
9. Oparil, S. and Haber, E.: The renin-angiotensin system I. New Engl.J. Med. Medical Progress 291(8):389, 1974. The renin-angiotensin system II, New Engl. J. Med. Medical Progress 291(9):476, 1974.
10. Laragh, J.H.: Hypertension Manual. New York, Yorke Medical Books, Dun-Donnelly Publishing Corp. New York, 1974.
11. Laragh, J.H.: The renin system and hypertension. in Proceedings of the First SCOR-Hypertension Conference The Renin System 3/7/80 New York Hospital-Cornell Medical Center, New York, NY Conference. Directors J.H. Laragh and J.E. Sealey pp.1-13.
12. Krakoff, L.R. and Laragh, J.H.: The renin system in the diagnosis of hypertension Ed. Siegel, L. Directions in Cardiovascular Medicine. Published by Hoechst-Roussel Pharmaceuticals, Sommerville, New Jersey 19
13. Case, D.B., Wallace, J.M., Keim, H.J. et al: Estimating renin participation in hypertension. Superiority of converting enzyme inhibitor over Saralasin. Am.J.Med. 61:790, 1976.

14. Gavras, H., Gavras, I., Hadzinikolaou, P. and Brunner, H.R.: Inhibition of angiotensin conversion:its role in treatment of hypertension and congestive heart failure. Cardiovascular Med.5:327, 1980.
15. Friedman, A., Chesney, R.W., Ball, D. and Goodfriend, T.: Effective use of captopril (angiotensin I-converting enzyme inhibitor) in severe childhood hypertension. J.Pediatr.97:664, 1980.
16. Brunner, H.R. et al: Oral angiotensin-converting enzyme inhibition in long-term treatment of hypertensive patients. Ann.Intern.Med. 90:19, 1979.
17. Bumpus, F.M.: Angiotensin antagonists in relation to hypertension. Hospital Practice, May 1974, p.80.
18. Laragh, J.H.: Vasoconstriction-volume analysis for understanding and treating hypertension:The use of renin and aldosterone profiles. Am.J.Med. 55:261, 1973.
19. Laragh, J.H., Sealey, J.E., Buhler, F.R. et al: The renin axis and vasoconstriction volume analysis for understanding and treating renovascular and renal hypertension. Am.J.Med. 58:4, 1975.
20. Sealey, J.E.: Clinical Plasma Renin Activity Measurements, in Proceedings of the First SCOR-Hypertension Conf. The Renin System 3/7/80. New York Hospital-Cornell Medical Center, New York, Directors, J.H. Laragh and J.E. Sealey, pp.13-22.
21. Wallach, L., Nyarai, I. and Dawson, K.G.: Stimulated renin:A screening test for hypertension. Ann.Intern.Med.82:27, 1975.
22. Grim, C.E., Luft, F.C., Fineberg, N.S. and Weinberger, M.H.: Responses to volume expansion and contraction in categorized hypertensive and normotensive man. Hypertension 1:476, 1979.
23. Stalker, H.P., Holland, N.H., Kotchen, J.M. and Kotchen, T.A.: Plasma renin activity in healthy children. J.Pediatr.89:256, 1976.
24. Sassard, J., Sann, L., Vincent, M. et al: Plasma renin action in normal subjects from infancy to puberty. J.Clin.Endocrinol.Metab.40:524,1975.
25. Hiner, H., Sann, L., Vincent, M. et al: Plasma renin action in normal children. J.Pediatr. 89:258, 1976.
26. Van Acker, K.J., Scharpe, S.L., Deprettere, A.J.R. and Neels, H.M.: Renin-angiotensin-aldosterone system in the healthy infant and child. Kidney Int. 16:196-203, 1979.
27. Goldberg, S., Krishan, I., Hames, C.B., Knight, M. and Spierto, F.W.: Elevated renin levels in normotensive adolescents. Pediatrics 54:596, 1974.
28. Weidmann, P., Beretta-Piccoli, C., Ziegler, W.H., Keusch, G., Gluck, A. and Reubi, F.C.: Age versus urinary sodium for judging renin, aldosterone, and catecholamine levels:Studies in normal subjects and patients with essential hypertension. Kidney Int. 14:619, 1978.
29. Laragh, J.H., Letcher, R.L. and Pickering, T.G.: Renin profiling for diagnosis and treatment of hypertension. JAMA 241(2):151, 1979.
30. Grim, C.E., Weinberger, M.H., Higgins, J.T. and Kramer, N.J.: Diagnosis of secondary forms of hypertension. A comprehensive protocol. JAMA 237(13):1331, 1977.
31. Brenner, H.R., Kirshman, J.D., Sealey, J.E. et al: Hypertension of renal origin:Evidence for two different mechanisms. Science 174:1344,1971.
32. Case, D.B. and Laragh, J.H.: Renin release and identification of renovascular hypertension. in Proceedings of the First SCOR-Hypertension Conference The Renin System 3/7/80, New York Hospital-Cornell Medical Center, New York, Directors, J.H. Laragh and J.E. Sealey, pp.79-80.

33. Vaughan, E.D.,Jr., Buhler, F.R., Laragh, J.H. et al: Renovascular hypertension:Renin measurements to indicate hypersecretion and contra-lateral suppression estimate renal plasma flow and score for surgical curability. Am.J.Med. 55:402, 1973.
34. Hiner, L.B., Gruskin, A.B., Baluarte, H.J., Cote, M.L., Sapire, D.W. and Levitsky, M.D.: Plasma renin activity and intrarenal blood flow distribution in a child with a pheochromocytoma. J.Pediatr. 89:950, 1976.
35. Hung, W., August, G.P.: Hyperreninemia and secondary hyperaldosteronism in pheochomocytomas. J.Pediatr. 94:215, 1979.
36. Vetter, H., Vetter, W., Warnholz, C. et al: Renin and aldosterone secretion in pheochromocytoma. Effect of chronic alpha-adrenergic receptor blockade. Am.J.Med. 60:866, 1976.
37. Warshaw, B.L., Anand, S.K., Olson, D.L., Grushkin, C.M., Heuser, E.T. and Lieverman, E.: Hypertension secondary to a renin-producing juxtaglomerular cell tumor. J.Ped. 94:247, 1979.
38. Chrysant, S.G., Kastagir, B.K., Stevens, L.E., Klinkmann, H. and Kolff, W.J.: Plasma renin activity in hypertension after renal homo-transplantation. Angiology 25(3):172, 1974.
39. Conn, J.W.: Plasma renin activity in primary aldosteronism. Importance in differential diagnosis and in research of essential hypertension. JAMA 190:222, 1964.
40. Godard, C., Riondel, A.M., Veyrat, R., Megevand, A. and Muller, A.F.: Plasma renin activity and aldosterone secretion in congenital adrenal hyperplasia. Pediatrics 41:883, 1968.
41. Davis, W.W., Newsome, H.H.,Jr., Wright, L.D. et al: Bilateral adrenal hyperplasia as a cause of primary aldosteronism with hypertension, hypokalemia and suppressed renin activity. Am.J.Med. 42:642, 1967.
42. Powell, H.R., Rotenberg, E., Williams, A.L. and McCredie, D.A.: Plasma renin activity in acute poststreptococcal glomerulonephritis and the haemolytic-uraemic syndrome.Arch.Dis.Child.49:802, 1974.
43. Amsterdam.E., Albers, W.A., Christlieb, A.R. et al: Plasma renin activity in children with coarctation of the aorta. Am.J.Cardiol.23: 396, 1969.
44. Ribeiro, A.B. and Krakoff, L.R.: Angiotensin blockade in coarctation of the aorta. New Engl.J.Med. 295:148, 1976.
45. Sealey, J.E., Buhler, F.R., Laragh, J.H. et al: The physiology of renin secretion in essential hypertension. Am.J.Med.55:391, 1973.
46. Burnner, H.R., Laragh, J.H., Baer, L. et al: Essential hypertension. Renin and aldosterone heart attack and stroke. N.Engl.J.Med. 286:441, 1972.
47. Gruskin, A.B., Linshaw, M., Cote, M.L. and Fleisher, D.: Low renin essential hypertension - another form of childhood hypertension. J.Pediatr. 78:765, 1971.
48. Kilcoyne, M.M.: Adolescent hypertension. II Characteristics and response to treatment. Circulation 50:1014, 1974.
49. Linshaw, M., Stapleton, F.B. , Gruskin, A.B., Baluarte, H.J. and Harbin, G.L.: Traction related hypertension in children. J.Pedatr.95:994, 1979.
50. Prebis, J.W., Polinsky, M.S., Gruskin, A.B., Baluarte, H.J., Ferguson, R.K. and Vlasses, P.H.: Delayed antihypertensive response to Captopril (CAP) (oral angiotensin converting enzyme inhibitor) because of clonidine (CLON) rebound. Pediatr.13:517, 1979.

HIGHLIGHTS: INITIAL ALTERATIONS OF RENAL FUNCTION IN CHILDREN WITH ACUTE STREPTOCOCCAL GLOMERULONEPHRITIS

Gustavo Gordillo-Paniagua, M.D., Felipe Mota-Hernandez, M.D., and René Feiman, M.D.

Hypervolemia is the most common pathophysiologic derangement observed initially in acute post-streptococcal glomerulonephritis(AGN). The major risk of hypervolemia is hypertension, frequently complicated with acute pulmonary edema or hypertensive encephalopathy. Reports in the literature show a 0.5 to 6% mortality due to these complications.

Plasma renin activity and serum aldosterone have been measured in AGN and found within normal limits. Information in the literature regarding modifications of renal handling of sodium in children with AGN is scarce; therefore, we undertook this study in the initial stages of the disease, trying to make a correlation with hypertension.

MATERIALS AND METHODS

Forty-one children with AGN and hypertension admitted to the Department of Nephrology in the Hospital Infantil de Mexico, were included into the study. Diagnostic criteria included previous streptococcal infection in association two weeks later with the appearance of manifestations of renal lesion of acute onset, hypervolemia and hypertension.

The patients were three to 12 years old; 25 were males. Dyastolic blood pressure varied from 85 to 130 mm Hg and all were above the 95th percentile.

The antecedent of B-hemolytic streptococcal infection, found in 41 cases, was documented by ASO titer elevation in 38 cases (93%), scarlet fever in 29 cases (71%) and positive throat cultures in 9 cases (21%).

The first sign of renal involvement was edema of the eyelids in 31 cases (76%), hematuria alone in 6 (15%), and both signs in 4 (10%). Except for one patient, all of them showed hypocomplementemia of 25 $\pm$ 16 mg/dl (normal 86 $\pm$ 17). The time of evolution between the onset of the infection and the appearance of the first sign of renal involvement was 5-32 days (average 14 $\pm$ 7). The time of evolution between the appearance of the first sign of renal lesion and admission to the study varied from 1 to 15 days (average 7 $\pm$ 4 days).

The following indices were made on urine to plasma ratios (U/P) of urea, osmolality, sodium, creatinine, fractional excretion of filtered sodium (FENa) and renal failure index (RFI).

RESULTS

Initial results were U/P osm 1.9 ± 0.8, U/P urea 29 ± 20.5, U/P sodium 0.53 ± 0.41, U/P creatinine 143 ± 148, RFI 1.1 ± 1.15 and FENa 0.8 ± 0.85. Due to the great dispersion observed in all values, a correlation with the time of evolution of the disease was attempted. The changes observed in all the indices were in direct relationship with the time of evolution. The patients were divided into three groups according to the time of evolution. Eighteen patients had one to five days of evolution at the time of admission (Group 1); fifteen had six to 10 days (Group II) and eight had 11-15 days (Group III).

Average FENa in G I was compared to G II and G III; no statistically significant difference was found between G II and G III. RFI showed similar values to FENa, but the actual figures were slightly higher in all three groups.

Average U/P creatinine in G I was 245; 61 in G II and 69 in G III, with p value < 0.01 when comparing G I with G II and G III. The difference found was in relationship with creatinine urinary concentration. Average U/P sodium in G I was 0.4; in G II 0.6 and G III 0.7, with p value < 0.02 comparing G I with G III.

Average U/P osmolality was 2.2 in G I and 1.65 in G II and G III with p value 0.05 comparing G I with G II. U/P urea in G I was 29, in G II 25 and 36 in G III; no statistical difference was found between the three groups. There was no difference in age, degree of hypertension, hemoglobin and hematocrit levels between the three groups.

DISCUSSION

The results of this study show differences in the renal function indices and renal handling of sodium which are related with the time of evolution of AGN. FENa increased progressively along with the time of evolution.

Low values of FENa during the first five days of evolution were correlated with increased U/P creatinine, which in turn was due to increased urinary creatinine concentration; serum creatinine remained constantly elevated. Increased U/P osmolality values, reported also by other authors, suggest maximal tubular water reabsorption during this period. All this could mean decreased FENa and could explain the poor correlation found between the degree of sodium retention and the changes in GFR. The fall in GFR before clinical manifestations appear could be the factor responsible for sodium retention initially,due to decreased filtered load as well as increased fractional reabsorption of the filtered sodium. Both circumstances may contribute to extracellular volume expansion and development of hypertension.

The variability of the renal function indices found early in the course of AGN suggests integrity of the tubular function since glomerulotubular balance was observed during the first five days of evolution, and tubular capacity to increase FENa in the presence of persistent hypervolemia was observed afterwards.

DISORDERS OF URATE METABOLISM IN CHILDREN AND ADULTS

James W. Prebis, M.D. , Alan B. Gruskin, M.D., H, Jorge Baluarte, M.D. and Martin S. Polinsky, M.D.

Gout has plagued man for centuries with evidence of gouty arthritis dating back to the ancient Egyptians. Over the years, numerous disease states have been described in children and adults which result from abnormalities in uric acid metabolism. This review will consider three aspects of urate metabolism: First, a brief description of disorders associated with altered uric acid homeostasis; secondly, the current understanding of uric acid metabolism occurring in healthy man; thirdly, an in depth consideration of the hyperuricemia found in hypertensive adults and children.

In man, uric acid is the end product of purine degradation and once formed, does not undergo further biochemical transformation. About two-thirds of the daily uric acid excretion occurs through the kidneys and the remainder via the gastrointestinal tract.[1] If there is a decrease in renal function, a proportionately greater increase in urate excretion will occur via the gastrointestinal tract. Elevations in serum uric acid can, therefore, be viewed as a result of either an overproduction of uric acid and/or a decrease in urate excretion.

In general, an increase in uric acid production is associated with either an abnormally rapid rate of cellular turnover (secondary hyperuricemia) or a genetically determined enzyme defect in purine biosynthesis (primary hyperuricemia).[2] (Table I, Part I)

Table I: Classification of Hyperuricemia

I. Increased production

A. Primary Hyperuricemia (enzyme defect)

Deficiency of hypoxanthine-guanine phosphoribosyl transferase
(Lesch-Nyhan syndrome)
Deficiency of glucose-6-phosphatase
(von Gierke disease)
Increase in phosphoribosyl pyrophosphate synthetase

B. Secondary Hyperuricemia
(Increased nucleic acid turnover)

Hemoglobin S-C disease
Hemolytic anemias

Infectious mononucleosis
Leukemia
Lymphoma
Multiple myeloma
Pernicious anemia
Polycythemia Vera
Sickle Cell disease
Thalassemia

Secondary hyperuricemia which is encountered more commonly by the practicing physician occurs in association with hemotologic disorders such as leukemia, polycythemia vera, Sickle Cell disease, and other chronic hemolytic anemias. Examples of primary hyperuricemia include a number of inborn errors of metabolism which result in an increase of purine biosynthesis and include a partial or complete deficiency of the enzyme hypoxanthine-guanine phosphoribosyltransferase (HGPRT). This enzyme deficiency is inherited in a sex-linked recessive manner and the complete absence of this enzyme results in the childhood Lesch-Nyhan syndrome which is characterized by choreoathetosis, spasticity, mental retardation, self mutilation and renal stones. Other inherited enzymatic defects producing hyperuricemia are an increase in the activity of the enzyme phosphoribosyl pyrophosphate synthetase (PRPP) or a deficiency in glucose-6-phosphatase (glycogen storage disease type I)

Elevations in serum uric acid are often the result of a decrease in the renal excretion of urate. This situation is typically seen in patients with a diminished glomerular filtration rate or in some patients with proximal tubular dysfunctions. Other disorders in which hyperuricemia results in part or in total from a decrease in the renal excretion of urate are tabulated in the following Table:[2,3]

Table I (Part II): Classification of Hyperuricemia

II. Decreased Excretion

Alcoholism
Bartters syndrome
Chronic beryllium disease
Diabetes ketoacidosis
Drugs: diuretics, salicylates, pyrazinamide, nicotinic acid, ethambutal
Hereditary fructose intolerance
Hyperparathyroidism
Hypertension
Lactic acidosis
Lead nephropathy
Maple syrup urine disease
Nephrogenic diabetes insipidus
Primary hyperoxaluria
Sickle cell anemia
Toxemia of pregnancy

Individuals with clinical gout can be classified into two heterogenious sub-groups; 1) metabolic over-producers of uric acid, or 2) the under-excreters of uric acid. Boss and Seegmiller have proposed a physiologic classification of hyperuricemia and gout based on the 24-hour urinary uric acid excretion.[4] Since normal adult males ingesting a purine free diet excrete less than 600 mg of urate per day, they classify a hyperuricemic man as an "overproducer" of urate if he excretes more than 600 mg of urate per day, while receiving a purine free diet. An "underexcreter" of urate is the hyperuricemic individual who excretes less than 600 mg of uric acid per day. Based on this classification, 10-20% of individuals with primary gout are "overproducers" while the remaining 80% are "underexcreters". In order to avoid the inherent difficulties of collecting a 24-hour urine specimen, studies in hyperuricemic adults[5] and children[6] have demonstrated that an elevation in the ratio of uric acid to creatinine (U.A/Cr) in a spot, morning urine specimen indicates a relative overexcretion of urate. In such situations the patient's hyperuricemia is secondary to an increase in uric acid production.

RENAL TRANSPORT OF URATE

A knowledge of the renal handling of uric acid is helpful in understanding the pathogenesis underlying hyperuricemia and can serve as a guideline for possible therapeutic intervention. A significant proportion of the data on the renal transport of urate in man is extrapolated from micropuncture studies in animals. Evidence from many animal species indicate that there is a bidirectional transport of urate, i.e., tubular reabsorption and secretion of filtered uric acid. The degree to which reabsorption vs secretion determines the final rate of urate excretion varies from species to species. In birds, reptiles and the dalmation coach hound the interaction of these two processes results in a net rate of urate secretion, while in monkeys and man, the net effect is one of reabsorption.[7] This point should be remembered when one extrapolates data from animal studies to clarify the mechanisms of urate transport in man.

The present concept for the renal handling of uric acid in man is based on a four component model: 1) Sodium urate is completely filtered at the glomerulus (filtration); 2) essentially all of the filtered urate is actively reabsorbed in the early proximal tubule (reabsorption); 3) urate is then secreted into the proximal tubular lumen (secretion); 4) varying quantities of luminal urate are then reabsorbed back into the peritubular blood resulting in a net excretion of 6-10% of the filtered load (post secretory reabsorption).

This model has evolved from the contributions of numerous investigators over the last 30 years. A brief review of the scientific developments leading to the formulation of this model will provide a clearer understanding of the factors controlling urate homeostasis. In 1950, Berliner and associates[8] conducted one of the first systematic investigations of the renal mechanisms controlling urate excretion in healthy man. They produced hyperuricemia by infusing lithium urate and measuring the rates of urate filtration and excretion. They concluded that tubular reabsorption occurred through an active carrier mediated mechanism of limited capacity. They calculated the tubular maximum (Tm) for urate reabsorption in man to be about 15 mg/min/1.73m^2 and felt that the reabsorption capacity for urate was so great that it rarely, if ever, became saturated under normal physiologic circumstances.

The first report of urate secretion occurring in man appeared in 1950 when Praetorius and Kirk described a patient with hypouricemia whose rate of urate excretion exceeded the filtered load by 46%.[9] These data were interpreted as indicating a net rate of urate secretion. Several years later, Gutman and Yü conducted extensive studies in patients with mild renal insufficiency conclusively demonstrating that urate secretion does occur in man.[10] Gutman and Yü proposed the classical "three component model" for urate transport, i.e., 1) plasma urate is filtered by the glomerulus; 2) filtered urate is reabsorbed by active tubular transport, 3) urate is then secreted by an active tubular transport mechanism.[11,12] At that time, it was not clear if reabsorption or secretion was the predominant factor determining the net rate of urate excretion. Later investigations by Steele et al[13] utilizing pyrazinamide which is known to specifically inhibit urate secretion at low doses without significantly affecting reabsorption, permitted further clarification of the renal mechanisms controlling urate transport: 1) the Tm for urate reabsorption is much higher than initially determined by Berliner and there is a proportional increase in urate reabsorption with increases in the filtered load of urate; 2) the rate of urate secretion is also enchanced by increases in plasma uric acid concentration. These data lead to the conclusion that in healthy man there is bidirectional transport of urate (reabsorption and secretion) which can be augmented by elevations in serum uric acid. Further studies utilizing pyrazinamide demonstrated that the primary factor controlling urate excretion was a change in the rate of urate secretion.

On the basis of in vitro experiments conducted in animals and several studies performed in man, it appears that urate secretion is an active carrier mediated process occurring along the peritubular plasma membrane of the proximal tubule.[3] This secretory mechanism is very similar, if not identical to that utilized by other weak organic anions such as para-aminohippurate. There is evidence to suggest that urate and PAH are in fact secreted by the same carrier in some animal species.[14] Regarding man, most studies indicate that hippurate and urate are transported by separate carriers.[15] Nevertheless, data from human and animal studies indicate that a number of organic acids may compete with uric acid for the same secretory carrier and thereby result in a decrease in urate secretion. This secretory competition may explain in part the hyperuricemia found in several disease states associated with increased concentrations of lactic acid[16] and other endogenous organic acids, for example alcoholism,[17] branch chain ketoaciduria (maple syrup urine disease),[18] Type I glycogen storage disease,[19] diabetic ketoacidosis[20] and chronic renal failure.[21]

In 1973, Diamond[22] and Steele[23] extended and revised the three component model of Gutman and Yü by identifying a fourth component for urate transport, i.e., post secretory reabsorption. The exact location and significance of this post secretory reabsorption is not clear at this time. Rieselbach and Steele[24] have proposed a very elegant model for the renal handling of urate which incorporates all four components of urate transport (Figure 1). As in earlier models, plasma urate is totally filtered and undergoes virtually complete active reabsorption in the early proximal tubule Secretion and post secretory reabsorption occur in the late proximal tubule. It is possible that the location of the post secretory reabsorptive process is the same as that for secretion, but most studies suggest a location further down stream. Experiments imply that the post secretory reabsorptive mechanism is also an active transport system but its Tm is much lower than that of the presecretory reabsorption of urate. Since essentially all urate is filtered and initially reabsorbed the factors which determine the daily fluctuations in urate excretion are the secretory and post secretory reabsorptive mechanisms. Rieselbach proposes that there may be a continuous balancing interaction between this secretion and post secretory reabsorption permitting "glomerulo tubular balance" of urate to occur. Thus, moderate alterations in rates of secretion could be modified by appropriate changes in the magnitude of post secretory reabsorption such that the daily fractional excretion of urate remains between 6-10%. This secretory-reabsorptive balance could adjust to major alterations in either the secretion or post secretory reabsorption of urate. Disruption of the secretory-reabsorptive balance can be demonstrated in disorders associated with hypo or hyper uricemia. As mentioned earlier, significant decreases in urate secretion are partially responsible for the hyperuricemia found in lactic acidosis, alcoholism and several other disease states. An abnormal decrease in post secretory reabsorption may explain the hypouricemia encountered in some patients with Wilson's disease[25] and Hodgkin's disease.[26] There is also a report suggesting that increases in post secretory reabsorption are responsible for an inheritable form of hyperuricemia.[27]

Model of Urate Transport

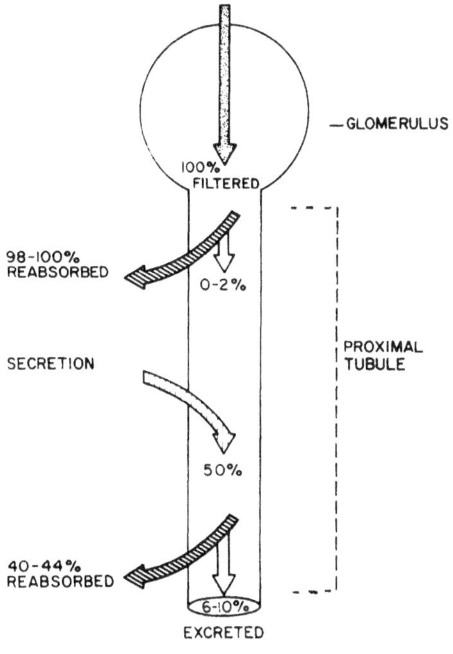

Figure 1

HYPERURICEMIA AND HYPERTENSION

The association of hyperuricemia with adult renovascular and essential hypertension has been recognized for decades.[28,29] Studies indicate that hyperuricemia occurs in 25-35% of untreated adults with essential hypertension.[30,3] The incidence of elevated serum uric acid increases to 50-58% when evaluating those adults receiving therapy for their hypertension or those with renovascular hypertension.[29-31] For years there has been debate over the issue whether hypertension contributes to the development of hyperuricemia or whether elevated serum uric acid produces vascular and renal damage which contribute to the later development of hypertension. Proponents of this latter theory point to the fact that 25-50% of patients with gout develop hypertension[32] and there is also an increased incidence of hypertension in patients with asymptomatic hyperuricemia.[33,34] It is possible that the chronic deposition of monosodium urate crystals in the renal medullary interstitium of these hyperuricemic patients results in nephrosclerosis and hypertension.[35] A recent animal study has shown that the urate loading of normotensive rats resulted in a significant increase in their blood pressure.[36] Further research is needed in this field since it is still not clear if hyperuricemia does influence the development of elevated blood pressures and, if so, by what physiologic mechanisms.

The possibility that hypertension could influence the development of metabolic derangements such as hyperuricemia and hyperlipidemia has intrigued investigators for years. Although there are numerous reports dealing with the incidence and pathophysiology of hyperuricemia in hypertensive adults, there is an obvious paucity of information which addresses the subject of uric acid metabolism in hypertensive children and adolescents.

We recently evaluated serum uric acid levels and the renal handling of urate in 31 hypertensive pediatric patients ranging in age from 3½ to 18 years.[37] All of these children had essential hypertension and none had received therapy for their elevated blood pressure prior to their inhospital evaluation. Serum uric acid levels were measured in these hypertensive children while they were receiving an unrestricted sodium diet and compared to serum values from healthy age-matched controls.[38] Thirteen of 31 or 42% of these children with essential hypertension were hyperuricemic (serum uric acid 2 standard deviations above the age appropriate mean value) (Figure 2). Prior reports by Breckenridge[30] and Cannon[31] has demonstrated that their hypertensive hyperuricemic adults had reduced uric acid clearances compared to hypertensive normal uricemic adults. They suggested that their patients' hyperuricemia was secondary to a renal tubular abnormality in the handling of uric acid. In order to determine if a decreased urate clearance also existed in our hypertensive hyperuricemic children, their uric acid and creatinine clearances were measured. From this data, the fractional excretion of uric acid (FeUA) was calculated ($C_{ua} \div C_{cr} \times 100$) and compared to the patient's serum uric acid level (Figure 3). A significant inverse correlation existed between the serum uric acid level and the FeUA of both normal uricemic and hyperuricemic hypertensive patients. This indicated that the hyperuricemic patients did in fact have a reduction in urate clearance compared to the normouricemic patients. Since all these hypertensive children had normal glomerular filtration rates this diminished urate clearance was probably secondary to either a decrease in the tubular secretion of urate and/or an increase in the pre or post secretory reabsorption of urate. Further studies are needed to clarify this point.

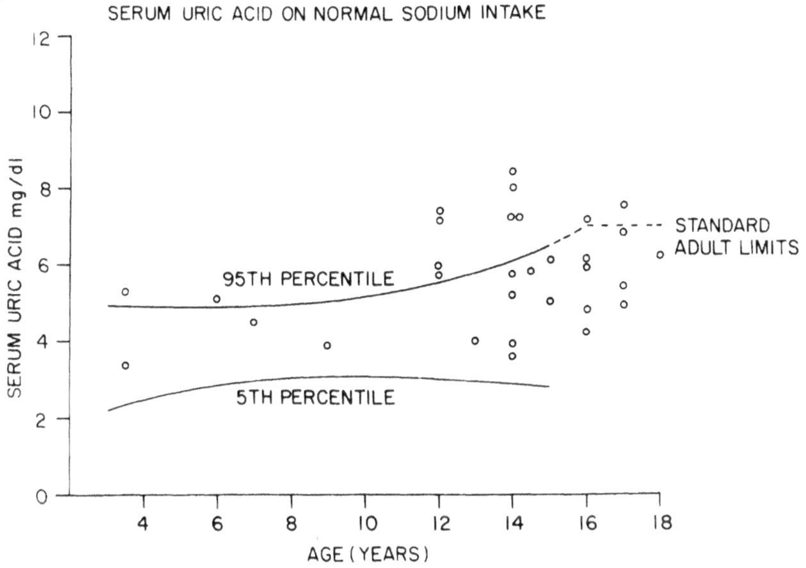

Figure 2. (Reprinted with permission of J.Ped.)

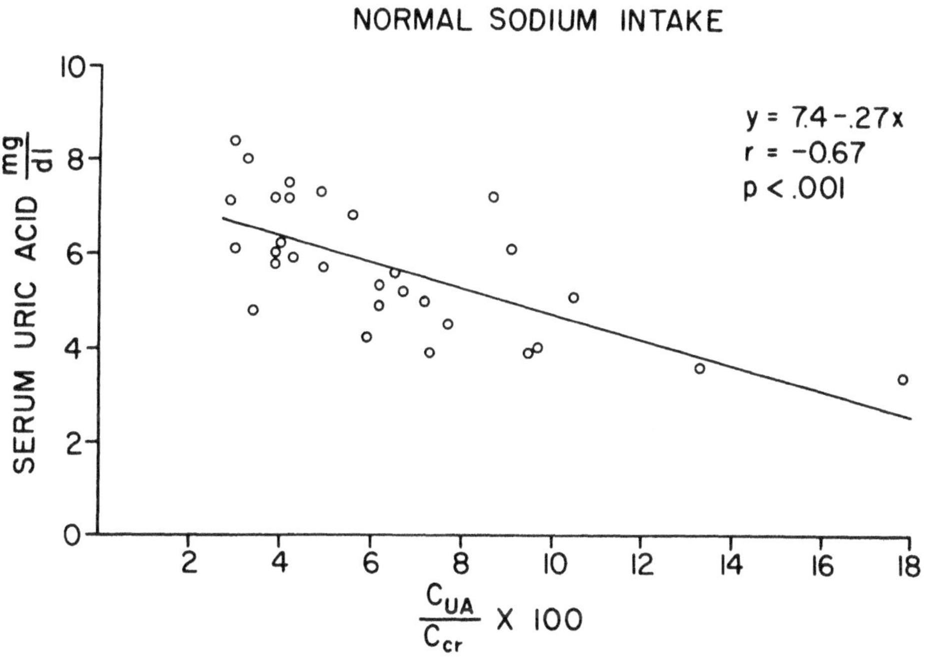

Figure 3. (Reprinted with permission of J. Ped.)

After the above studies were completed these same 31 children were given a 200 mg sodium diet for three days to determine if sodium restriction would have any effect on uric acid metabolism. Using the same standards to define hyperuricemia as described earlier, 17 of 31 or 55% of the hypertensive children and adolescents were hyperuricemic after completing the low sodium diet (Figure 4).

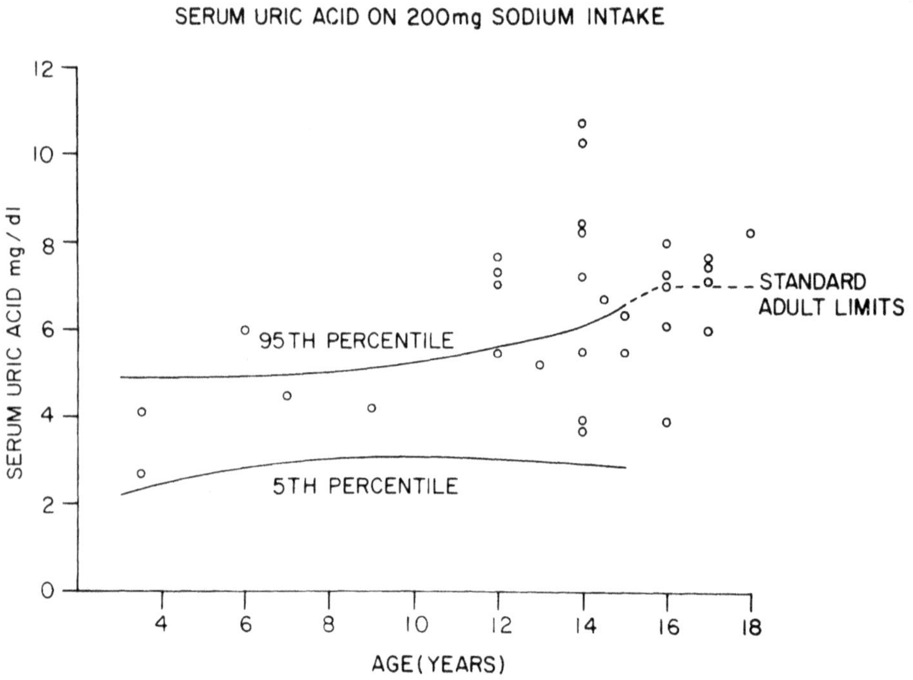

Figure 4

Nearly half of these children had serum uric acid levels higher than 7 mg/dl and several were as high as 10-11 mg/dl. The sodium restricted diet did produce a degree of volume contraction which was reflected by a mean weight loss of 1.8 ± 0.9 kg. The FeUA was again measured after the children had completed the low sodium diet. A comparison of the serum uric acid level vs the FeUA again revealed a strong inverse correlation for all these hypertensive patients (Figure 5). Following the 200 mg sodium diet the mean FeUA for all these subjects significantly decreased from 6.40% to 5.12%, yet there was no significant change in their creatinine clearance. These data indicate that the increase in serum uric acid following the restricted diet was due to a decrease in urate excretion.

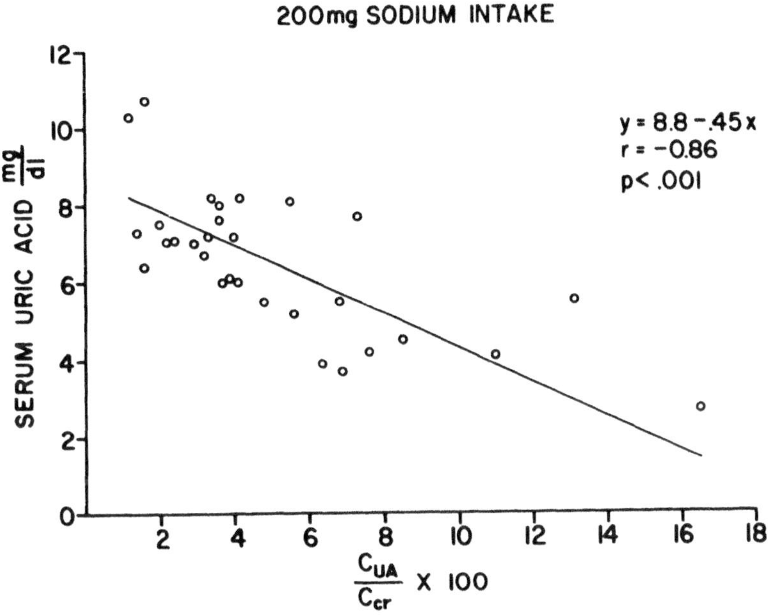

Figure 5. (Reprinted with permission of J. Ped.)

There are several possible explanations for this reduced urate clearance. It is unlikely that alterations in the patient's glomerular filtration rate had any role in the reduced urate clearance since there was no significant change in the endogenous creatinine clearance of these patients while ingesting a normal sodium intake (creatinine clearance=109±26 ml/min/ $1.73m^2$) vs a low sodium intake (creatinine clearance = 101±23 ml/min/$1.73m^2$) (p=0.15). The low sodium diet did produce variable degrees of volume contraction in all the children and adolescents as reflected by a mean weight loss of 1.8±0.9 kg. A number of studies have shown that chnages in extracellular volume can alter the proximal tubular reabsorption of solutes including sodium,[39] bicarbonate,[40] phosphorus,[41] glucose[42] and uric acid.[43-45] It is unlikely that this mechanism alone produced the diminished excretion of uric acid since 98-100% filtered uric acid is normally reabsorbed in the proximal tubule and this total reabsorption will increase with increasing filtered loads of uric acid up to serum uric acid levels of 16 mg/dl.[13] Other studies have indicated that volume contraction may also decrease the excretion of urate by diminishing its secretion in the proximal tubule. Experiments by Weinman[44] and Steele[45] have demonstrated that the hyperuricemia occurring in association with the use of diuretics is secondary to volume contraction with the resultant increase in the proximal tubular reabsorption of urate as well as decrease in secretion. Another mechanism which could theoretically contribute to the decreased clearance of urate would be an increase in the post-secretory reabsorption. A hypothetical model which could explain the diminished excretion of uric acid following volume contraction is depicted in Figure 6. The initiating event of this process would be a decrease in active secretion of urate with continued post-secretory reabsorption which would result in an increase in serum uric acid. Hyperuricemia would then be maintained by the complete proximal reabsorption of all filtered urate. When the volume contraction has been corrected, there would be a concommitant increase in urate secretion which would increase urate excretion and thereby return serum uric acid levels to normal values.

Model of Urate Transport

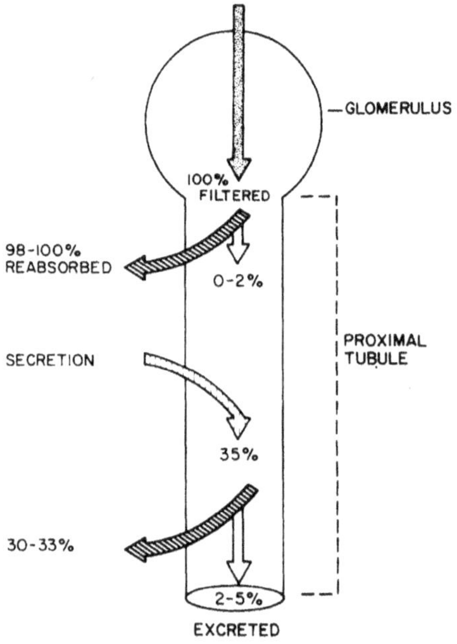

Figure 6

As mentioned earlier several investigators have shown that the hyperuricemia found in hypertensive adults is due to a decrease in urate excretion. Whether this decreased excretion is secondary to a tubular defect in urate reabsorption and/or secretion is unclear. In order to determine if there was evidence of an abnormality in the tubular secretion of urate in our hyperuricemic patients, data obtained as part of a furosemide stimulation test were used to compare the relative secretory function of the hyperuricemic vs normouricemic hypertensive children. The rationale for this study is the following:

Furosemide is an organic acid whose diuretic properties are based on its ability to block the reabsorption of chloride and sodium in the ascending limb of the loop of Henle.[46] Its diuretic action is due to the presence of this drug within the tubular lumen rather than the peritubular blood. It has also been demonstrated that furosemide gains access to its site of action primarily by secretion at the proximal tubule via the transport pathway for organic acids. The higher the concentration of furosemide within the lumen of the tubule the greater the rate of excretion of sodium, chloride and water.[47-50]

As indicated earlier, plasma urate is secreted by an active carrier mediated mechanism which is similar if not identical to that utilized by other weak organic acids. Clinical states have already been described where an elevation in serum organic acids can result in a decrease in urate secretion secondary to the organic acid competing with uric acid for the same secretory carrier. Since the organic acids furosemide and uric acid are both secreted into the proximal tubule via similar organic acid transport pathways,[14,15,48,49] we theorized that if there was a decrease in the secretion of uric acid in the hypertensive hyperuricemic patient, there may also be a decrease in the secretion of furosemide which would be reflected by a diminished rate of excretion for sodium, chloride and water. In order to test this hypothesis, 1 mg/kg of furosemide was administered orally to 21 children with essential hypertension. Eight of these children were hyperuricemic for age and none of the subjects had received medication for their hypertension prior to the study. After the patient had received furosemide his urine was collected for five consecutive hours and measured for electrolytes and volume. The hyperuricemic, hypertensive children and adolescents excreted statistically less sodium, chloride and urine compared to the normal uricemic hypertensive subjects (Table 2).[51]

Table 2: Response to Furosemide

	Sodium excretion (μEq/5 hr/1.73m^2)	Chloride excretion (μEq/5 hr/1.73m^2)	Urine output (ml/5 hr/1.73m^2)
Normouricemic child	190	240	1700
Hyperuricemic child	139	180	1300
	$p<.03$	$p<.02$	$p<.02$

Several preliminary conclusions can be based on these data. First, there was a statistically significant reduction in the diuretic response to furosemide in the hyperuricemic patients as demonstrated by the decreased excretion of sodium, chloride and urine. Second, there is probably a reduction in the secretion of the organic acid furosemide into the proximal tubule of the hyperuricemic children since the diuretic response to furosemide is directly related to its concentration in the renal tubule. Third, an abnormality in the tubular secretion of furosemide could reflect a similar abnormality in the tubular transport of uric acid in hyperuricemic patients. These data, therefore, support the concept that the decrease in uric acid excretion seen in hypertensive hyperuricemic children and adolescents is due to a reduction in uric acid secretion.

In conclusion, studies indicate that hyperuricemia occurs in a significant number of untreated adults and children with essential hypertension. It appears that in the majority of hypertensive patients, hyperuricemia is the result of a decrease in the renal excretion of urate. Our furosemide studies suggest that the reduced urate excretion is in part due to a reduction in the tubular secretion of urate. The presence of tubular dysfunction in hypertensive patients is not a new concept when one considers that in 1944

Goldring demonstrated abnormalities in tubular function as well as decreased glomerular filtration rate and renal plasma flow in adults with chronic hypertension.[52] It is possible that persistent hypertension has a pathogenic role in the development of these tubular dysfunctions. The presence of hyperuricemia in hypertensive children and adolescents may then be one of the earliest manifestations of organ damage secondary to elevated blood pressure.

Future longitudinal studies will be needed to answer the following questions: Does hyperuricemia worsen the long term prognosis of the hypertensive child or adolescent? Will the early detection and treatment of hypertension in children and adolescents prevent or reverse these abnormalities in the renal handling of urate?

REFERENCES

1. Sorenson, L.B. and Levison, D.J.: Origin and extrarenal elimination of uric acid in man. Nephron. 14:7, 1975.
2. Wyngaarden, J.B. and Kelley, W.N.: Gout, in the Metabolic Basis of Inherited Disease. New York, 1978, McGraw-Hill Book Company, p.916.
3. Chonko, A.M. and Grantham, J.J.: Disorders of urate metabolism and excretion, in Brenner, B. and Rector, Jr. M., editors: The Kidney, Philadelphia, 1981, W.B. Saunders Company, p. 1023.
4. Boss, G.R. and Seegmiller, J.E.: Hyperuricemia and gout. N.Engl.J. Med. 300:1459, 1979.
5. Simkin, P.A., Hoover, P.L., Paxson, C.S. and Wilson, W.F.: Uric acid excretion: quantitative assessment from SPOT, midmorning serum and urine samples. Ann.Intern.Med. 91:44, 1979.
6. Kaufman, J.M., Greene, M.L. and Seegmiller, J.E.: Urine uric acid to creatinine ratio - a screening test for inherited disorders of purine metabolism. J.Pediatr. 73:583, 1968.
7. Zins, G.R. and Weiner, I.M.: Bidirectional urate transport limited to the proximal tubule in dogs. Am. J. Physiol. 215:411, 1968.
8. Berliner, R.W., Hilton, J.G., Yü, T.F. and Kennedy, T.J.,Jr.: The renal mechanism for urate excretion in man. J.Clin.Invest.29:396, 1950.
9. Praetorius, E. and Kirk, J.E.: Hypouricemia:With evidence for tubular elimination of uric acid. J.Lab.Clin.Med. 35:856, 1950.
10. Gutman, A.B., Yü, T.F. and Berger, L.: Tubular secretion of urate in man. J.Clin.Invest. 38:1778, 1959.
11. Gutman, A.B. and Yü, T.F.: A three component system for the regulation of renal excretion of uric acid in man, Trans.Assoc.Am.Physicians 74:353, 1961.
12. Gutman, A.B.: Significance of the renal clearance of uric acid in normal and gouty man. Am.J.Med. 37:833, 1964.
13. Steele, T.H. and Rieselbach, R.E.: The renal mechamism for urate homeostasis in normal man. Am.J.Med. 43:868, 1967.
14. Moller, J.V.: The relation between secretion of urate and p-amino-hippurate in the rabbit kidney. J.Physiol. 192:505, 1967.
15. Boner, G. and Steele, T.H.: Relationship of urate and p-amino-hippurate secretion in man. Am.J.Physiol. 225:100, 1973.
16. Yü, T.F., Sirota, J.H., Berger, L., Halpern, M. and Gutman, A.B.: Effect of sodium lactate infusion on urate clearance in man. Proc.Soc.Exp. Biol.Med. 96:809, 1957.

17. Lieber, C.S., Jones, D.P., Losowsky, M.S. and Davidson, C.S.: Interrelation of uric acid and ethanol metabolism in man. J.Clin. Invest.41:1863, 1962.
18. Schulman, J.D., Lustberg, T.J., Kennedy, J.L., Museles, M.I. and Seegmiller, J.E.: A new variant of maple syrup urine disease (branch chain ketoaciduria). Am.J.Med. 49:118, 1970.
19. Jakovcic, S. and Sorenson, L.B.: Studies of uric acid metabolism in glycogen storage disease associated with gouty arthritis. Arthritis Rheum. 10:129, 1967.
20. Goldfinger, S., Klinenberg, J.R. and Seegmiller, J.E.: Renal retention of uric acid induced by infusion of beta-hydroxybutyrate and acetoacetate. N.Engl.J.Med. 272:351, 1965.
21. Orringer, E.P., Weiss, F.R. and Preuss, H.G.: Azotemic inhibition of organic anion transport in the kidney of the rat:mechanisms and characteristics. Clin.Sci. 40:159, 1971.
22. Diamond, H.S. and Paolino, J.S.: Evidence for a postsecretory reabsorptive site for uric acid in man. J.Clin.Invest. 52:1491, 1973.
23. Steele, T.H. and Boner, G.: Origins of the uricosuric response. J.Clin.Invest. 52:1368, 1973.
24. Rieselbach, R.E. and Steele, T.H.: Influence of the kidney upon urate homeostasis in health and disease. Am.J.Med. 56:665, 1974.
25. Wilson, D.M. and Goldstein, N.P.: Renal urate excretion in patients with Wilson's disease. Kidney Int. 4:331, 1973.
26. Bennett, J.S., Bond, J., Singer, I. and Gottlieb, A.J.: Hypouricemia in Hodgkin's disease. Ann.Intern.Med.76:751, 1972.
27. Stapleton, F.B., Nyhan, W.L., Borden, M. and Kaufman, I.A.: Renal pathogenesis of familial hyperuricemia:studies in two kindreds. Ped.Res., Oct., 1981 (In Press).
28. Kinsey, D., Walther, R., Sise, H.S., Whitlaw, G. and Smithwick, R.: Incidence of hyperuricemia in 400 hypertensive patients. Circulation 24:972, 1961.
29. Dollery, C.T., Duncan, H. and Schumer, B.: Hyperuricemia related to treatment of hypertension. Brit.Med.J. 2:832, 1960.
30. Breckinridge, A.: Hypertension and hyperuricemia. Lancet 1:15, 1966.
31. Cannon, P.J., Stason, W.B., DeMartini, F.E., Sommers, S.C. and Laragh, J.H.: Hyperuricemia in primary and renal hypertension. N.Engl.J.Med. 275:457, 1966.
32. Wyngaarden, J.B. and Kelley, W.N.: Gout, in the Metabolic Basis of Inherited Disease, New York, 1972, McGraw-Hill Book Company, p.931.
33. Fessel, J.W.; High uric acid as an indicator of cardiovascular disease. Am.J.Med. 68:401, 1980.
34. Fessel, J.W., Siegelaub, A.B. and Johnson, E.S.: Correlates and consequences of asymptomatic hyperuricemia. Arch.Int.Med.132:44, 1973.
35. Emmerson, B.T.: Gout, uric acid and renal disease. Med.J.Aust.1:403,1976.
36. Wexler, B.C. and Greenberg, B.P.: Effect of increased serum urate levels on virgin rats with no arteriosclerosis versus breeder rats with preexistant arteriosclerosis. Metabolism 26:1309, 1977.
37. Prebis, J.W., Gruskin, A.B., Polinsky, M.S. and Baluarte, H.J.: Uric acid in childhood essential hypertension. J.Pediatr.98:702, 1981.
38. Stapleton, F.B., Linshaw, M.A., Hassanein, K. and Gruskin, A.B.: Uric acid excretion in normal children. J.Pediatr. 92:911, 1978.
39. Spitzer, A. and Windhager, E.: Effect of peritubular oncotic pressure changes on proximal tubular fluid reabsorption. Am.J.Physiol.218: 1188, 1970.

40. Slatopolsky, E., Hoffsten, P., Purkerson, M. and Bricker, N.S.: On the influence of extracellular fluid volume and of uremia on bicarbonate reabsorption in man. J.Clin.Invest. 49:988, 1970.
41. Suki, W.N., Martinez-Maldonado, M., Rouse, D. and Terry, A.: Effect of expansion of extracellular fluid volume on renal phosphate handling. J.Clin.Invest. 48:1888, 1969.
42. Robson, A.M., Srivastava, P.L. and Bricker, N.S.: The influence of saline loading on renal glucose reabsorption in the rat. J.Clin.Invest. 47:329, 1968.
43. Steele, T.H.: Evidence of altered renal urate reabsorption during changes in volume of the extracellular fluid. J.Lab.Clin.Med. 74:288, 1969.
44. Weinman, E.J., Eknoyan, G. and Suki, W.N.: The influence of extracellular fluid volume on the tubular reabsorption of uric acid. J.Clin.Invest. 55:283, 1975.
45. Steele, T.H. and Oppenheimer, S.: Factors affecting urate excretion following diuretic administration in man. Am.J.Med.47:564, 1969.
46. Seely, J.F. and Dirks, J.H.: Site of action of diuretic drugs. Kidney Int. 11:1, 1977.
47. Chennavasin, P., Seiwell, R., Brater, D.C. and Liang, W.M.: Pharmacodynamic analysis of the furosemide-probenecid interaction in man. Kidney Int. 16:187, 1979.
48. Deetjen, P.: Micropuncture studies on site and mode of diuretic action of furosemide. Ann.N.Y. Acad.Sci.139:408, 1966.
49. Hirsch, G.H., Pakuts, A.P. and Bayne, A.J.: Furosemide accumulation by renal tissue. Biochem.Pharmac.24:1943, 1975.
50. Bowman, R.H.: Renal secretion of furosemide and its depression by albumin binding. Am.J.Physiol.229(1):93, 1975.
51. Prebis, J.W.: Uric acid regulation in hypertensive children. Proc.Fifth Int.Ped.Neph.Symp. (In Press).
52. Goldring, W. and Chasis, H.: Hypertension and hypertensive disease. New York, 1944, Commonwealth Fund.

DISCUSSION

José Strauss, M.D., Moderator

MODERATOR: We shall now entertain questions or comments.

QUESTION: I have a couple of naive questions. Could someone comment on the significance of extremely high renin levels in the neonatal period--what that might mean. My second question is, what might be the significance of high renin in an end-stage renal disease patient despite volume expansion. The third, if the study on adults with hyperuricemia and hypertension was regressional analysis applied to the data of hyperuricemia as a marker for hypertension, was it isolated for it?

RESPONSE: First, about the regression analysis. Somebody has very elegantly looked at the business of uric acid in terms of age, obesity, ponderal index, multifactorial analysis of variance, etc. All those statistics that none of us understands very well--especially myself--despite the fact that there are all the things except the uric acid component, and reading his articles, they are rather convincing. So, I think he has done it. Question number two: the high renin levels in patients with end-stage renal disease. My view is that there are certainly a number of patients on dialysis who, despite the fact that you dialyze them adequately, remain hypertensive. Other patients who, when you volume deplete them at the end of dialysis, despite the fact that you may even give them drugs, their blood pressures go up. There are some renin measurements to suggest that even with a small shrunken kidney, renin levels may hyper-respond with volume contraction. Some people suggest that if you have patients with end-stage renal disease with high renins whom you cannot adequately control with antihypertensive therapy, that this is the group of patients that you ought to seriously consider for a nephrectomy.

COMMENT: I am going to present some data later on on the prevalence of this condition. There are a number of studies in adult dialysis patients, end-stage renal disease patients, and our own study in children. In most series the incidence of hyper-reninemia runs about 5-15%. I have always considered, perhaps naively, that these are patients who, because of their intrarenal pathology, perhaps have arteriolar narrowing and so have a primary hyper-reninemic state due to the pathology. Most of them are patients with glomerulonephritis. So yes, these patients have renin-dependent hypertension although they also may have volume dependent hypertension even though they have a primary outpouring of renin. Because of this intrarenal pathology, when they retain fluid between dialysés and become overloaded, they also have a volume component to their hypertension, too. These patients do respond to bilateral nephrectomy and they respond to renin suppressing drugs to treat their hypertension. But it is a small percent--5 to 15%--and I think they have intrarenal pathology which explains the high renin levels and so they don't have a normal renin-volume response mechanism, as was shown on the board with his teeter-toter effect. It's lacking because of some intrarenal pathology.

COMMENT: The other thing, of course, that people talk about is the lack of vasodepressors because of a shrunken kidney mass. Nobody knows what role this may play. Another comment, you hear people talk about it but I don't think we give it its due. It is, the patient with chronic renal disease is almost invariably volume expanded, even after most dialyses. The fact that they have "renin levels" in the normal range tends to support this conclusion. The whole concept of inappropriate relationships between renin and volume, some people think this is very important in the end stage renal disease. Other people think it is less important. But, we have really two types of excessive renin activity. Numbers that are super-high by anybodys criteria, and then the so-called whole concept of inappropriately high for whatever (volume balance, and so on). Probably both are operative to some degree.

COMMENT: We have some patients with renal hypoplasia who are at the end-stage. They went on dialysis with moderate hypertension. After being volume depleted, they became more hypertensive. This probably can be explained also because they are renin dependent and maybe the volume expansion masks the situation. Then, they pass from a volume dependent hypertension to a renin dependent hypertension after dialysis. Those cases are the ones who are subjected to nephrectomy in order to be able to go on dialysis.

COMMENT: With the application of continous ambulatory peritoneal dialysis (CAPD) which is so good for the control and balance of the dialyzed patient that usually got into complications with hemodialysis, I wanted to know if in the data presented, the renin levels of patients who are on CAPD were compared to those of patients who are hemodialyzed and continuously have a high renin state.

COMMENT: No. We haven't really done that but I would respond that almost all patients on any form of dialysis are volume expanded because they can't put out the urine, and gain weight between dialyses. Almost every patient on any kind of dialysis tends to have volume dependent hypertension. Again, a small percentage of those patients may also have renin dependent hypertension because I think there is some form of intrarenal pathology that causes it. But, they are almost all volume dependent and CAPD just happens to be a better technique for controlling volume than hemodialysis - at least in my hands and I think in other people's also. So, we find that children on CAPD are easier to control with their blood pressure because we can take off more volume but I have not looked at what percentage of high renin hypertension there is among that group.

COMMENT: The adult data on CAPD would suggest that blood pressure control over the long haul is probably best on CAPD versus intermittent peritoneal dialysis (IPD) versus hemodialysis. That may be due to, among other reasons, the volume business. Another possibility is that the peritoneal membrane is probably a more effective membrane for removing larger molecular weight compounds and whatever that might mean in terms of hypertension, the patient on CAPD would have more of that removed.

COMMENT: We studied 13 patients in our dialysis unit with end-stage renal disease and on hemodialysis. We looked at renin levels two hours post-dialysis and correlated this with blood pressure, volume depletion and also catecholamines level. We are doing some further studies but did not find a correlation between renin levels and hypertension. However, there was a correlation between volume depletion and hypertension.

QUESTION: What about catecholamines?

RESPONSE: We are still pending on that.

COMMENT: Later on I'll present material on that. We do have a correlation between hydrogen levels and hypertension. It's not like correlation coefficients; it's like grouping data. Patients with high renins have higher blood pressures than ones with normal renins.

MODERATOR: The question about nephrectomies was raised. At one point a few years ago we were nephrectomizing patients who had uncontrollable hypertension. Lately, we feel that we can manage them with such potent drugs that nephrectomy has not been necessary. We even submitted a paper about a patient who had been nephrectomized and one of the reviewers thought that that was criminal. Since some of the panel will not be here for the Session on Treatment, maybe we can touch on that subject now. Do we have a position, a recommendation, or are we still in the same situation in which we used to be?

RESPONSE: Yes. With the more potent anti-hypertensive drugs, the situation has changed. The only one I have had experience with is Minoxidil; we have not had Captopril available to us in our center. With Minoxidil we have been able to do away with nephrectomies in the vast majority of these patients with high renin hypertension.

COMMENT: I would agree that most patients no longer need nephrectomies. I would simply say that last week a parent made us remove a transplanted kidney which wasn't doing very well, had been on a lot of steroids and had some of the side effects of Minoxidil with hair all over the face and over the body. Granted it was a peculiar situation. But for a combination of reasons they made us take out this child's kidney. Her creatinine was only 3 mg/dl. She had been in another hospital with seizures, coma, etc. So, there's that aspect, although by no means should it be the most important aspect. Another problem you run into is that after transplant with multiple drugs you do see some patients who despite the fact that they are on two, three, four or five drugs including small doses of Minoxidil, remain hypertensive and you get caught. Is it the new kidney? Is it the old kidney? In an immuno-suppressed patient, trying to get renins out of the renal veins of three kidneys is not the easiest or best thing to do. Again, most of the time, it is not necessary and I think the incidence is sufficiently small that it does not justify doing nephrectomies. An interesting question which arises is the impending release of Captopril which is supposed to be out in the market. It is one of the renin inhibitors (of the converting enzyme). Is that going to solve a lot of problems?

It will at least remove the renin component from all types of hypertension. I am sure the company hopes so but that remains to be seen.

MODERATOR: Related to transplantation, we are still nephrectomies but prophylactically, if you want, by protocol. All patients receiving a live related kidney get bilateral nephrectomies and splenectomy. That's the protocol here in Miami. The results are really super, among the best in the world. Are there any reactions to that approach? Not yet. I also wanted to comment on the patient just mentioned who was on Minoxidil and had all the hair problem. I am told that the patient is a boy. In boys you could have sold to the parents the idea that he would be very successful with girls with all that hair and hypermale appearance. So, maybe they could put up with the problem. Really it's terrible that the kidney had to be taken out. I don't know whether that falls within the extremes of child abuse. I would think that it may have been a consideration to forbid the parents to get that kidney removed. The question of what is the right of the family versus what is right for the child always comes up.

COMMENT: This particular child has been in the intensive care unit with hypertensive encephalopathy twice, has been on a sodium nitroprusside drip for thirty days and obviously it's a very unusual story but it's worth commenting. There was a great deal of discussion about that very subject among the nephrologists and staff. Most people who have seen the child, knew the family, and were involved, agreed. We had a biopsy which showed that a good part of the kidney was on its way to chronic rejection and when we added it all up, we supported the family's position, given this particular set of circumstances. Are you doing bilateral nephrectomies in your live related transplants?

RESPONSE: No. Nor splenectomies.

COMMENT: We are in the middle. We don't do splenectomies but we have tended--although we don't do that many live related transplants--to do a bilateral nephrectomy in live related transplants.

QUESTION: Why is it done only in live related transplants?

MODERATOR: That has been a subject of discussion, arguments, so on. We thought that we wouldn't go along with the splenectomies. We thought that bilateral nephrectomy in a live related donor made sense because those kidneys were not going to perform any function; we were taking an organ from a healthy subject, and the risks involved seemed to be greater with the recipient's kidneys left in place. Therefore, one might want to increase the chances that there would not be complications like intractable hypertension. The cadaver kidneys, though valuable, may not justify the drastic preparation of the recipient. Still, when possible, even the cadaver kidney recipients have bilateral nephrectomy but it is not as strict a requirement as for the live related recipient. When specifically indicated, the recipient's own kidneys are taken out regardless of type of kidney donor. The splenectomy is a subject that keeps being discussed and argued. All recipients, regardless of type of kidney donor are subjected to a splenectomy. Recently, there was a speaker here from a major transplant center. He gave the group here the highest rating, stating that the results in Miami are the best in the world. The only difference he could really see was the splenectomy. I wonder whether the panel, with all the reports and statistics that they provide, read and compile, can tell us whether there is any pattern to this - whether groups that do bilateral nephrectomy and/or splenectomy do seem to have any better results than the other groups.

RESPONSE: I think that's the line of choice of the institution. If you have good data, for how long? Everybody has good results the first year. The important thing is to follow through and see how well they are going to do. What was the age at the time of splenectomy? That would also make a difference. But at this stage of the game, personally, I feel better with removing the kidneys, but not as good with removing the spleen. That's personally. If your statistics are good and they remain good, then you are doing the right thing. In the majority of the cases, in most of the data I find, people do not remove the spleen and their data can be also superb; there was also a time when those people were not removing the kidneys either. Let it be because of shock absorber effect of the transplanted kidney or be just for the erythropoetin that is left for the anemia of the children. That's a matter of an institution.

QUESTION: One of the problems in renin profiling adults is their lack of consistency. A patient might have a high renin, then the test is repeated several weeks, months later and it might be normal or low. Did you have the chance of repeating them in children?

RESPONSE: No, but that's a very valid question. How persistent is a specific abnormality in renin profile? There's actually a paucity of data in adults as to how reproducible renin profiling is over time. I'm aware only of a couple of papers. I just forget the numbers. I think somewhere between a quarter and a third maybe even 35-40% change renin profile when people go back and do it again. So, there is a fair number who do change. Again, the question arises in an adult who is aging, along with all the rest of us; is a child a better model to look at? I don't know. That's one of the things we propose to do. It's a very important question. The other corollary question is that as I pointed out, it appears as though our hyper-reninemic patients also have high uric acids. We, for example, have not yet looked at the serum creatinine systematically to see if there are some differences. Do all the markers change? When you measure them all together, do only some of them? For example, in the adult data where the renin status changes, does the EKG change? The echocardiogram? Does the uric acid change? Lipids change? It's hard to sort it all out but the renin profile does change.

MODERATOR: Along those lines, I was thinking about the daily variations that you were mentioning in the plasma renin activity and how little sense it makes, in a way, to attempt to correlate with a 24-hr urinary sodium excretion. Wouldn't it be better to attempt sodium excretion-creatinine clearance concomitant with the draining of the blood for plasma-renin. Could half an hour, one hour collection after water ingestion be not preferable because you are correlating the urinary excretion with plasma renin which may be fluctuating along the points you were talking about.

RESPONSE: The question is, first of all, is a 24-hr urine a valid indicator? That changes from day to day. Some people feel you ought to get three measurements of 24-hr urines, that the average is a better indicator. When you get down to the practicality of doing things, and in general, sodium excretion overall reflects volume status, but by no means in a perfect manner. It's a scheme that people have worked out that seems to have a practical use. There are some data, looking at the first morning urine and does that reflect the day's urine? Shorter urine collections? It doesn't seem to blend together quite as well. The other thing,about the time of the day you get your renin. I think the reason people tend to use the four hour upright renins, you've been walking around for a while and you stimulate your renin system and you've tended to move it into a range where you can measure it better. Some of the problems with drawing renins supine first thing in the morning is that they are much lower. Then the ability to separate out values becomes much harder. There's another scheme that people are using that we hope to begin to look at as a way of looking more to high renins. It's the concept of acute volume expansion and what is the renin response. Of course, one of the reasons we are looking at the Lasix stimulation test is we're going in the other direction and that's acute volume depletion. What is the relative degree of renin increase? At least in our adolescent population, it is very difficult if not impossible to recognize a low renin without some form of stimulation. The high renins are fairly easy to recognize in terms of a 24-hr excretion. It gets down to defining normal, setting arbitrary criteria, setting nomograms, and then applying them, and using them. There may be much better methods. For example, the whole business of throwing all of this out and just giving renin inhibitors and seeing what happens. That may tell you as much as all the rest of this. The state of the art now, in Pediatrics at least, in terms of what is renin profiling all about is a decade behind the state of the art in adults. What we're trying to do is get some handle on it as to what it means, what its relative value is.

COMMENT: First of all, I'd like to ask you a question and be a little bit critical. I was a little surprised on your data relating renin to age. Actually, when you put all the data together and do a correlation coefficient, although it is statistically significant, it is not a very good correlation coefficient. In fact, it was .219. If you do what was mentioned earlier as appropriate and you square that, you come out with the effect of age on renin as contributing only 5%; .22 comes out to be .05. You only have an effect of age on renin of 5%.

RESPONSE: If you look at that same sort of thing, with a better renin method, it comes better. The particular method we were using at that time was a method that gave low values, and started off with a low value to begin with and you got lower. For example, a two or three year old;data I showed was 2-3 ng/ml/hr while our current adolescent values are 4 ng/ml/hr plus or minus a standard deviation of 2; so, you have a much bigger range. If you use that method. Although we haven't done it, other people have. And you go back to age related correlation; the slope is steeper. So, I think that part of this may have been the particular method we were using at the time. A number of people looked at the age related changes and it starts at birth and diminishes evidently until 80 or 90 years of age. Nobody yet has a very good explanation as to why it changes. I think one of the problems of adult studies is that people are mixing up 20 year olds and 50 year olds and 70 year olds, although now they are going back and attempting to separate them out by age.

COMMENT: I think your work looking at children--I guess these were mostly essential hypertension--is intriguing and most valuable. Could I ask, how much of a work-up did these children have to say they were essential hypertensives rather than secondary hypertensives?

RESPONSE: All our children, because they are in a protocol, have had at least renal scans done, looking for differences in each side. They have had Addis Counts done, a whole school of chemistries, including some renal chemistries. They had ultrasound studies, EKG's, eye exams, etc.

QUESTION: How about arteriography?

RESPONSE: No, they have not had arteriographies. We talked about going back. Some of our high renin essential hypertensives have mild hypertension, don't have a change on renal scan, and the question arises, should we go back and do a renal arteriogram? We have been a little edgy in the child who is an adolescent with a blood pressure of 145 to 150 mm Hg over 94 to 98 mm Hg, to submit him to an arteriogram, based on the current state of the art. Although maybe we should. I would hope you would agree.

RESPONSE: I would agree.

COMMENT: There are many pitfalls with renin profiling. One that has not been terribly emphasized in this Discussion is that the antihypertensive therapy that has been used has an effect on plasma renins as well. There are those drugs that stimulate renin much as the vasodialators and the diuretics, and those that suppress renin such as the beta blockers and other sympatholytic agents. So, that's another variable in the equation of numerous influences that come to bear on plasma renin activity - the state of antihypertensive treatment. Another comment or really a re-affirmation of what was presented before as an approach to the work-up of the individual with hypertension, I would like to reaffirm because it makes good sense for individuals who are in a primary care realm. That is, with a fairly limited work-up, I dare say you can cover probably 95% at least of the usual secondary causes of hypertension, using fairly simple measures. It is only for a very small minority of limited individuals that one has to get into more sophisticated, invasive diagnostic methods.

MODERATOR: Would you like to stop for a minute and take up that subject? Would someone like to?

RESPONSE: I really have nothing further to add except that I am in complete agreement. Just a physical, urinalysis and a simple chemical panel does it.

MODERATOR: Would you like to comment on the staging of a work-up? Sometimes I am called to consult on a problem and I find that a renal arteriogram has been done but there is no creatinine clearance. Sometimes maybe a urinalysis has not been done. We have to spend time then, going through the ABC's. Do you have any comment on that?

RESPONSE: To reiterate what we've already said, if you get an SMA 12 or 20 (different people have different SMA panels), this will give you your electrolytes, BUN, and creatinine - I'm not a great believer in creatinine clearances because even in the best of hospitals, there are collection errors and I don't think it adds too much to a serum creatinine. You do the simple tests of renal function, urinalysis and probably urine culture. Certainly you should not go along to the more sophisticated tests until you have done the simpler ones. The simpler ones will identify the secondary causes of hypertension-- probably 95% of the cases. So I agree wholeheartedly that a history and physical and simple evaluation of the renal system with urinalysis and a chemistry panel are what's needed.

MODERATOR: Also, in terms of the marked discrepancies among the different series, in the incidence or prevalence of renal hypertension, probably the panel has some thoughts about this also. Last year at this Seminar, we heard the incidence of renal hypertension in Paris, France; considering that it was from a referral center, it was as high as 30-40%. Then, we had the figures from London where practically renal hypertension seems to be non-existent. Do you think that the series are comparable, that there is enough systematization that we can say that it happens in different populations in different ways, or is it all up for grabs?

COMMENT: I think the explanation is simple. Maybe I am simplistic. If you look at asymptomatic children who have been found because of screening, who have mild hypertension, a lot of them are going to have essential hypertension. But, if you look at symptomatic patients referred to centers with high blood pressures, almost all of them are going to have a cause and the vast majority are going to be renal. I think it's a simple matter of severe hypertension versus mild hypertension. That's what I tried to portray. In the older studies looking at referrals with severe hypertension, they all found the cause was usually renal. Now, the screening studies of asymptomatic children who are picked up by routine taking of blood pressure, they usually have mild hypertension and there usually is not a cause found. I think we are just looking at two ends of the spectrum. At the low end of the spectrum, there is no cause; at the high end of the spectrum, there is a cause, usually renal.

COMMENT: We pretty much see all of the hypertension at our institution because of our interest in people with this problem. We also have an end-stage renal disease clinic. If you look back over our experience of the last six, eight, ten years, as we have gotten more interested in the general subject of hypertension, we have moved more and more away from secondary causes and are seeing progressively more and more children with primary or essential hypertension. The referring physicians are taking more blood pressures and Medical Clinics are taking more blood pressures. About a year ago, we crossed over in terms of our total population from more secondary forms with chronic renal disease to more primary forms. If you play the statistical game, that 1% of adolescent population and three readings spread out over time, will have fixed diastolic hypertension, then certainly that exceeds the reported incidence for the secondary forms. So that you've got to, almost by definition, if you are seeing any at all, see more primary hypertension. This has been what our experience is. I think it's a question of where, who refers, etc.

COMMENT: I think if people are aware that adolescents per se are having higher blood pressure than the usual population on first examination, then you will avoid a lot of people being labeled hypertensives because no one brings this into consideration. Most of the time, on the first physical examination, adolescents will have slight increases in diastolic blood pressure.

RESPONSE: I would agree. If anybody calls me and says, "I have someone in my office with high blood pressure, do you want to see him?", what we say is that, if it's mild numbers, take their blood pressure for the next three months. If it's still high, send them back, and most of them, you never hear from again. We've been involved with one tract study. It's a black adolescent urban ghetto population where again, the first go-around 10-12% had high readings. The second go-around, 4%, and the third, about 1½%. So, before one does much of anything, one ought to be sure that those numbers at least are remaining elevated, given the current state of the art.

COMMENT: We don't have this disease until we get set up and start looking for it; then, we start finding it. In some places there is more prevalence of secondary hypertension than in others. For instance, in my hospital, there are important cases of hypertension. Among thousands of cases with secondary hypertension I can remember only one or two with essential hypertension. But, if in the Outpatient Department the doctors start to take blood pressures more and more, I'm sure that they will have more cases of essential hypertension, as I can see in my private practice. They will refer to me more cases with essential hypertension. They are not very important cases of hypertension, that is why they don't go to the hospital first. I agree with what has been said. There are more differences among the secondary causes; they are due to different geographical prevalences. We have more renal arteriosclerosis, mainly caused by non-specific arteritis. For example, in Japan, Kawasaki has more of these cases than other countries. The hypertension secondary to acute glomerulonephritis is more important to us because we haven't been able to eradicate the streptococcus; it is a very important cause. We have discrepancies among the physicians diagnosing hypertension due to pyelonephritis. I don't think pyelonephritis per se has very much to do with hypertension except in end-stage renal disease. But in most of these cases, what causes the hypertension is something subjacent like hypoplastic kidney or some other alterations in the kidney but not the infection or obstruction.

COMMENT: Reference was made to the Muscatine study. I don't think from that data we are entitled to conclude that the incidence of essential hypertension is 26% or whatever. I think all they can say is that there has been a subset of a very small group of individuals in whom there is no apparent secondary cause of hypertension who have a borderline reading, and I think it's important to perhaps refrain from even using the term, labeling the child as having hypertension. I had occasion to ask one researcher recently the outcome of this particular subset of individuals, the ones who continued to have the 95% high readings or a bit above it, despite weight reduction and so forth. Not a single individual has required pharmacotherapy for elevated blood pressure. So, I don't know if we can yet even say that they are going to be essential hypertensives later as young adults. I think that that remains an open question. They obviously need fairly long term follow-up.

COMMENT: We were talking in my simultaneous workshop in this Seminar about the fact that we walk around and say "greater than 95% confidence limits, you are hypertensive. Ergo that is bad." What we were talking about is that blood pressure is probably a continuum. Let's look at some of the life insurance actuarial data; remember they bet on whether you live or die and they make money. If you start with a young adult with a blood pressure of approximately 110/70 mm Hg, for every increment of a few mm Hg from mass population, sloppily taken blood pressures, the higher your blood pressure goes from that number on, the shorter your life span. So, although we set arbitrary criteria, we are talking about what we see in the United States. We are not talking about people in the deserts of Brasil who have a much lower blood pressure, etc. Maybe we ought to think much more in terms of a continuum. One of the things we have battered around is, is there such a thing as relative hypertension? What does it mean if someone goes from the 20th percentile to the 90th percentile? Does this mean anything epidemiologically? Disease wise? We saw an adolescent who was in the 20th percentile. We had one high reading of his sport's physical exam. But then the rest of his readings were sort of about the 95th confidence limits; his family physician used dipsticks in the urine and found some protein. We did an IVP and found an unusual looking right kidney. We worked this child up and concluded that he had had trauma as a football player and had a hematoma compressing the kidney. He had the kidney removed and his blood pressure fell from approximately the upper limits all the way back down. Was that child hypertensive? Does it mean anything? We don't know. It's another valid consideration in terms of tracking of individual patients. Probably other people have similar kinds of stories.

COMMENT: Another thing that we are forgetting is that we have quite an obvious number of adolescents who are taking contraceptives without the knowledge of parents or primary physicians. We tend to find two things that are really worrisome when we see them in practice. Sometimes they have high blood pressure and they have a positive antinuclear factor. Immediately there is a cause to call a nephrologist. The first thing I ask them is, have you been taking birth control pills? Sometimes I have to leave the room because I am afraid the lightning is going to strike me, they lie so blatantly. Once they give in to your confidence, they tell you that they have been taking them. They went to the free clinic and they were given these things and most of the time they have high prednisone content and they go into these peaks of hypertension for a short time while they are taking the pills. We have removed the birth control pills for four months, repeated the studies for blood pressure, and the blood pressure has dropped and so has the ANA. It has disappeared. I find this in some of my female patients - hypertension because someone forgot to gain their confidence so they would tell that they did take birth control pills. That is now one of the biggest things that I find-- an increased blood pressure from the pills.

MODERATOR: Regarding the tracking that was touched upon, the recommendations of the task force on hypertension for NIH are that once you feel satisfied that the patient is hypertensive, that you start with the thiazide directly. The question was related to the administration of the thiazide diuretic, to see if the tracking changes, if indeed there is a tracking. The question that I have pertains to treatment; if one is giving a diuretic to stimulate the production of renin, does it make sense to give a diuretic to modify slight hypertension? Under what circumstances (if ever) do you think that renin overproduction is actually induced by the diuretic?

RESPONSE: I think it's an open question. The adult data with the use of thiazides are mixed. Obviously, in some patients the renin goes up. What we haven't mentioned is that there are some studies in adults that with thiazides, lipids go up. There are other studies in which lipids do not go up. When you take this data back into childhood years, if some of these responses (the renin response, the elevated uric acid, etc.) with thiazide, really are physiologic volume responses, then theoretically you should be OK. But, the question arises, if you cramp something up in a human body that is a physiological response and you leave it that way for five or six or ten years, does it then perpetuate itself? Again, we have no way of knowing. I think from a physiologic perspective, if you can identify some kind of a marker, it would perhaps make more physiologic sense to try and provide a specific drug that would inhibit that response. What do I mean by that? If you have high renin hypertension, although lowering volume would lower blood pressure, would you be better off giving a renin inhibitor? If you have low renin hypertension (where people think you have an excess volume and maybe some sort of adrenal hormone) would you be better off giving a volume depleter? Then, what happens five, ten, fifteen years later? On the other hand, when you get into the therapy business, all of these drugs have responses associated with them which tend to correct themselves. Again, looking at some of the thiazide data, some people will tell you six, 12, 20 months later, the volume is back to normal. If the patient's blood volume is back to normal and he still has a high renin, a high uric acid, and a high lipid - again, what does this mean? I don't know; but, when you talk about treating children and dealing with the whole hypertension problem in terms of prevention, I think we should go very carefully and see what happens in selected populations before we make any sweeping recommendations.

MODERATOR: The subject of treatment is going to be discussed more thoroughly later in the Seminar. As you see, it is a juicy subject. Would anyone like to comment further now?

RESPONSE: I agree with what has been said. The thought of the use of thiazide diuretics in mild hypertension is one of the examples of just empiric, non-specific therapy. As was pointed out, you may give a thiazide diuretic to a patient who has high renin. In fact, some of my internist colleagues who have patients with renal artery stenosis and mild hypertension, they may still use a thiazide diuretic as their first line of treatment. It's completely nonspecific therapy. We like to use specific therapy where we can. But, nevertheless, with the thiazide diuretics there's the first line where you really just fall back on empiricism. They've been used for a number of years now and they are effective. The side effects, in general and at least over the short term, are not devastating. It's effective treatment when given for a mild hypertension and a relatively harmless drug at least over the short term.

COMMENT: For whatever value, we got involved in systematically comparing a new diuretic agent (which has uricosuric properties) with thiazides in terms of their effect on uric acid, one of our areas of interest. When the new diuretic agent became released for general large scale use, although all the initial studies were very good, it ran into a number of toxic side effects resulting in removal of the drug from circulation. I think when you translate that down to children, if you are talking about treating somebody six months or a year, it's probably not going to make any real difference. But, if you are thinking about 20, 30, 40 years of therapy, a good drug that's worth anything can have a lot of side effects. The more you use it, the more you find out about it. Until we know what childhood hypertension is, we should do like the older pediatricians who have always been conservative in recommending therapy. It usually has turned out right by doing no harm.

QUESTION: Have you seen hyperglycemia in any of your patients on hemodialysis who have been using propranolol?

RESPONSE: No, but we don't look for it.

COMMENT: I'm aware of a child elsewhere who was on peritoneal dialysis who got some Inderal and developed hyperglycemia.

COMMENT: I have not seen any children but I have reviewed the data in the adult dialysis unit. There were four cases that coming off dialysis had cardiac standstill, were taken to the emergency room and the only finding was a glucose of less than 50 mg/dl. Two of the patients were black. We could not trace any enzymatic defect that could explain that problem. It was worrisome that such a thing would occur within a six month period. The only thing we could trace back was the propranolol dosage. There was no clear relationship between dosage and effect because the dose was between 40 and 120 mg.

COMMENT: Pertaining to small kidneys, we have information that we presented to the American Academy of Pediatrics meeting. We got interested in looking at small kidneys for a variety of reasons, not only the ones that are bilateral and go on to end-stage disease. This may not seem to relate very generally to the theme of this session but I think there's a relevance for people in practice. What I'm really talking about is the diagnosis of pyelonephritis in women as the cause of end-stage renal failure where it has been bilateral or where there has been a unilateral small kidney and hypertension. That's a common association. Sometimes it's associated with renal artery lesion but not always. Oftentimes these are ascribed to hypoplastic developmentally small kidneys but that's difficult to prove. We were interested in this and went back and looked at our museum collection of small kidneys. These were children who had either unilateral or bilateral small kidneys, maybe presenting with hypertension, and who went on to renal failure treatment. Where we could document a voiding cystogram was done, we had a very high rate of discovery of reflux. Now, this has been reported in the past from San Francisco as well as other places. I dare say that the vast majority if not all cases of so-called pyelonephritis have as their antecedent in women and in infant girls, reflux. This may not be apparent. One has to ask a very complete history in terms of, "Did your child have unexplained febrile illnesses as an infant?", because in many cases you don't get a clear history of urinary tract infection. In any case, I think what we are seeing far down the road is this ordinarily benign disease, urinary tract infection, but not benign in the setting of reflux. For that reason, as has been emphasized before, the occurrence of urinary tract infection should be an indication to delve further; further investigation to establish whether or not reflux is present. If there is a role for prevention, it is to discover these cases very early because reflux nephropathy, which is a name now for pyelonephritis associated with reflux, appears to occur early in life. Once the damage is done, by age five, six, or seven, there isn't too much we can do to prevent further progression to occur. This kind of discovery has to be made very early in life, if not in infancy. Then, if we do find reflux and employ the surgery that seems appropriate or chemoprophylaxis, then we should prevent hypertension later in life due to the small kidney or end-stage renal failure.

COMMENT: It's worth pointing out that there are some families that have been recorded where there is a genetic incidence of reflux nephropathy. So that, if one has a history of a mother with this, it is something that should be considered after the child is born. We have seen a couple of families with members who have reflux nephropathy.

MODERATOR: We probably need to summarize some points of agreement in particular with reference to the previous comments. We could say that the urinary tract infection should be taken as an excuse to evaluate patients. I think we all agree that we should do a work-up --an intravenous pyelogram or renal scan and a voiding cystourethrogram by iodinated contrast material or by radionucleide, with the first infection. At the same time, I think we need to be careful in concluding that we need to operate on those refluxes. The answers are not there yet. We have a proposal from one of the panel members to do a Latin American evaluation of this problem. There is a European study going on now, and probably we will find out what is the role of reflux in clinical settings as opposed to the experimental setting of others. In general, it is very important to identify those patients. What one should do with them is not clear. Sometimes they do well just with observation and that is what we need to know. Also, those patients who seem to benefit from antibiotic or antimicrobial treatment, what role are we, indeed, playing?

Now, for those who would like to stay a little longer and informally share information about grant applications, we shall spend some time with this subject. Thank you. (See Appendix for grant information).

IV

TREATMENT MODALITIES

SYNDROME OF INAPPROPRIATE SECRETION OF ANTIDIURETIC HORMONE

Michael Freundlich, M.D. and José Strauss, M.D.

Antidiuretic hormone (ADH) plays a prominent role in the control of volume and osmotic homeostasis. ADH, or arginine vasopressin, is secreted in the hypothalamus, travels down the hypothalamic-hypophysial tract coupled to a protein called neurophysin, and is stored in the posterior aspect of the hypophysis. From there, it eventually is liberated in the blood stream. The changes occurring in osmolality or volume are sensed by intracranial osmoreceptors and pressure or volume receptors located at the carotid and aortic sinuses, and left atrium, respectively. Once vasopressin enters the circulation, it follows a course to its specific receptor site on the contraluminal (blood) side of the collecting duct cells of the kidney where it initiates a chain of intracellular events through activation of cyclic AMP. This reaction brings about a striking increase in the luminal-cell membrane permeability to water, urea, sodium and other solutes (1). These biochemical events may be inhibited or enhanced by a host of circumstances and might lead to derangements in body fluids.

Essentially ADH is closely integrated with the thirst stimulatory mechanism. Under normal circumstances, fluid osmolality is kept in a very narrow range despite large variations in the amount of water and solute intake. Figure 1 depicts the activation of the mechanism involved in ADH secretion as two parallel loops, as well as the role played by the kidney.

The major factors that regulate ADH release are osmotic pressure of plasma and volume of circulating blood. Although many studies have been addressed to the issue of dominant influence of either osmolar or volume factors on the rate of ADH secretion, it is currently believed that both factors mutually interact without "dominance" of one over the other (2). A two or three percent increase in plasma osmolality results in a three to fivefold increase in plasma ADH and an eventual 500 to 600 percent increase in urine osmolality (3,4). A similar increase in plasma ADH has been reported with a decrease of 8-10% in blood volume (5). An excessive secretion or release of ADH, inappropriate for the serum total osmolality or the volume of circulating blood has been described as the Syndrome of Inappropriate Antidiuretic Hormone (SIADH) (6).

An increasing awareness of the existence of clinical situations associated with ADH excess, has made possible their diagnosis and appropriate management. The course of such a patient with several typical features of SIADH is graphically presented in Figure 2 and herein described.

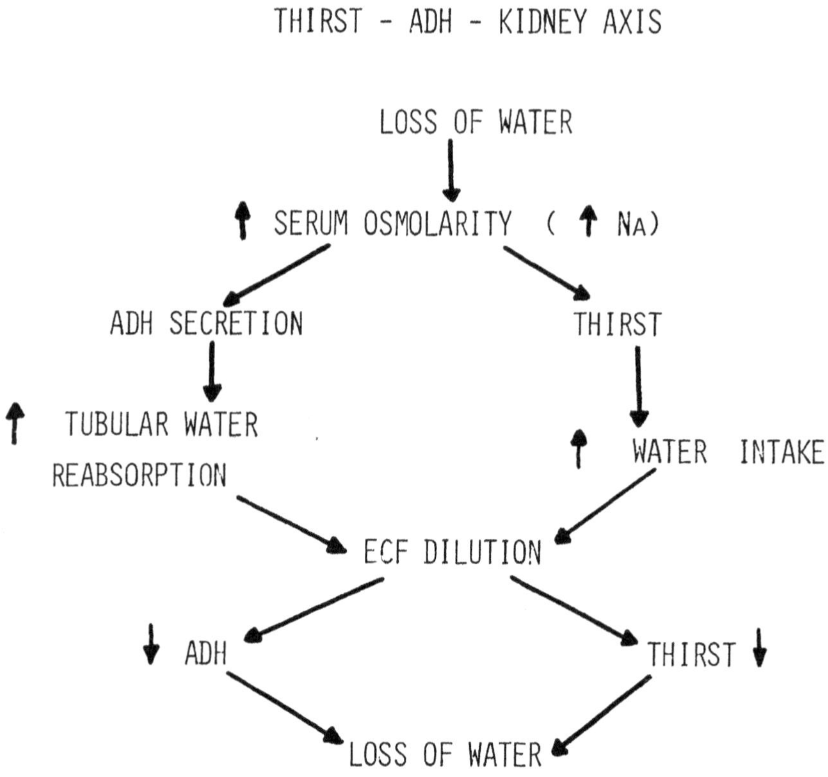

FIGURE 1. Interrelationships of thirst, ADH secretion and kidney response.

Case Presentation

A seven-year-old boy presented with coma and left hemiparesis. He had been treated with corticosteroids and multiple blood components for four months because of a bone marrow aplasia. His initial examination revealed a BP of 130/90 mm Hg, diffuse petechial and ecchymotic lesions, and a semicomatose state with left hemiparesis. A brain CT scan showed a hemorrhagic area in the right cerebral area. Pertinent laboratory data: BUN 20 mg/dl, creatinine 0.8 mg/dl, serum Na 124 mEq/L, K 3.7 mEq/L, and Cl 98 mEq/L. CVP was 6 cm H_2O. During the initial

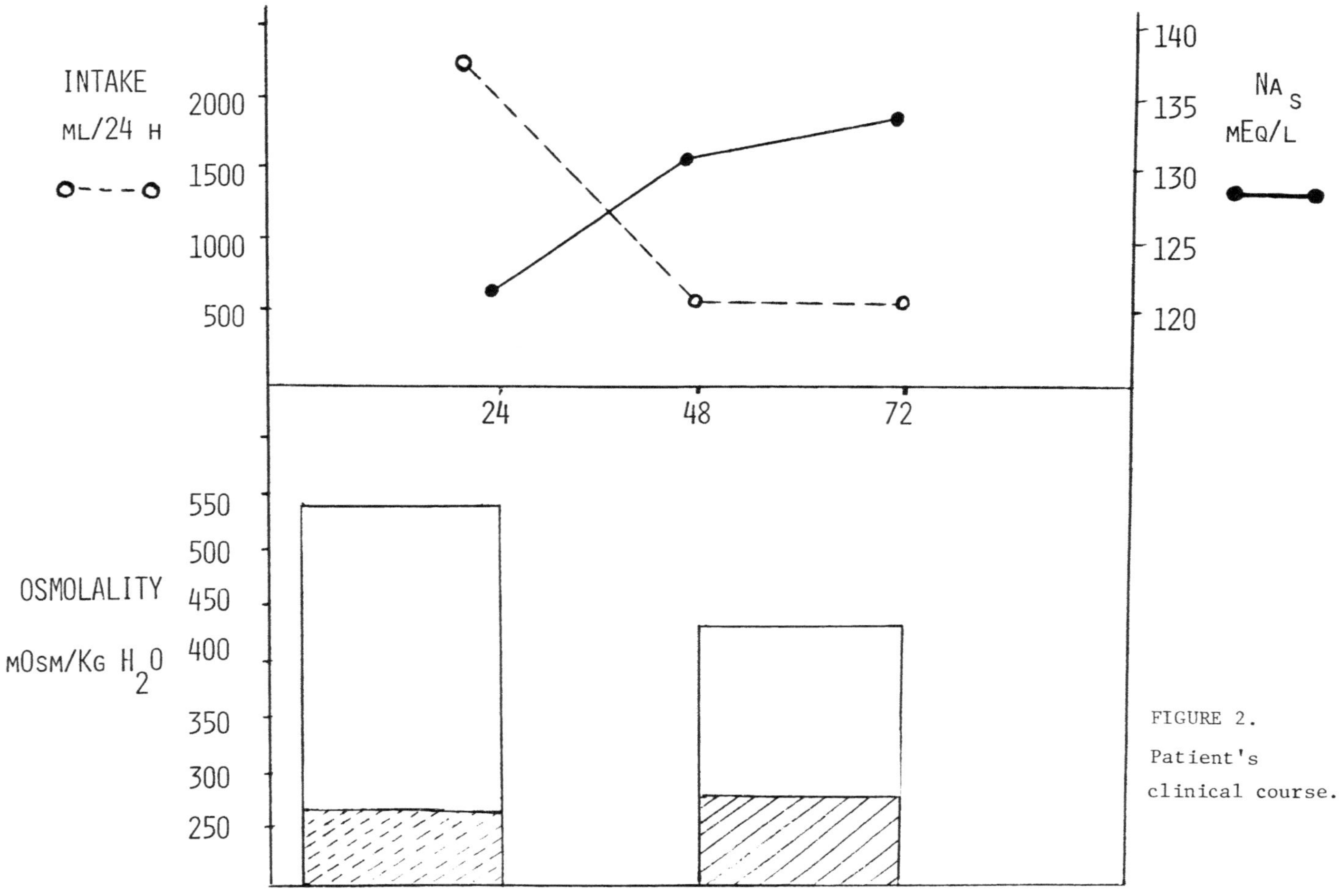

FIGURE 2. Patient's clinical course.

24 hours he was given 2060 ml fluids and 240 mEq sodium. The following day the serum sodium was 124 mEq/L and the osmolality 262 mOsm/kg. Urinary sodium was 118 mEq/L and total osmolality 537 in mOsm/kg with a total urine volume of 2140 ml in the preceding 24 hours. At this point, the amount of fluids administered was restricted to 500 ml/day and no sodium was added. By the third day, the serum sodium concentration had risen to 132 mEq/L and the patient started to become alert.

Comment

As noted, the patient presented with hyponatremia, and without evidence of hypovolemia as reflected by a normal CVP reading. Despite the hyponatremia, the total daily urinary sodium excretion (247 mEq) was essentially identical to the amount of sodium administered (240 mEq). These findings coupled to the presence of serum hypotonicity with a urine that is not maximally dilute and a urine osmolality that is not less than that of the serum, establishes the diagnosis of inappropriately excessive ADH secretion.

The cardinal features of SIADH are depicted below in Table 1. The series of events leading to the hypotonicity as well as to the compensatory mechanisms remain somewhat speculative. The degree of hyponatremia and the hyposmolality cannot be quantitatively accounted for by the increase in body water and loss of urinary sodium. The discrepancies in osmolality could be explained if in addition to sodium, other body cations were lost during the development of hyposmolality and regained during its correction; however, balance studies have failed to confirm this possibility (6,7). Bartter and Schwartz (7) have postulated that "inactivation of cell solutes" occurs within the cell and prevents the movement of water into the cells; the mechanism of this "inactivation" remains unexplained. The persistent natriuresis despite hyponatremia is presumably related to the expansion of the extracellular fluid and the resultant decrease in sodium reabsorption (increased fractional sodium excretion) by the renal proximal tubule due to the influence of a so-called "third-factor" (glomerular filtration rate and aldosterone are referred to as first and second factor, respectively). A series of experiments pioneered by de Wardener et al, paved the way for the search for a humoral factor with natriuretic properties. Recent studies by Bourgoignie et al. of uremic patients and animals (8,9) have characterized a substance capable of producing an increase of 10-15% in the fractional excretion of sodium. This substance may play a role in the persistent natriuresis and in the prevention of further total body water expansion. The lack of edema usually noticed in patients with SIADH could thus be explained.

TABLE 1. Clinical Features of SIADH

Hyponatremia with serum hyposmolality
Inappropriately elevated urine osmolality
Persistent natriuresis
No evidence of volume depletion
Normal renal-adrenal-thyroid functions
Lack of diuretic administration
Hypouricemia (?)

A more recent observation has been the finding of serum uric acid equal to or less than 4 mg/dl in 16 of 17 patients with SIADH. The hypouricemia was clearly related to the volume expansion state and the serum uric acid concentration rose after a period of water restriction (10). The establishment of hypouricemia as a frequent finding in pediatric patients with SIADH warrants further studies.

A variety of clinical circumstances has been noticed to be associated with SIADH at all ages (Table 2); however, in pediatrics the most frequent are meningitis, pneumonia, surgery, head trauma, assisted ventilation, neonatal hypoxia, and hemorrhage. Several drugs, some used frequently, have potential effects on the secretion rate and action of ADH (Table 3).

The clinical manifestations of the syndrome depend upon the underlying disease and reflect the degree of hyponatremia or hypotonicity. Symptoms include: lethargy, apathy, disorientation, muscle cramps, anorexia, nausea, agitation. Signs include: abnormal sensorium, hyporeflexia, Cheyne-Stokes respiration, hypothermia, Babinsky reflexes, pseudobulbar palsy, seizures, coma.

Many clinical conditions in pediatrics can resemble SIADH, but since hyponatremia is the most constant finding, we have found that an effective way to make a differential diagnosis is to follow a rational pathophysiologic sequence as in Table 4. As shown, SIADH represents a state of hyponatremia accompanied by an increased total body water and persistent natriuresis.

The management of patients with SIADH has included several therapeutic modalities; however, fluid restriction by itself will correct the hyponatremia and prevent further expansion in the majority of patients (6,7,9, 11).

We limit the amount of fluid given initially to insensible water loss and half of the urinary output. If after 24 hours the serum sodium has not shown an upward trend, further fluid restriction to only insensible water loss is instituted. Treatment of the underlying disease

TABLE 2. Clinical Entities Associated with SIADH

1. Tumors
   Ca lung, duodenum, pancreas, lymphoma

2. C.N.S.
   Meningitis, encephalitis, abscess, trauma, hemorrhage, Guillain-Barre, S.L.E.

3. Intrathoracic
   Infection: pneumonia, TBC, abscess.
   Left Atrial Pressure; pneumothorax, atelectasis, asthma, cystic fibrosis, PDA ligation, mitral commissurotomy

4. Stress
   Post-op, anesthesia, pain

5. Drugs

6. Idiopathic

TABLE 3. Drug Interactions with ADH

	↑ADH Secretion	↑Action	↓Secretion	↓Action
Chlorpropamide	+	+		
Tolbutamide		+		
Diguanide		+		
Vincristine	+			
Cyclophosphamide	+			
Carbamazepine	+			
Chlofibrate	+			
Morphine	+			
Phenothiazine	+			
Ara-A	+			
Acetaminophen	+	+		
Indomethacin		+		
Diphenylhydantoin			+	
Lithium				+
Demeclocycline				+

eventually will bring about the resolution of all the derangements of the syndrome. However, rapid correction of the hyponatremia is required in the patient who shows prominent symptomatology such as lethargy, coma or seizures.

We have successfully used hypertonic saline and furosemide administration following the protocol suggested by Hantman et al. (12); in several patients a dramatic response occurred within hours. The rationale behind this approach is the inducement of a negative water balance with a concomitant replacement of the urinary sodium and potassium losses. This requires careful monitoring of urinary volume and electrolyte losses every two hours and frequent determination of serum electrolytes and osmolality. In this manner, urine electrolytes are replaced exactly as lost in the urine while urine volume is not replaced until the desired negative water balance is achieved.

An example of a 40 kg patient who has a serum sodium of 120 mEq/L and plasma osmolality of 245 mOsm/kg is given,using an estimated total body water content of 60% of body weight and a desired plasma osmolality of 280 mOsm/kg.

1) (weight in kg) (60%) = total body water

$$(40)\ (0.6) = 24$$

2) (total body water) (plasma osmolality) = miliosmols of total body solute

$$(24)\ (245) = 5880$$

3) $$\frac{\text{total body solute}}{\text{x liters}} = \frac{\text{desired plasma osmolality}}{\text{1 liter}}$$

$$\frac{5880}{x} = \frac{280}{1}$$

HYPONATREMIA

1		Deficit of total body water and larger deficit of total body sodium	Excess total body water	Excess total body sodium and larger excess of total body water
	ECF volume depletion		Modest ECF volume excess (no edema)	Profound ECF volume excess (edema)
2	Renal Losses - Diuretic Excess, Adrenal insufficiency, salt-losing nephritis, renal tubular acidosis with bicarbonaturia	Extrarenal losses - Vomiting, Diarrhea, "third space"-burns, pancreatitis, traumatized muscle	Hypothyroidism, pain, emotion, drugs, syndrome of inappropriate ADH secretion	Nephrotic Syndrome, cirrhosis, cardiac failure
3	urinary sodium concentration > 20 mEq/L	urinary sodium concentration < 10 mEq/L	urinary sodium concentration > 20 mEq/L	urinary sodium concentration < 10 mEq/L
4		isotonic saline	water restriction	water restriction

NORMONATREMIA

TABLE 4. Diagnosic and therapeutic approach to hyponatremia.
Reproduced with permission from Schrier, R.W. and Berl, T.: Disorders of Water Metabolism. In Schrier, R.W.(Ed.): Renal and Electrolyte Disorders. New York: Little, Brown and Co., 1976, p. 36.

4) total body water - x = desired negative water balance
24 - 21 = 3 liters

Additional therapeutic modalities in the management of SIADH have included lithium (13), demeclocycline (14,15), urea (16), furosemide (17) and phenytoin (18). Although their use in pediatrics is not desirable, more careful analysis of their usefulness is warranted.

SUMMARY

We have reviewed several physiologic and pathophysiologic aspects related to antidiuretic hormone with particular reference to SIADH. This syndrome can be associated with multiple clinical circumstances, and is basically characterized by a state of serum hypotonicity (and hyponatremia) with persistent natriuresis and elevated urine osmolality. Although several therapeutic modalities are available, water restriction remains the cornerstone in the successful management of most patients.

REFERENCES

1. Hays, R.M.: Antidiuretic Hormone. N. Eng. J. Med. 195:659, 1976.
2. Weitzman, R.E.: Factors regulating the secretion and metabolism of arginine vasopressin (antidiuretic hormone). In Brenner, B.M. and Stein, J.H.: Hormonal Function and the Kidney. Contemporary Issues in Nephrology. Vol. 4. New York: Livingston, 1979, p. 146.
3. Robertson, G.L., Mahr, E.A., Athar, S. et al.: Development and clinical application of a new method for the radioimmunoassay of arginine vasopressin in human plasma. J. Clin. Invest. 52:2340, 1973.
4. Friedman, A. and Segar, W.E.: Antidiuretic hormone. J. Pediatr. 94:521, 1979.
5. Dunn, F.L., Brennan, T.J., Nelson, A.E., et al.: The role of blood osmolality and volume in regulating vasopressin in the rat. J. Clin. Invest. 52:3212, 1973.
6. Schwartz, W.B., Bennett, W., Curelop, S. et al.: A syndrome of renal sodium loss and hyponatremia probably resulting from inappropriate secretion of antidiuretic hormone. Am. J. Med. 23:529, 1957.
7. Bartter, F.C. and Schwartz, W.B.: The syndrome of Inappropriate Secretion of Antidiuretic Hormone. Am. J. Med. 42:790, 1967.
8. Bourgoignie, J.J., Hwang, K.H., Espinel, C. et al.: A natriuretic factor in the serum of patients with chronic uremia. J. Clin. Invest. 51:1514, 1972.
9. Fine, L.G., Kaplan, M. and Bricker, N.S.: Disturbances of salt and water metabolism in chronic renal failure. In Edelman, C. Jr. (ed.): Pediatric Disease. Boston: Little, Brown and Co., 1978, p. 348.
10. Beck, L.H.: Hypouricemia in the syndrome of inappropriate secretion of antidiuretic hormone. N. Eng. J. Med. 301:528, 1979.
11. Kaplan, S.L. and Feigin, R.D.: Syndrome of Inappropriate Secretion of Antidiuretic Hormone in Children. In Barness, L. (ed.): Advances in Pediatrics. Chicago: Yearbook Medical Publishers, 1980, vol. 27, p. 247.

12. Hantman, D., Rossier, B., Zohlman, R. et al.: Rapid correction of hyponatremia in the syndrome of inappropriate secretion of antidiuretic hormone. Ann.Inter. Med. 78:870, 1973.
13. Baker, R.S., Hurley, R.M. and Feldman, W.: Treatment of recurrent syndrome of inappropriate secretion of antidiuretic hormone with lithium. J. Pediat. 90:480, 1977.
14. Forrest, J.N., Cox, M., Hong, C. et al.: Superiority of demeclocycline over lithium for the treatment of chronic syndrome of inappropriate secretion of antidiuretic hormone. N. Eng. J. Med. 298:173, 1978.
15. Schrier, R.W.: New treatments for hyponatremia. Editorial, N. Eng. J. Med. 298:214, 1978.
16. Decaux, G., Brimioulle, S., Gennette, F. et al.: Treatment of the syndrome of inappropriate secretion of antidiuretic hormone by urea. Am. J. Med. 69:99, 1980.
17. Decaux, G., Waterlot, Y., Gennette, F. et al.: Treatment of inappropriate secretion of antidiuretic hormone with furosemide. N. Eng. J. Med. 304:329, 1981.
18. Sordillo, P., Matarese, R.A., Novich, R.K. et al.: Specific modalities of therapy for inappropriate antidiuretic hormone secretion. Clin. Nephr. 15:105, 1981.

MANAGEMENT OF NEPHROTIC EDEMA

G. Zilleruelo, M.D. and José Strauss, M.D.

Edema is one of the cardinal features of the nephrotic syndrome (NS) (1), and can be mild or severe, localized or generalized. Although presence or severity of the edema does not correlate well with the renal histopathology or prognosis, it may present several clinical problems (Table 1). Severe, generalized edema or anasarca may be associated with circulatory collapse due to an important decrease in the effective arterial blood volume (2,3). Respiratory distress may result from increased pulmonary interstitial fluid (ITF), mechanical compression from pleural effusion, or ascitic fluid interference with diaphragmatic movement (4,5). Skin distension with rupture can be observed in the lower extremities and abdomen which could be the entry site for skin infections and/or cellulitis (6).

Primary peritonitis and vascular thrombosis are seen in patients with active nephrosis and edema (7,8). Peritonitis usually is due to a single organism. Although Streptococcus pneumonia has been most frequently implicated, organisms such as E. coli, H. influenza and other gram negatives may be involved (9). Prednisone therapy, low serum level of IgG and impaired phagocytosis have been proposed as predisposing factors (10). However, clinical signs of active nephrosis with edema and ascites have been the single most constantly present factor (11). Thromboembolic complications have been observed in approximately 20% of patients with NS, especially in those with membranous nephropathy (12). Use of corticosteroids, persistent proteinuria, hypercoagulable state, and overuse of diuretics have been described as predisposing factors (13,14). However, as with

TABLE 1. Clinical Properties Associated with Nephrotic Edema

Circulatory Collapse
Respiratory Distress
Skin Rupture and Infections
Peritonitis
Vascular Thrombosis
Patient Discomfort and Depression

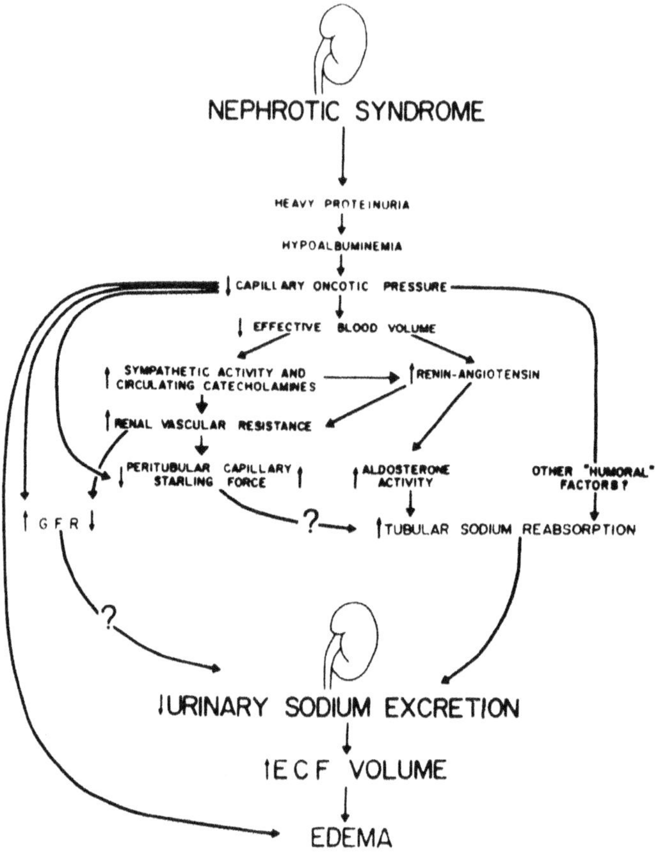

FIGURE 1. Pathophysiology of edema formation in Nephrotic Syndrome. Reproduced with permission from Schrier, R.W.: Renal sodium excretion, edematous disorders and diuretic use. In Schrier, R.W. (ed.): Renal and Electrolyte Disorders. Boston: Little, Brown and Co., 1976.

any other complication of edema, causal relationships are not well established because of the multiple variables involved. Many times the patient demands some form of treatment for the edema because of discomfort or esthetic reasons. The decision as to whether the treatment should be aimed specifically at correction of the edema or a part of the general management of the nephrotic patient, is difficult. The various treatments used for NS most times are sufficient to relieve the edema and prevent complications. If not, the edema itself should be treated. This decision and the treatment modality chosen should be based on thorough knowledge of the possible pathogenesis of the edema.

PATHOPHYSIOLOGY OF EDEMA

There have been several reviews and hypotheses about the pathophysiology of edema in NS (15-18). All emphasize the sequence of massive proteinuria, hypoalbuminemia and decrease in plasma oncotic pressure which finally lead to an imbalance of the Starling forces at the capillary level. This supposedly results in accumulation of fluid in the interstitial space and contraction of plasma volume (PV). Efforts to demonstrate a consistent reduction in blood or plasma volume have been unsuccessful (19). However, in cases with "normal" plasma volume, evidence of increased sympathetic activity with high plasma levels of norepinephrine has been suggestive of a decrease in "effective" PV (20). The decrease in effective PV triggers several mechanisms which induce an increase in renal tubular reabsorption of filtered sodium and water in excess of that required for maintenance of the extracellular fluid (ECF). The result is a positive balance of sodium and water with increased ECF volume and edema (Fig. 1). For edema to appear, ITF pressure must become positive (21). In fact, edema usually is not clinically detectable until the ITF volume has risen to about 30% above normal (22). In severe edema, ITF volume increases to several hundred percent above normal (Fig. 2). If mild to moderate edema persists for a few days or weeks, even a 1-2 mm Hg interstitial pressure rise can cause severe edema (22).

Although the primary event postulated in the mechanism of edema formation is the decrease in colloid osmotic pressure (COP) inside the capillary, there is no available information about these changes in nephrotic children. The COP estimated from total protein has a good correlation with that measured but only if albumin is not administered for several days prior to the blood letting (Fig. 3) (23).

In NS there is an important leakage of protein in the ITF space which increases tissue COP. The extravascular pool of albumin can be as high as 30-50% of the total ECF albumin (24). This promotes increased ECF volume and edema. The lymphatic drainage becomes crucial since there is no other route through which excess ITF protein can return to the circulatory system (25).

Presence of edema before appearance of proteinuria has been observed occasionally at the onset of NS (26). Conversely, we have seen children with severe hypoalbuminemia and no edema (27). It is clear that there are factors other than decreased COP regulating the capillary dynamics and exchange of fluid at this level. We have studied the vascular permeability factor(s) supposedly present in lymphocyte culture supernatant from these children (28). Intradermal injection of NS serum in the abdominal skin of guinea pigs, followed by an IV injection of Evans blue dye, induced an

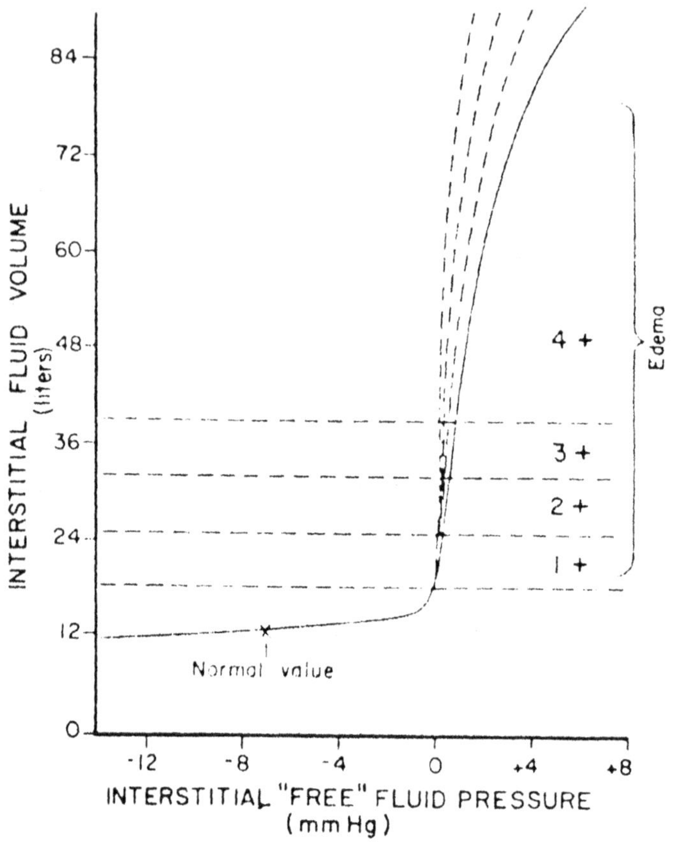

FIGURE 2. Relationship of edema to the pressure-volume curve of the interstitial spaces. The dash curves show the effect of prolonged edema on the pressure-volume curve. Reproduced with permission from Guyton, A.C.: The lymphatic system, interstitial fluid dynamics, edema and pulmonary fluid. In Guyton, A.C. (ed.): Textbook of Medical Physiology. Philadelphia: W.B. Saunders Co., 1981.

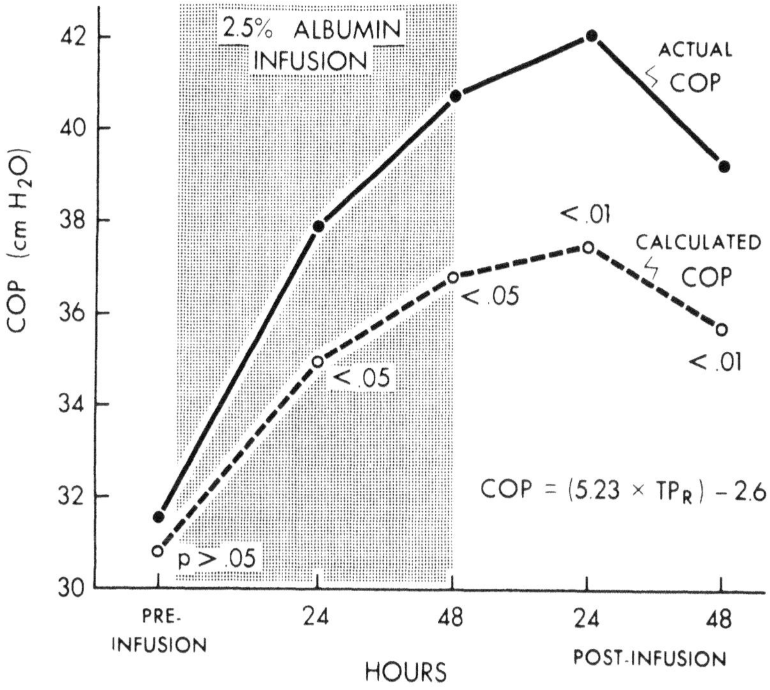

FIGURE 3. Effect of albumin infusion in the correlation of total protein and colloid oncotic pressure. Reproduced with permission from Rowe, M.I., Lankau, C. and Newmark, S.: Clinical evaluation of methods to monitor colloid oncotic pressure in the surgical treatment of children. Surg. Gynecol. Obstet. 139:889, 1974.

increased extravasation of dye in the skin as compared to controls (guinea pigs injected normal human serum followed by Evans blue dye). Our results are in agreement with reports by others (29). The presence of this factor(s) apparently is not related to the histologic type of glomerular disease (Fig. 4) (29). The increase in vascular permeability has been shown in vivo with the use of radiolabelled albumin extravasated after application of a tourniquet to an extremity (Fig. 5) (29).

TREATMENT OF EDEMA

Numerous therapeutic modalities have been applied to patients with NS in order to decrease or eliminate edema. They have included prednisone, diet manipulation, diuretics, volume expanders and water immersion.

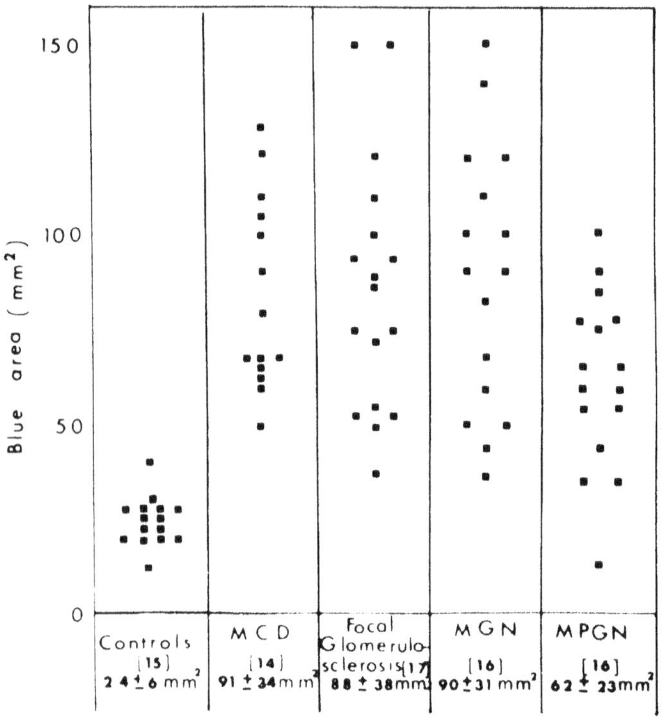

FIGURE 4. Demonstration of vascular permeability factor(s) in different types of glomerular diseases. Positive results represent extravasation of Evan's blue dye in guinea pig skin. Reproduced with permission from Sabel, A., Heslan, J.M, Branellec, A. et al.: Vascular permeability factor produced by lymphocytes of patients with nephrotic syndrome. In Hamburger, J., Grossnier, J., Grumfeld, J.P. et al. (eds.): Advances in Nephrology, vol. 10. Chicago: Year Book Medical Publishers, Inc., 1981.

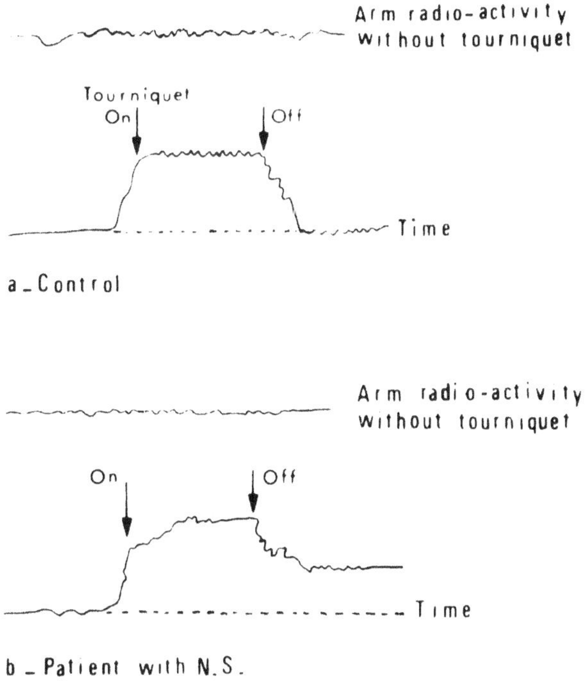

FIGURE 5. Demonstration of vascular permeability factor(s) in vivo with the use of radio-labeled albumin extravasated after application of a tourniquet to an extremity. Reproduced with permission from Sobel, A., Heslan, J.M., Branellec, A. et al.: Vascular permeability factor produced by lymphocytes of patients with nephrotic syndrome. In Hamburger, J., Grossnier, J., Grumfeld, J.P. et al. (eds.): Advances in Nephrology, vol. 10. Chicago: Year Book Medical Publishers, Inc., 1981.

Prednisone

It is well known that prednisone induces remission of the primary event of minimal change NS (MCNS), namely proteinuria. Once proteinuria decreases or stops, the edema usually subsides (6). However, it has been observed that diuresis may occur and edema resolve before proteinuria decreases. Initially, prednisone may induce a worsening of sodium retention and of edema (30). It is possible that prednisone has a direct action in the capillary permeability and/or at the renal tubule by an anti-ADH-like effect (31).

A recent study has shown the importance of the renín sodium profiling in patients with NS (32). Two groups of nephrotics were found, one with high renin and another with low renin. The high renin group showed evidence of central volume depletion and responded to corticosteroids with diuresis, natriuresis, and normalization of the high renin and aldosterone blood levels. In two patients with high renin nephrosis, the prednisone effect on renin and aldosterone excretion preceded the onset of diuresis, natriuresis, and the correction of proteinuria (Fig. 6). The mechanism involved was postulated to be a decrease of capillary leakage of protein. Patients with NS sometimes do not respond to corticosteroid therapy or they respond after a prolonged period. Therefore, other modalities of management of the edema are sometimes necessary.

Diet

Whatever the fundamental physiologic imbalance is in edematous patients, an altered ability to excrete sodium occurs in most of them. Water retention generally appears to be a secondary phenomenon (33). Therefore, the use of sodium restricted diets to approximately 1 g Na^+/m^2/day is recommended. Further restriction is not practical and would affect total food intake, as well as further decrease the appetite of these patients. The diet should contain an adequate amount of proteins.

Observations in patients with hypoproteinemic edema not associated with renal disease frequently have shown edema resolution with bed rest on a low sodium diet (34). We have seen the same result with fasting for a few days; diuresis and decrease in proteinuria were acutely induced in at least 50% of the patients studied (35). Fluid restriction should not be excessive since it may exaggerate the hypovolemia and its complications, and eventually lead to a decrease in glomerular filtration rate (GRF). Depending on the degree of edema, fluid intake should replace part of or the whole urine output. It is important to realize, however, that the ability to excrete solute free water in the urine is impaired during the phase of edema formation (36). Once diuresis starts, fluid intake should be liberalized and even sodium restriction may not be necessary anymore.

Diuretics

The temptation to treat mild asymptomatic edema with diuretics should be resisted. Diuretics used alone in nephrotics are unpredictable and have serious potential side effects (2,37). Repeated administration of powerful diuretics may further reduce the plasma volume and the GFR. Therefore, their use should be strictly individualized to help those children who are not able to follow a sodium restricted diet and have a very low urine sodium excretion.

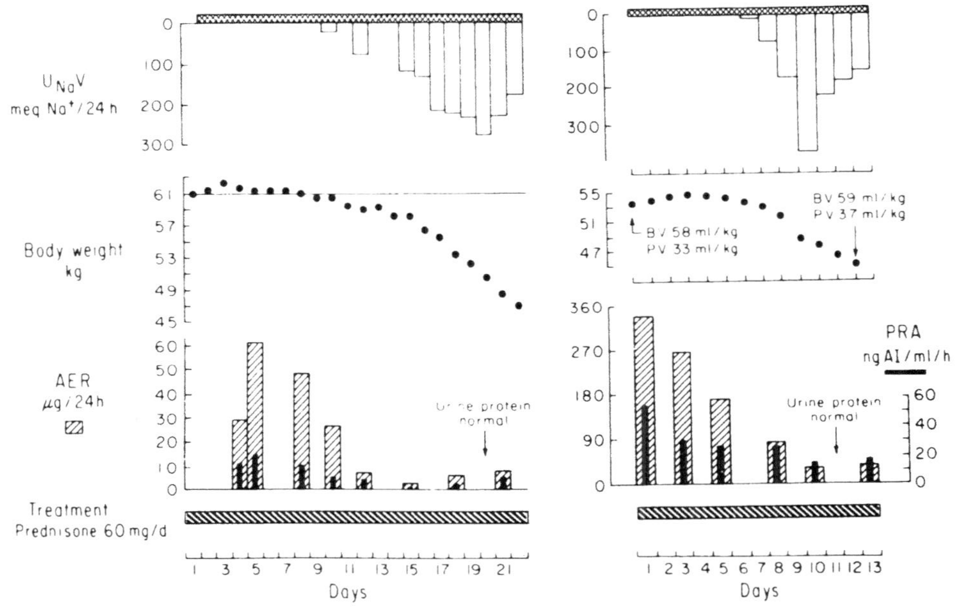

FIGURE 6. Effect of prednisone on plasma renin activity (PRA) and aldosterone excretion rate (AER) in two patients with high renin nephrosis. Reproduced with permission from Meltzer, J.I., Keim, H.J., Laragh, J.H. et al.: Nephrotic Syndrome: vaso-constriction and hypervolemic types indicated by renin-sodium profiling. Am. Intern. Med. 91:688,1979.

The initial response to diuretic therapy in these patients often is good. This is especially true with the use of potent loop action diuretics such as furosemide alone or in combination with spironolactone. Diuretic resistance seems to be determined by the severity of hypoproteinemia (37). Nephrotic adults receiving chronic diuretic therapy were invariably found to have decreased ECF, PV, and GFR, and increased BUN (38,39). These variables corrected themselves without harm after cessation of diuretic therapy. We must emphasize, however, that we are not aware of reports on the use of diuretic therapy alone in children with MCNS. Because of the potential side effects including renal vein thrombosis and hypovolemic shock (2), prolonged use of diuretics without previous volume expansion should be avoided.

Volume expanders

An ideal plasma volume expander should have certain desirable properties (Table 2). None of the available alternatives for volume expansion fulfill all the ideal requirements. These alternatives include: Plasma Protein Fraction 5%, human serum albumin 25%, Dextran, and Mannitol 20%. All have been reported to be successful in inducing a diuretic response in NS (37, 40-43).

Mechanisms involved in the production of diuretic response by volume expansion probably are diverse. Albumin infusion has been postulated as being effective by inducing changes in COP and moving extracellular fluid from the interstitium to the vascular space (44). The sequence of events occurring after albumin infusions is illustrated in Figure 7. There is a rise in COP with rapid dilution of plasma; PV also increases, and there is a transient increase in serum sodium. Maximum increase in GFR and Na^+ excretion follows 30 min to 2 hours after starting the infusion. A notable water diuresis with increase in urine flow may occur one hr after infusion is started and be associated with an increase in urine sodium excretion. Large excretion of potassium, nitrogen, phosphorus and calcium also occurs (40). Infusion of hyperoncotic albumin has been shown to significantly decrease plasma ionized calcium with an increase in parathyroid hormone followed by an increase in phosphate clearance and a decrease in proximal tubule sodium reabsorption (45). Increase in urine volume is usually greatest on the first day of therapy, falls off during succeeding infusions, and returns to baseline when therapy is discontinued. It must be emphasized that the effect of albumin is only transient since the primary effect on plasma albumin concentration is quickly dissipated because of increase in urine albumin excretion. Therefore, the goal of therapy is not to return serum albumin to normal but to increase the COP transiently in order to interrupt the vicious cycle of hypoalbuminemia-edema, thus allowing for an increase in PV and urine output.

TABLE 2. Desirable Properties of an Ideal Plasma Volume Expander

Oncotic pressure similar to plasma
Remain in the circulation for certain period of time
Subject to excretion and/or metabolic degradation
Should not affect adversely any visceral function
No antigenic, allergenic or pyretic effect
Pharmacologically inert
No interference with blood typing and cross-matching
Easily sterilized
Adequate viscosity and solubility

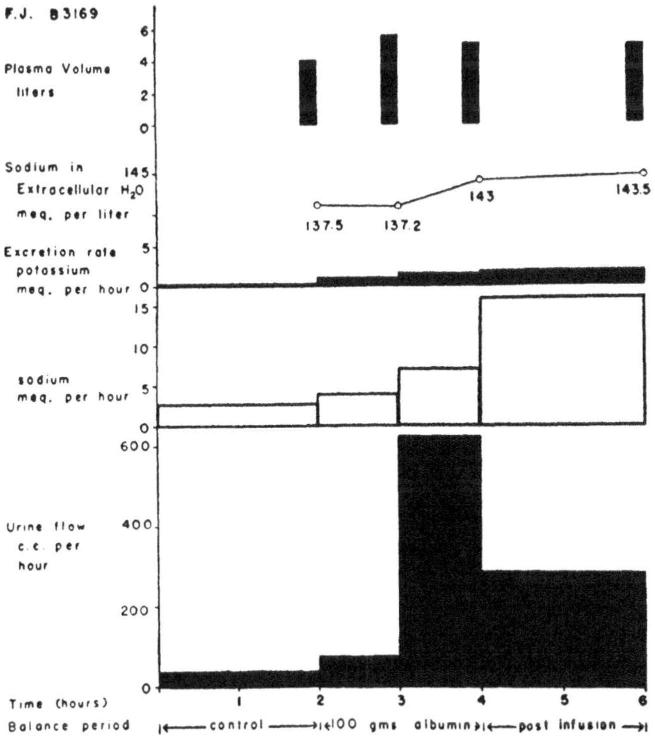

FIGURE 7. Sequence of events occurring after albumin infusion in the nephrotic syndrome. Reproduced with permission from Orloff, J., Welt, L.G., and Stowe, L.: The effects of concentrated salt-poor albumin or the metabolism and excretion of water and electrolytes in nephrosis and toxemia of pregnancy. J. Clin. Invest. 29:770,1950.

In a previous study (43) we compared the acute (48 hs) effect of the infusion of albumin 25% versus mannitol 20%. Both were administered at a dose of 1 g/kg over 2 hours and followed by an i.v. bolus of furosemide 1 mg/kg. Both regimens elicited a good diuretic response with important natriuresis. There were no clear differences in serum or urine osmolarity or electrolytes. However, blood hematocrit showed a trend to decrease with albumin and increase with mannitol. We concluded that mannitol, with its osmotic diuretic effect and without increased oncotic pressure (and concomitant pull of interstitial water to be intravascular space), may be potentially harmful if used repeatedly in already hypovolemic patients.

There are well known effects of the use of concentrated albumin in nephrotics. However, there are other unknown effects which may be as important. Transient hypertension is probably one of the most common side effects; it occurs in approximately half of the patients (46). This complication could be overcome by giving solutions more slowly or with simultaneous antihypertensive therapy. We have seen several patients develop gross hematuria immediately after albumin infusions; the significance of this event is not clear (47). Also, an increase in serum creatinine has been observed in 25% of the patients receiving these infusions (46). In some (mainly those with focal and segmental glomerular sclerosis), the increase in serum creatinine was not reversible; this observation is based on a small number of patients and will require further confirmation. Sudden hypotension has been observed with the use of Plasmanate which contains a high percentage of pre-kallikrein activator (48). Anaphylactic reactions, hypovolemic shock, and congestive heart failure, although rare, have been reported with albumin infusions (49). In patients who have recently undergone renal biopsy, there is a potential for bleeding at the site of renal biopsy after plasma volume expansion (50). Hypercatabolism and depletion of albumin-bound substances are potential side effects which require further study to determine their significance. In summary, plasma volume expansion should be contraindicated or done with extreme caution in patients with severe hypertension, anuria or renal failure, and congestive heart failure.

Dextran also has been used to produce diuresis in NS with good results (42). This substance is a bacterial polysaccharide with long branched chains of glucose units (M.W. 40,000 - 70,000). When injected, the larger molecules are further broken down and excreted as smaller fractions or slowly metabolized (51). The infusion of dextran probably induces plasma oncotic changes similar to those following albumin infusion (42). In the same line of products, hydroxyethyl starch (Hespan) and other polymers with high molecular weight are promising for use either alone or in combination with albumin infusions.

EXPERIMENTAL APPROACHES

Other therapeutic modalities are being sought to induce diuresis in NS patients. Although all have theoretical bases, only future trials will prove their efficacy. One of particular interest is head-out immersion in warm water. The physiological effects of this modality have been studied in detail in normal subjects and cirrhotic patients (52,53). The external hydrostatic pressure gradient obtained with immersion in 1.3 m of water up to the neck in a seated position caused central hypervolemia, apparently resulting from the squeezing of extracellular fluid from the lower limbs and trunk; this hypervolemia resulted in decreased vasopressin and aldosterone secretion. The result and decrease in renal tubular sodium reabsorption was associated with an important diuresis with natriuresis and kaliuresis (53). Possible mechanisms involved in this response are presented in Figure 8 (54). Since nephrotic patients with edema also have a decreased effective arterial blood volume with secondary hyperaldosteronism, the beneficial effects of water immersion are potentially important. A recent publication has suggested that water immersion is effective in inducing diuresis in adult nephrotics and could be considered as a therapeutic agent in cases not responding to conventional therapy (55).

CONCLUSION

We have reviewed the pathophysiologic bases for a rational approach in the management of nephrotic edema. The decision of when and how to treat edema should be carefully evaluated in each patient. From the several therapeutic modalities available, the one that best fits a particular patient should be selected and the response closely evaluated. In this manner, clinical problems associated with severe edema will be prevented and complications due to overtreatment hopefully will be avoided.

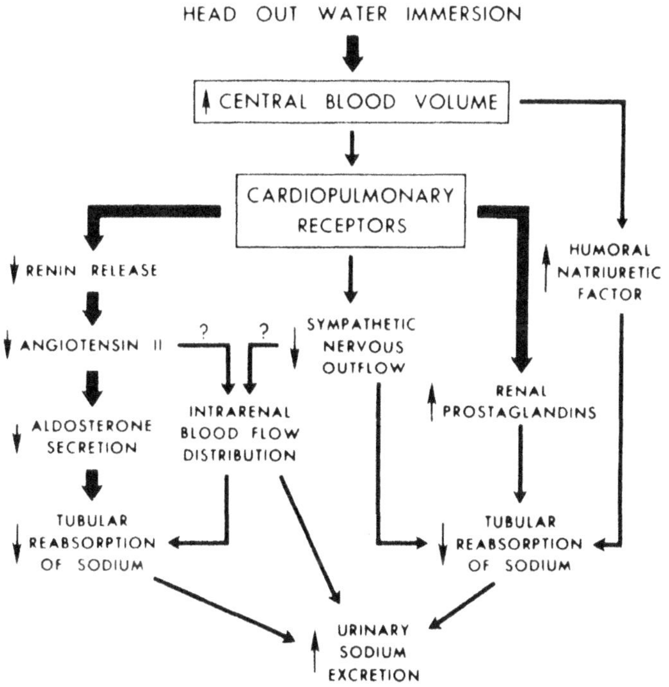

FIGURE 8. Mechanisms involved in the natriuresis of head-out water immersion. Reproduced with permission from Bourgoignie, J.J., Pennell, J.P. and Jacob, A.I.: Sodium metabolism and volume regulation. In Gonick, H.C. (ed.): Current Nephrology. Boston: Houghton Mifflin Professional Publishers, 1979.

REFERENCES

1. Schrier, R.W.: Renal sodium excretion, edematous disorders and diuretic use. In Schrier, R.W. (ed.): Renal and Electrolyte Disorders. Boston: Little Brown and Co., 1976, p. 45.
2. Yamauchi, H. and Hopper, J. Jr: Hypovolemic shock and hypotension as a complication in the nephrotic syndrome. Ann. Intern. Med. 60:242, 1964.
3. Egan, T.J., Kenny, F.M., Jarrah, A. et al.: Shock as a complication of the nephrotic syndrome. Amer. J. Dis. Child. 113:364, 1967.
4. Gaar, K.A. Jr., Taylor, A.E., Owens L.J. et al.: Effect of capillary pressure and plasma protein on development of pulmonary edema. Amer. J. Physiol. 32:547, 1970.
5. Wyllie, R., Arasu, T.S. and Fitzgerald, J.F.: Ascites: Pathophysiology and management. J. Pediatr. 97:167, 1980.
6. Rance, C.P., Arbus, G.S. and Balfe, J.W.: Management of the nephrotic syndrome in children. Pediatric Clinics of North America 23:735, 1976.
7. Speck, W.T., Dresdale, S.S. and McMillan, R.W.: Primary peritonitis and the nephrotic syndrome. Am. J. Surg. 127:267, 1974.
8. Bennett, W.W.: Renal vein thrombosis in nephrotic syndrome. Ann. Intern. Med. 83:577, 1975.
9. Harken, A.H. and Shochat, S.J.: Gram-positive peritonitis in children. Amer. J. Surg. 125:769, 1973.
10. O'Regan, S., Mongeau, J. and Robitaille, P.: Primary peritonitis in the nephrotic syndrome. Int. J. Ped. Nephrol. 1:216, 1980.
11. Zilleruelo, G., Galindez, R., Gorman, H. and Strauss, J.: Peritonitis in nephrotic children. Manuscript in preparation.
12. Llach, F., Papper, S. and Massry, S.G.: The clinical spectrum of renal vein thrombosis: acute and chronic. Amer. J. Med. 6o:819, 1980.
13. Kendall, A.G., Lohmann, R.E., Dossetor, J.B. et al.: Nephrotic syndrome: a hypercoagulable state. Arch. Intern. Med. 127:1021, 1971.
14. Lieberman, E., Heuser, E., Gilchrist et al.: Thrombosis, nephrosis and corticosteroid therapy. J. Pediatr. 73:320, 1968.
15. Eder, H.A., Lauson, H.D., Chinard, F.P. et al.: A study of the mechanisms of edema formation in patients with the nephrotic syndrome. J. Clin. Invest. 33:636, 1954.
16. Levy, E.J.: The pathophysiology of nephrotic edema. In Strauss, J. (ed.): Pediatric Nephrology: Current Concepts in Diagnosis and Management. New York: Plenum Press, 1976, vol. 3, p. 321.
17. Metcoff, J. and Janeway, C.A.: Studies on the pathogenesis of edema of nephrotic syndrome. J. Pediatr. 58:640, 1961.
18. Roberti, R.E., Muñoz-Arizpe, R. and Gordillo-Paniagua, G.: Pathophysiology of edema in the nephrotic syndrome. In Strauss, J. (ed.): Pediatric Nephrology: Nephrotic Syndrome. New York: Garland Press, 1979, vol. 5, p.49.
19. Eisenburg, S.: Blood volume in persons with edema and the nephrotic syndrome. Am. J. Med. Sci. 255:320, 1968.
20. Kelsch, R.C., Light, G.S. and Oliver, W.J.: The effect of albumin infusion upon plasma norepinephrine concentration in nephrotic children. J. Lab. Clin. Med. 79:516, 1972.

21. Guyton, A.C.: Interstitial fluid pressure: II. Pressure volume curves of interstitial space. Circ. Res. 16:452, 1965.
22. Guyton, A.C.: The lymphatic system, interstitial fluid dynamics, edema and pulmonary fluid. In Guyton, A.C. (ed.): Textbook of Medical Physiology. Philadelphia: W.B. Saunders Co., 1981, p. 397.
23. Rowe, M.I., Lankau, C. and Newmark, S.: Clinical evaluation of methods to monitor colloid oncotic pressure in the surgical treatment of children. Surg. Gynecol. Obstet. 139:889, 1974.
24. Gitlin, D., Janeway, C.A. and Farr, L.E.: Studies on the metabolism of plasma proteins in the nephrotic syndrome. I. Albumin, Gammaglobulin and iron-binding globulin. J. Clin. Invest. 35:44, 1956.
25. Sterns, E.E.: Current concepts of lymphatic transport. Surg. Gynecol. Obstet. 138:773,1974.
26. Schreiner, G.E.: The nephrotic syndrome. In Strauss, M.B. and Welt, L.G. (eds.): Diseases of the Kidney, 2nd ed. Boston: Little, Brown and Co., 1971, vol. 1, p. 503.
27. Strauss, J., Personal Communication.
28. McLeod, T., Personal Communication.
29. Sobel, A., Heslan, J.M., Branellec, A. and Lagrue, G.: Vascular permeability factor produced by lymphocytes of patients with nephrotic syndrome. In Hamburger, J., Grossnier, J., Grumfeld, J.P. and Maxwell, M. (eds.): Advances in Nephrology, Chicago: Yearbook Medical Publishers, Inc., 1981, vol. 10, p. 315.
30. Gorman, H.M., Zilleruelo, G., Galindez, R. et al.: The side-effects of glucocorticoids and alkylating agents in the nephrotic syndrome. In Strauss, J. (ed.): Pediatric Nephrology, Nephrotic Syndrome. New York: Garland Press, 1979, p. 247.
31. Lindeman, R.D., Van Buren, H.C., and Raisz, L.G.: Effect of steroids on water diuresis and vasopressin sensitivity. J. Clin. Invest. 40:152, 1961.
32. Meltzer, J.I., Keim, H.J., Laragh, J.H. et al.: Nephrotic Syndrome: Vasoconstriction and hypervolemic types indicated by Renin-Sodium Profiling. Ann. Intern. Med. 91:688, 1979.
33. Chonko, A.M., Bay, W.H., Stein, J.H. et al.: The role of renin and aldosterone in the salt retention of edema. Am. J. Med. 63: 881, 1977.
34. Shear, L., Ching, S., and Gabuzda, G.J.: Compartmentalization of ascites and edema in patient with hepatic cirrhosis. N. Engl. J. Med. 282:1391, 1970.
35. Strauss, J., Zilleruelo, G., McLeod, T. et al.: Food manipulation and minimal change nephrotic syndrome. Abstract, Ped. Res. 14:1001, 1980.
36. Gur, A., Adefuin, P.Y., Siegal, N.J. et al.: A study of the renal handling of water in lipoid nephrosis. Ped. Res. 10:197,1976.
37. Davison, A.M., Lambie, A.T., Verth, A.H. et al.: Salt-poor human albumin in the management of nephrotic syndrome. Brit. Med. J. 1:481, 1974.
38. Jewkes, R.F., Burki, N. and Guz, A: Observations of renal function in patients undergoing therapeutic diuresis with furosemide. Clin. Sci. 38:439, 1970.

39. Garnett, E.S., and Webber, C.E.: Changes in blood volume produced by treatment in the nephrotic syndrome. Lancet II, 78:9, 1967.
40. Luetscher, J.A. Jr., Mall, A.D., and Kremer, V.L.: Treatment of nephrosis with concentrated human serum albumin. II. Effects on renal function and on excretion of water and some electrolytes. J. Clin. Invest: 29:896, 1950.
41. Orloff, J., Welt, L.G. and Stowe, L.: The effects of concentrated salt-poor albumin on the metabolism and excretion of water and electrolytes in nephrosis and toxemia of pregnancy. J. Clin. Invest. 29:770, 1950.
42. James, J., Gordillo, G., and Metcoff, J.: Effects of infusions of hyperoncotic dextran in children with the nephrotic syndrome. J. Clin. Invest. 33:1346, 1954.
43. Zilleruelo, G., Galindez, R., Weiss, M. et al.: Effect of Albumin-Furosemide or Mannitol-Furosemide in nephrotic children. Abstract, Ped. Res. 13:522, 1979.
44. Chinard, F.P., Lauson, M.D., Eder, H.A. et al.: Plasma volume changes following the administration of albumin to patients with nephrotic syndrome. J. Clin. Invest. 32:629, 1953.
45. Knox, F.G., Schneider, E.G., Willis, L.R. et al.: Proximal tubular reabsorption after hyperoncotic albumin infusion. Role of parathyroid hormone and dissociation from plasma volume. J. Clin. Invest. 53:501, 1974.
46. Sherwinter, J., Weiss, R., Simpson, E. et al.: Effects of albumin and furosemide (A-F) in nephrotic patients with severe edema. Abstract, Ped. Res. 13:520, 1979.
47. Unpublished observations
48. Aloing, B.M., Hojima, Y., Pisano, J.J. et al.: Hypertension associated with prekallikrein activator in plasma protein fraction. N. Engl. J. Med. 299:66, 1978.
49. Rice, C.L. and Moss, G.S.: Blood and blood substitutes, Current Practice: Adv. Surg. 13:106, 1979.
50. Unpublished observations.
51. Mudge, G.H.: Agents affecting volume and composition of body fluids. In Goodman, L.S. and Gilman, A. (eds.): The Pharmacological Basis of Therapeutics. New York: McMillan Publishing Co., Inc., 1980, p. 848.
52. Epstein, M. and Saruta, T.: Effect of water immersion on renin-aldosterone and renal sodium handling in normal man. J. Appl. Physiol. 31:368, 1971.
53. Epstein, M., Levinson, R., Sancho, J. et al.: Characterization of the renin-aldosterone system in decompensated cirrhosis. Circ. Res. 41:818, 1977.
54. Bourgoigne, J.J., Pennell, J.P. and Jacob, A.I. Sodium metabolism and volume regulation. In Gonick, H.C. (ed.) : Current Nephrology Boston: Houghton Mifflin Professional Publishers, 1979, p. 1.
55. Berlyne, G.M., Brown, C., Adler, A. et al.: Water immersion in nephrotic syndrome. Arch. Intern. Med. 141:1275, 1981.

HIGHLIGHTS: RENAL FUNCTION MODIFICATIONS INDUCED BY FUROSEMIDE IN CHILDREN WITH ACUTE POST-STREPTOCOCCAL GLOMERULONEPHRITIS

Ricardo Muñoz-Arizpe, M.D., René Feiman, M.D., and Gustavo Gordillo-Paniagua, M.D.

Hypertension was the most frequent and risky presenting symptom of patients with acute post-streptococcal glomerulonephritis (AGN) admitted to the Hospital Infantil de Mexico. We intended to determine in this study the renal function parameters involved in the development of hypertension, and if these could be corrected by furosemide administration.

Fifteen AGN patients aged 4-12 years were studied. Evolution from the clinical onset to the time of the study ranged from two to 12 days. Average initial BP was 137 ± 15/105 ± 15 mm Hg. Furosemide was given initially 5-10 mg/kg/dose orally, and repeated at 6 hr intervals, depending upon the patient's response; the total number of doses varied from patient to patient. Renal function parameters were evaluated prior to and after furosemide administration; the time that elapsed between the latest dose of furosemide given and the second renal function evaluation was variable. According to this time interval, the patients were divided into two groups: I ($<$ 9 hours) and II ($>$ 9 hours). Group III included nine healthy adult volunteers studied prior to and four hours after a single oral dose of furosemide 1 mg/kg. The following parameters were evaluated: U/P urea, creatinine, osmolality and sodium ratios; fractional excretion of the filtered sodium (FENa), and renal failure index (RFI). There was no significant difference in any parameter between groups I and II during the initial evaluation, but there was a significant difference when compared to group III. After furosemide administration, a significant difference between groups I and II was noticed in all parameters except U/P sodium, due to the longer time elapsed between the last given dose and the second evaluation in group II. Significant difference was observed between groups I and III before and after furosemide administration, mainly due to a decreased U/P osmolality and U/P creatinine ratios, secondary to enhanced water excretion. The significant increase of FENa was due to increased urinary sodium concentration, as well as decreased urine creatinine concentration that followed increased water excretion. Serum levels of Na, K and creatinine were unchanged. The functional changes described above were accompanied by a parallel reduction of BP to average values of 110 ± 10/80 ± 10 mm Hg suggesting that the development of hypertension was due to diminished FENa during the pre-clinical stages of AGN.

PHARMACOTHERAPY OF HYPERTENSION

Eliseo Perez-Stable, M.D. and Barry J. Materson, M.D.

Pharmacological treatment of hypertension continues to be the most effective and perhaps only practical management of hypertension. There is a rising tide of sentiment in this country for managing hypertension and other chronic diseases with diet, exercise, and a variety of behavioral modification techniques, including relaxation response, biofeedback, and transcendental meditation to the exclusion of drugs. There is no convincing evidence from well-controlled studies that any of these various techniques have a permanent or prolonged antihypertensive effect (1).

Isotonic exercise, when done properly and regularly, reduces arterial pressure to 5 to 10 mm Hg but cannot be seriously considered as a replacement for drug therapy. Salt restriction in the diet to 75 mEq of sodium (4.5 grams of salt) daily is the most effective of the non-pharmacological modalities of therapy in reducing the arterial pressure. In hypertensive patients with diastolic between 90 and 105 mm Hg a reduction of salt intake to less than 6 grams daily would drop the diastolic to less than 90 mm Hg in probably 75% of the patients (2). However, most patients are not able to maintain this dietary modification for more than a few months. Weight reduction is also effective in dropping diastolic and systolic pressure, but until now, only in individuals with 20% or more of overweight and if the weight loss is in the range of 20 to 30 pounds (3).

No study has been published demonstrating a lasting effect of all of these non-pharmacological modalities of therapy in the treatment of hypertension. Even more, some patients who do not comply with these recommendations of changing their life-style, may become embarrassed and may elect to drop out of therapy and thus they become lost to follow-up. Adherence to a dietary regimen may be much more difficult than is adherence to a pharmacological regimen. The young patient with labile or mild hypertension, for whom dietary therapy has the most to offer, often has great deal of difficulties following a diet. Their life-style is inextricably linked to Pizza Hut, McDonald's, Wendy's or T.V. dinners. Only a few highly motivated will make the effort to adhere to diets limited in sodium and calories.

INDICATIONS

The first (4) and second (5) Veterans Administration Studies on antihypertensive drugs demonstrated a decrease in morbidity and mortality in hypertensive patients with diastolics between 105 to 129 mm Hg whose blood pressure was reduced with antihypertensive drugs in comparison with a control group treated with placebos. The recently published investigation of the Hypertension Detection and Follow-up Program (HDFP) (6) has demonstrated the beneficial effects of lowering the diastolic pressure in patients with mild hypertension, whose diastolic is between 90 to 104 mm Hg. This large multicenter project screened more than 150,000 persons to identify 10,940 hypertensive patients, which were randomized in two groups. In the Stepped Care (SC) group the medical care was free, the patients were treated by nurse practitioners and they were intensively followed-up. In this group the medication was increased step-wise to bring the diastolic pressure (DP) to 90 mm Hg or less. In the Referral Care (RC) group, the patients were treated by private physicians or community resources, there was fee for service or third-party payment and there was no deliberate follow-up. Control of BP was consistently better for the SC than for the RC group. Five years mortality from all causes was 17% lower for the SC group compared to the RC group and 20% lower for the SC group with entry DP of 90 to 104 mm Hg compared to the corresponding RC group. The frequency of coronary artery disease was 26% less in the SC group.

The HDFP study provides a rationale for aggressively treating all patients with hypertension, including those with mild forms of the disease. However, the design of the study, comparing two groups of patients in different settings, invites to criticism, that factors other than control of high blood pressure might have contributed to the results.

The Australian therapeutic trial (7) in mild hypertension, also demonstrated the beneficial effects of drug therapy in mild hypertension. The results showed a significant reduction in mortality in the actively treated group. There was also a significant reduction in the incidence of non-fatal trial end-points. However, there was little overall difference in ischemic heart disease. Only the HDFP study has shown reduction in coronary disease with drug therapy.

TREATMENT

Chemotherapy is the only practical solution to the hypertension problem. The impact of an extensive work-up of patients for curable hypertension in reducing morbidity and mortality in the hypertensive population has been minimal. Worse than doing too little work-up before starting therapy is to delay antihypertensive chemotherapy until an extensive work-up is completed. A complete history and physical examination, urinalysis, biochemical profile, chest X-ray and an electrocardiogram are all that is needed in most instances. We do not do routine renin profiles or IVP's.

Prior to beginning a course of life-long treatment, the patient with mildly elevated blood pressure should be seen on at least three separate visits to document fixed hypertension.

The goal of therapy is to lower the blood pressure to normal or to the lowest level that the patient will tolerate. Usually a diastolic pressure of 90 mm Hg or lower may be achieved without serious side effects. To this end, a "stepped care" (8) approach has been developed as a logical guide to treatment. This is a series of recommendations which has proved to be useful for the majority of patients, is simple to implement and can be readily used by paramedical personnel. In essence, "stepped-care" begins all patients who require drug therapy with a diuretic drug (Step 1). If goal blood pressure (usually 140/90 or less without symptoms) is not reached a Step 2 antiadrenergic drug is added to the diuretic. If goal pressure is still not attained, a Step 3 vasodilator drug is added to the first two. Guanethidine is used as a Step 4 drug.

Polypharmacy is scientifically justified and often necessary because frequently a single drug will not reduce blood pressure without also inducing prohibitive untoward effects. Since many drugs produce their hypotensive effect by different mechanisms, they can be combined so that their therapeutic effects are additive. Also, two drugs may be combined in order to counteract their individual side-effects. For example, a direct vasodilator induces a reflex tachycardia which can be suppressed by agents which depress the activity of the adrenergic nervous system.

Antihypertensive drugs can be divided into four groups according to their mechanisms of action: 1. Diuretics; 2. Agents which decrease the activity of the adrenergic nervous system; 3. Direct vasodilators; 4. Drugs which interfere with the renin-angiotensin system.

Diuretics

Thiazide derivatives are the most frequently used. Their antihypertensive action is related to a natriuretic effect with a consequent fall in body weight, plasma volume and cardiac output. Roughly 1 to 2 liters of extracellular fluid are excreted and this loss is more or less maintained as long as the patient remains under treatment. Several weeks after starting diuretic therapy, the cardiac output tends to return to normal and the peripheral resistance tends to decrease. The dose of thiazide varies from 25 to 100 mg daily of hydrochlorothiazide or its equivalent. There are numerous different benzothiadiazine preparations which all have essentially the same properties as hydrochlorothiazide although some are longer acting than others. Generic hydrochlorothiazide is the least expensive and is usually satisfactory for routine antihypertensive use. Other non-thiazide drugs which have a similar effect in the renal cortical diluting segment (and a minor effect in the proximal tubule) re chlorthalidone, quinethazone and metolazone. The blood pressure lowering properties of this entire class of drugs is similar. Usually one can expect a reduction of at least 10 mm Hg in 60% or more of the patients treated. The systolic pressure reductions are on the order of 15 to 30 mm Hg and 10 to 20 mm Hg for the diastolic. All of the diuretic drugs potentiate the effect of the vasodilators and adrenergic nervous system inhibitory drugs. We have a preference for the longer acting diuretics such as chlorthalidone or metolazone to enhance compliance. The thiazide diuretics tend to lose their effectiveness as GFR declines. Metolazone, however, appears to be effective (although the dose may have to be increased) even in the face of moderate renal failure.

The use of "loop" diuretics, such as furosemide or ethacrynic acid does not offer any advantage unless there is marked reduction of glomerular filtration rate. Higher than usual doses are generally required. Loop diuretics and thiazide-related drugs have in common the induction of hypokalemia, hyperuricemia, hypereninemia and some decrease in carbohydrate tolerance. They have been used in combination with potassium sparing diuretics such as spironolactone and triamterene to prevent potassium depletion.

The question of potassium depletion and replacement during the use of diuretic drugs for the treatment of hypertension has evoked controversy. There is fairly good evidence derived by whole body counting of naturally radioactive potassium that there is about a 10% absolute depletion of total body potassium following the administration of thiazides. Homeostatic mechanisms then prevail and a new steady rate is achieved. As long as there remains the stimulus of slight hypovolemia, and especially if this is coupled with a degree of hyperaldosteronism, it is unlikely that the exogenous administration of potassium (even potassium chloride) will make much of a dent in the total body deficit. It appears to be excreted just as in any other potassium load. Also, there is little evidence to suggest that in asymptomatic patients serum levels of potassium as low as 3.0 mEq/L cause any harm. The current recommendations are: 1) restrict dietary sodium moderately to reduce potassium loss, 2) do not routinely replace potassium when administering oral diuretic drugs for treatment of hypertension, 3) accept serum levels of potassium down to 3.0 mEq/L as long as the patients are asymptomatic and 4) be certain to perform serum potassium levels before the administration of thiazides. Extra caution is required for digitalized patients. Very recently published data (9) suggest that there may be an increase in ventricular irritability in diuretic treated hypertensive patients whose serum potassium is less than normal. This single study has been severely challenged and requires confirmation. However, should it be confirmed, it would then be necessary to revise the acceptable lower of serum potassium upward. Less common side effects of thiazides are related to hypersensitivity reactions and include rash and thrombocytopenic purpura. Diuretic therapy alone controls the hypertension in a great number of patients, but if, after its use, the blood pressure remains elevated, then one of the other types of agents should be added.

Agents acting on the adrenergic nervous system

These drugs can be divided into those which work primarily in the CNS (rauwolfia derivatives, methyldopa, clonidine), alpha-adrenergic blocking drugs (phenoxybenzamine, phentolamine, prazosin) beta-adrenergic blocking drugs (propranolol and many others), and sympathetic nerve blocking drugs (guanethidine).

Rauwolfia derivatives have an action peripherally through depletion of norepinephrine stores, but an important mechanism is on the central nervous system. The daily dose of reserpine should never exceed 0.25 mg. The starting dose should be 0.05 or 0.1 mg. Its unwanted reactions are depression in susceptible individuals, increased gastric motility and acidity and nasal stuffiness. Initial reports of an association with breast cancer in women have not been confirmed by subsequent studies.

Methyldopa interferes with the conversion of dopa to dopamine by competitive inhibition of the enzyme dopa decarboxylase and results in the formation of a weak transmitter of adrenergic stimuli. Methyldopa has a major effect in the central nervous system as an alpha-receptor agonist. The dose varies between 0.5 to 2.0 mg/day. A serious side effect of methyldopa is hemolytic anemia. Fortunately, it is quite rare, although the induction of a positive direct Coomb's test is fairly common. A type of hypersensitization reaction characterized by low grade fever, elevation of SGOT and jaundice has been described. Sleepiness and dry mouth are common secondary effects. Both rauwolfia derivatives and methyldopa in therapeutic doses decrease the peripheral resistance and do not affect the cardiac output.

Clonidine works mainly by CNS alpha-adrenergic stimulation which has an inhibitory effect on the sympathetic outflow from the brain. It has rapid onset of action and needs to be given only twice a day. Its major drawback in addition to dry mouth and drowsiness (35 to 40%), is that there may be a rebound hypertensive response upon sudden discontinuation of the drug. Patients should be warned not to stop the drug and physicians must withdraw their patients slowly from it.

When used alone, rauwolfia derivatives, methyldopa and clonidine tend to increase renal tubular reabsorption of sodium with a resultant expansion of plasma and extracellular fluid volume. In these circumstances, the antihypertensive effect is partially neutralized. This phenomenon explains some instances of drug resistance and can easily be overcome by the addition of diuretic drugs.

Prazosin is both an arteriolar and venous vasodilator which probably works by selective post-synaptic inhibition of alpha-1 receptors. Its use is not associated with the reflex tachycardia and palpitations seen with the other vasodilators. Important clinical side effects are postural hypotension and dizziness. The initial dose of prazosin should be 1 mg and the patients should be warned of possible orthostatic hypotension. Most patients respond to about 15-20 mg per day. Because it reduces both cardiac preload and afterload, it may be of special value in the treatment of hypertensive patients who also have congestive heart failure.

Propranolol is the prototypical beta adrenergic blocking agent. It blocks beta receptors in the heart and thus reduces the cardiac component of elevated blood pressure; it has been recommended for treatment of hypertensive patients with high cardiac output. By interfering with renin release in the juxtaglomerular apparatus, propranolol reduces PRA by more than 80%. Its use has been recommended in high renin forms of hypertensive states. However, the antihypertensive effect is not dependent upon its anti-renin effect. New evidence suggests that propranolol may also have a major central nervous system effect. Bronchial asthma and active peripheral arterial occlusive disease are absolute contraindications and congestive heart failure a relative contraindication to the use of propranolol.

The chemistry of beta-blocking agents has been intensively explored and many new drugs with specific characteristics have been introduced or are being prepared for introduction on the market in the United States. Nadolol is similar to propranolol in its general properties but differs in that it is extremely long acting. One dose daily is sufficient to provide beta-blockade for 24 hours. Timolol is also a broad spectrum beta-blocker but, because of its water solubility, it has been marketed in the form of eye drops for the treatment of glaucoma. The oral form of the drug acts similarly to propranolol except that, like the eye drops, it is capable of reducing intraoccular pressure when given systemically. Drugs such as metoprolol and atenolol block only the beta-1 receptors when given in low doses. The specific advantage is that they do not cause bronchial constriction to the extent that the nonselective beta-blocking agents do. They may also be of value in patients with insulin dependence diabetes mellitus. Drugs such as oxprenolol and pindolol possess intrinsic sympathomimetic activity (ISA). This partial agonist effect appears to limit the degree of bradycardia which is induced by doses of these drugs sufficient to lower the blood pressure.

Guanethidine is usually reserved for patients with severe forms of hypertension. This agent produces a depletion of the stores of norepinephrine in the nerve ending. Since it does not penetrate the blood-brain barrier and, therefore, has little adrenergic neuronal blocking activity within the central nervous system, depression does not occur. To become effective, guanethidine must utilize the "membrane-pump" of the sympathetic nerve ending to enter the nerve. Tricyclic antidepressants block the entry of guanethidine into the neuron and thus sharply interfere or reverse the action of the drug. Amphetamine and other drugs can competitively displace guanethidine from the neuron and reverse its antihypertensive effect. The hypotensive effect of guanethidine is mainly due to a decrease in cardiac output, with a minimal effect on the peripheral resistance. Retrograde ejaculation and postural hypotension are the two main complications. Diarrhea, especially when associated with an exaggerated gastrocolic reflex, may pose serious social problems.

Direct vasodilators

Hydralazine and minoxidil (10) are presently available for oral use. Both act directly on arteriolar smooth muscle with a resultant decrease in peripheral resistance. Since the sympathetic system is not directly affected, the decrease in blood pressure stimulates arterial baroreceptors inducing a reflex hyperactivity of the sympathetic system with increase in heart rate, stroke volume and myocardial oxygen requirement. Unfortunately, the increase in cardiac output neutralizes in part the hypotensive effect of decreasing peripheral resistance. Daily doses over 200 mg of hydralazine may precipitate a clinical state resembling disseminated lupus erythematosis. All manifestations of the latter, except the renal lesion, may occur. Combined use of a beta blocker with hydralazine or minoxidil prevents the reflex increase in cardiac output, thus enhancing their antihypertensive action. Many patients, especially older ones who are being treated with diuretic drugs, will not experience reflex sympathetic hyperactivity even though they enjoy a beneficial effect of hydralazine. Minoxidil also is an extremely potent retainer of salt and water and generally requires large doses of diuretic drugs to prevent congestive heart failure, edema, pleural effusions, and rarely, pericardial effusion. Minoxidil causes a markedly increased blood flow to the skin and thereby stimulates markedly the growth of hair. Generally this is of no concern to men, but women may find this intolerable to the extent that they may elect to die of their hypertension rather than accept treatment with Minoxidil.

Drugs which interfere with the renin-angiotensin system

Hypertension may be treated by interfering with the renin-angiotensin system at several different levels. The diuretic drug spironolactone is a steroid type drug which competes for receptor sites in the cytosol of renal tubular cells and antagonizes the effects of aldosterone. It will cause a substantial fall in blood pressure in the hypertensive states in which excess aldosterone presumably is the major cause of hypertension; i.e., primary aldosteronism due to adrenal tumor or hyperplasia.

Saralasin as mentioned above, is a competitive inhibitor at the arteriolar receptor sites for angiotensin-II.

Captopril, (11,12) this unique agent is an orally active inhibitor of converting enzyme. Initial experience with Captopril disclosed a high degree of antihypertensive efficacy with few side effects. The cardiovascular hemodynamic changes induced by the drug are characterized by a marked decrease in total peripheral vascular resistance without changes in cardiac output. The hemodynamic changes are not correlated with baseline plasma renin activity. The decrease in total peripheral resistance without changes in cardiac output pointed toward a vasodilator activity of Captopril at both arteriolar and venous level.

Initial experience with Captopril was very encouraging. There was a high degree of antihypertensive response with very few side effects. Also, thiazide diuretics enhance the antihypertensive effects. However, patients on long-term therapy may develop skin rashes and loss of taste that are mild and usually resolved with continued treatment. A more serious consideration is the development of proteinuria in some patients and the nephrotic syndrome, more rarely. Renal biopsies have revealed electron-dense deposits on the subepithelial side of the glomerular basement membrane and immunofluorescence studies have identified these deposits as immunoglomerulopathy induced by penicillamine and seems to be induced by the mercapto group presence in both substances. More recently, severe agranulocytosis, which has been found to be fatal in some instances, has been reported. There is hope that the development of second generation converting enzyme inhibitors without the mercapto group may be free of these serious complications.

HYPERTENSIVE CRISIS

Hypertensive crisis is a sudden, life-threatening elevation of blood pressure, usually, but not always, associated with diastolic pressure greater than 130 mm Hg, a situation in which it is necessary to lower the blood pressure rapidly and effectively.

Hypertensive emergencies may be classified into two groups:
1) Situations demanding immediate reduction in blood pressure (minutes to hours) as in hypertensive encephalopathy, hypertension with aortic dissection, hypertension with cerebral or subarachnoid hemorrhage and severe hypertension associated with rapid deterioration of renal function.
2) Situations that require prompt reduction in blood pressure, (hours to days) as in accelerated hypertension (hypertension associated with retinal hemorrhages and exudates), malignant hypertension (hypertension associated with hemorrhages, exudates, and papilledema) and severe hypertension associated with deterioration of renal function.

The treatment should be guided to lower the blood pressure as rapidly and as safely as possible. Once this is accomplished, the patient should be switched to an effective regimen of oral therapy for continued blood pressure control. The following drugs are useful in treating hypertensive crisis: Hydralazine, diazoxide and sodium nitroprusside are all direct vasodilators. Hydralazine may be given in "stat" doses of 10 mg I.M. to lower arterial pressure until a patent I.V. line can be set up or the patient moved to an intensive care area. It is usually given as a controlled I.V. infusion titrated to the arterial pressure. The pressure responses are somewhat slower than for the other agents (1 to 3 min for a response after the infusion rate is changed) and rapid infusion may cause severe chest pain indistinguishable from angina. Diazoxide may be given in repeated small intravenous doses (30 mg every 5 min) or given by drip infusion until the desired blood pressure reduction is achieved. Arterial pressure fall is usually rapid and may remain at the new level for twelve or more hours. Furosemide should be given concomitantly to avoid sodium retention and edema. Hyperglycemia is a known complication and should be watched for carefully, especially in patients with known carbohydrate handling problems. Both hydralazine and diazoxide cause an increase in cardiac work. They are less useful drugs for hypertension induced pulmonary edema and are not the drugs of choice for dissecting aortic aneurysm or intracranial bleeding associated with hypertensive crisis. Sodium nitroprusside is the most potent of the vasodilators. Its effect and cessation of effect are almost instantaneous and therefore, extremely responsive to changes of infusion rate. It is best used in the intensive care setting where an arterial pressure line can be monitored constantly and the rate of infusion adjusted accordingly. It must be mixed fresh, used within four hours and protected from light. Prolonged use is associated with increasing serum levels of thiocyanate which must be monitored closely after 48 hours. Hydroxycobalamine may be used to prevent this. Trimethaphan is a ganglionic blocking agent which has been an old and reliable mainstay for treatment of hypertensive crisis. It has a rapid response time and will produce hypotension if the rate is too rapid. Like nitroprusside, it must be used with arterial pressure monitoring in an I.C.U. setting. These last two drugs also lower the cardiac output so that they are the drugs of choice for treating dissecting aortic aneourysms associated with hypertensive crisis. Trimethaphan is the drug of choice for intracranial bleeding associated with severe hypertension.

REFERENCES

1. Shapiro, A.P., Schwartz, G.E., Ferguson, D.C.E. et al.: Behavioral methods in the treatment of hypertension: a review of their clinical status. Ann. Intern Med. 86:626, 1977.
2. Hunt, J.C., Margie, J.D.: The influence of diet on hypertension management. Hypertension Update: Mechanisms, Epidemiology, Evaluation, Management. Editorial Board of Dialogues in Hypertension. Bloomfield, New Jersey, Health Learning Systems, 1980, p. 197.
3. Reisin, E., Abel, R., Modan, M. et al.: Effect of weight loss without salt restriction on the reduction of blood pressure in overweight hypertensive patients. N. Engl. J. Med. 298:1, 1978.
4. Veterans Administration Cooperative Study Group on Antihypertensive Agents. Effects of treatment on morbidity in hypertension. I. Results in patients with diastolic blood pressures averaging 115 through 129 mm Hg. JAMA, 202:1028, 1967.
5. Veterans Administration Cooperative Study Group on Antihypertensive Agents. Effects of treatment on morbidity in hypertension. II. Results in patients with diastolic pressure averaging 90 through 114 mm Hg. JAMA, 213:1143, 1970.
6. Five-year findings of the Hypertension Detection and Follow-up Program. JAMA 242:2562, 1979.
7. The Australian therapeutic trial in mild hypertension. Report by the Management Committee. Lancet, June 14, 1261, 1980.
8. The 1980 Report of the Joint National Committee on Detection, Evaluation and Treatment of High Blood Pressure. Arch. Intern. Med., 140:1280, 1980.
9. Mitchell, H.C., Graham, R.M. and Pettinger, W.A.: Renal function during long-term treatment of hypertension with Minoxidil: Comparison of benign and malignant hypertension. Ann. Int. Med. 93:676, 1980.

10. Pettinger, W.A.: Minoxidil and the Treatment of Severe Hypertension. N. Eng. J. Med. 303:922, 1980.
11. Brunner, H.R., Gabars, H., Waeber, B. et al.: Oral angiotensin-converting enzyme inhibitor in long-term treatment of hypertensive patients. Ann. Int. Med. 90:19, 1979.
12. Bravo, E., Tarazi, R.C.: Converting enzyme inhibition with an orally active compound in hypertensive man. Hypertension 1:39, 1979.

DISCUSSION

José Strauss, M.D., Moderator

MODERATOR: Do we have any questions or comments?

QUESTION: From one of the papers I gather that intravenous mannitol is about as effective as intravenous albumin. I'd like to comment about that. There really has been very little increase in our understanding during the past 20 years. It's rather disappointing. There have been a lot of refinements but not much increase in our basic understanding.

RESPONSE: Regarding your question about the use of mannitol in nephrotic syndrome, in fact, there was no clear change in serum osmolality, pre- and post-infusion of mannitol and what we found more interesting was this trend toward an increase in the hematocrit. In spite of observing a good diuretic response, I would put a word of caution in the repeated use of mannitol in these already hypovolemic patients. In our experience, we did not observe any of these patients going into hemodynamic problems--shock, etc. Still, we would recommend at least alternating mannitol with some other way of plasma volume expansion that would persist, have a more prolonged effect on the plasma expansion. That's the way we have handled several patients,by alternating mannitol infusions and albumin infusions. Also, all patients must be closely monitored. A very practical way of estimating the plasma volume is by following the hematocrit levels pre- and post-infusion.

MODERATOR: If I may expand on that, without taking the comment on that material away, I would like to open the subject of possible complications of the treatment of nephrotic edema. The question has been raised repeatedly about possible complications which may be induced in patients receiving volume expanders--in particular albumin--followed by furosemide. People have observed the occurrence of thromboses of various vessels, in particular of veins, and in particular,renal; therefore, we have been very cautious with the inducement of a diuresis. When we saw that mannitol was actually increasing the hematocrit, we felt that it may be worsening the situation and may lead to the occurrence of thrombosis even though we had not seen it. We have not studied the various hematological aspects that may contribute to the formation of thrombi but we would like to know your opinion about those aspects and whether you have seen any complications or not, what are your thoughts, and any information on this subject which you want to share with all of us.

COMMENT: I want to point out these complications with thrombosis. I have seen in my visits to South America where people have employed furosemide to treat nephrotic edema, I have seen a couple of patients who developed arterial femoral thrombosis. One child having minimal change nephrotic syndrome had to be amputated because of these complications. Therefore, I would say that the use of furosemide or any one of these potent diuretics in patients with hypovolemia should be contraindicated. After using volume expanders like albumin, I haven't seen and I don't know about any complications. That is one of the reasons we were choosing in those rare cases in which it is necessary to get rid of the edema, to start using albumin. After that, we can use albumin or mannitol and after that use the diuretic. I haven't seen this sort of complication after albumin. I have not seen what was presented as a contraindication; that is, bleeding of the patient that had a renal biopsy. I think that that may happen not because of the albumin infusion but because the time elapsed from the moment the biopsy was done and the moment that they started to bleed. There are two points of danger after renal biopsy. One is during the first hours because of the direct lesion, and second, when the clot is going out. So, it happens about the fourth or fifth day after biopsy. I wonder if that was the case but then we don't have to implicate the albumin infusion. Now, it's better if you have to get rid of the edema, to do this before doing the renal biopsy and then you can have better results from the biopsy because if not, you will have a lot of edema in the biopsy sample. The other contraindication to the albumin infusion that was listed was focal and segmental sclerosis nephrotic syndrome. Well, it happens to be in those cases when we need to get rid of the edema because those are cases in which edema--for some reason which I don't know and I haven't seen an explanation--is more severe; and they get infected more often. These are probably the cases in which we need most to do this combination. So, I don't see this as a contraindication. Maybe these are the cases in which we have to get used to these pharmacologic tools to get rid of the edema.

COMMENT: I would like to comment on this concept. The question first of the albumin use alone or with furosemide has been raised. It is in fact well known that just with albumin infusion you can get an effect but it's not as good as if you add, following the expansion, a loop action diuretic such as furosemide. In fact, what we have observed in certain patients is that we have very good results in the initial infusion but after we continue, the second or third infusion in the same patient, we do not obtain the same results, even if the patient remains severely edematous. We have raised the possibility in those cases that by giving albumin we are in a way producing more leakage of albumin and therefore, increase further the colloid oncotic pressure of the interstitial fluid. This worsens the fluid trapping phenomenon. It has been shown in nephrotics that, if you can increase serum albumin by 30 or 50%, the main albumin pool will be extravascular. So that is a problem. The question of thrombosis, the risk of thrombosis: I reviewed thoroughly the literature published about thrombosis and the nephrotic syndrome. I could not find a single entity where there was a direct relationship with the use of albumin infusion associated with Lasix. The problem in the analysis of this information about thrombosis and nephrotic syndrome is that many variables are involved. They include: 1) the so-called hyper-coagulable state; 2) the excretion of a certain substance that would favor thrombosis has been recently described; 3) the large excretion in the urine of these patients of beta-2 thromboglobulin or antithrombin three which are factors that prevent the normal intravascular clotting mechanism; 4) other. To add another point, with mannitol it has been shown that there is improvement in circulation; it produces vascular dilatation. So, if it's used with caution, I don't think you should have those complications. In terms of biopsy and the explanation given, I agree. We had bleeding in a couple of patients in whom the albumin was used within 24 hours after the biopsy. We observed acute kidney pain and gross hematuria in a patient who did not have it before. The problem with focal segmental sclerosis is not settled. I only raised the question. It's just the type of patient where we are obligated to do something else besides prednisone. One distinguished group reported about 25 children with NS in whom they had used albumin infusion. Approximately 25% of those patients had an increase in serum creatinine; only in those with focal segmental sclerosis the elevated serum creatinine persisted with a further deterioration in renal function. I don't know the significance but I was thinking of the hypothesis about the overload of the mesangium in patients with proteinuria. By producing this artificially increased proteinuria, I wonder what effect we are having in those patients' glomeruli.

MODERATOR: The other question that has been alluded to, I would like to have it clarified even further, if at all possible. What about adding furosemide to the albumin infusion? It was stated that it was not needed and that whenever albumin has been given alone, enough diuresis was obtained and therefore, that an unnecessary risk was being created. Would you agree that that is the wrong thing to do or would you endorse that concept? We feel, as was mentioned, that albumin alone does not induce an adequate diuresis. And we feel, as was also mentioned, that if we proceed with the administration of furosemide after the albumin infusion or by another suitable volume expander, we are protecting the patient. Would you like to comment further on your approach to this problem?

COMMENT: Nowadays there is not such an entity as the resistant or the protracted edema. We can get rid of that in almost 100% of cases with severe edema. These are not ordinary cases so what we do is not a routine therapy. I have used in a patient, for instance, acetazolamide, mannitol infusion, mercurial diuretics and furosemide; I got rid of a very severe edematous state. But, I wouldn't do it in the next patient. Maybe once it was necessary, so we did it. These are individual patients and they require individual treatments. What I would prefer to do is to use just one agent. If it doesn't work, then I use the second agent. If it doesn't work, then I make some scheme with some diuretic that may be a volume expander and then a diuretic that works in the proximal tubule and then a diuretic that works in the loop of Henle or in the distal tubule. So, we have all these possibilities but these are for particular, very individualized treatments.

MODERATOR: Do you start with albumin alone?

RESPONSE: In the nephrotic syndrome, if it is very necessary, yes, I use it. But it is only in rare cases that I need it.

MODERATOR: Most frequently you use from the very beginning albumin plus a diuretic?

RESPONSE: No, I use albumin most times alone, but then some other times I use those other agents. I monitor all the infusions by means of the blood pressure and the blood hematocrit.

RESPONSE: We always give albumin and furosemide but I have no data to show that furosemide is needed. I'm not sure that we've done a study using albumin alone to see if it was effective. I'm sure we have given albumin alone to some patients in whom it was not effective; therefore, we added furosemide. Now albumin and furosemide is the standard therapy in our center.

MODERATOR: We have this study that was presented today. We could expand it to include albumin alone and compare the results with those obtained after using furosemide after albumin or mannitol.

COMMENT: I agree that there has been no convincing demonstration that there is any relationship between thrombosis and diuretic therapy. I've never seen any thrombosis and I have used a lot of diuretics. There aren't any reports that have been convincing in that regard since there are multiple things going on. It would be wrong to conclude that a diuretic was implicated. Let me say a word about the notion that there is a child with edema refractory to the usual pharmacotherapy. We've looked at this more critically recently. Over the years we also had been agressive in using albumin along with furosemide, knowing full well that its effect was supposed to be short lived, that the infused albumin was 100% recovered in the urine of the following 24-36 hours. So, its effect as a volume expander, therefore its effect as an adjunct to a diuretic, was really relatively short lived. For longer term management or to be given to an outpatient, it really was not a contribution to the pharmacologic approach to edema. There is some data in the pharmacology literature on this, and it's my understanding that for furosemide to be effective as a diuretic, it has to be delivered to the Loop of Henle's lumen and then interact with receptors. Furosemide is filtered to some extent but not greatly because it is protein bound. To a large extent it arrives in the distal tubule by virtue of proximal secretory process. There are data in nephrotics suggesting that one of the major problems in delivering enough free unbound drug is the fact that albumin is extensively filtered. It's present in the lumen, and therefore, rendering very little of the total amount available in free form. I can see where infusions of albumin would perhaps complicate the matter, especially with the knowledge that with repeated infusions it became increasingly difficult to achieve a diuresis. My experience more recently is that I have rarely found a patient who is truly refractory to just treatment with furosemide alone. For that reason, in recent years I have not used albumin at all. We tend to use furosemide along with spironolactone frequently. What we find is that we have to escalate the dose tremendously. Apparently this will provide enough free drug if the patient gets a high enough dose - enough free drug is delivered despite the filtration of albumin as well to the distal site. So, I think it's a question of dose, really. You do have to get into dosages that are well above those ordinarily used. We have used 500-600 mg/day of furosemide.

MODERATOR: You haven't had any complications from using just furosemide and at those doses?

RESPONSE: I haven't seen any yet, no. There is an occasional patient in whom we still are unable to get a very effective diuresis. We have had good luck with another diuretic, Natolozone, which has some of the proximal action as well. In combination with that I have yet in recent years to encounter a refractory patient and really have abandoned using albumin at all.

The other comment I wanted to make was related to the matter of a patient having problems with a very rigorous diuresis and going into hypovolemia, a hypovolemic crisis and so forth or acute renal failure after rigorous diuretic treatment. I should add parenthetically, the assumption we make about plasma volume in nephrotics is not borne out entirely in the literature. As one surveys the literature, there are very conflicting results as to what plasma volume means in nephrotics. They are not all "hypovolemic". In any case I have never seen a nephrotic have bad problems or go into shock with rigorous diuresis with the exception of some minimal lesion nephrotics in whom it happened in a few instances when we forgot to stop the furosemide. As they went into remission with prednisone, they then had a prednisone-induced remission concurrent with a pharmacologic type of diuresis due to furosemide; as they went into remission they just continued to diurese and diurese and got very dry. It's our practice now to stop pharmacologic agents in a child whose remission is imminent. When the urine protein is down to 2+ or so, we stop the furosemide at that point and allow the prednisone induced remission to proceed.

COMMENT: When we talk about complications, specific problems from complications, we think about the evident ones. What about the silent ones? We can have a patient with long-standing nephrotic syndrome, long-standing edema especially due to membranous nephropathy, to whom we give furosemide, and we feel happy. But, do we do a routine cavogram on these patients to see whether or not there is a renal vein thrombosis?

COMMENT: I think there have been very few studies done in a prospective way with this aspect. One was just recently published with the review of approximately 150 nephrotic patients who were followed prospectively. In many of them there was a baseline evaluation including venocavogram. What they found was development, in about 20% at one point or another, of renal vein thrombosis. They make the interesting point that the great majority of these renal vein thromboses were sort of silent, as you were saying-- not the acute, typical symptoms with flank pain, hematuria, hypertension, etc. So, this was detected just because these patients were followed in a prospective way. In 2/3 of the cases, the cause of the nephrotic syndrome was membranous nephropathy-- a well-known association. I think that what you said is true. We don't have the data; but, what is the cause-effect relationship? Is it a hypercoagulable state, corticosteroids, hypovolemia, or is it the diuretic treatment?

MODERATOR: What about the question as to whether or not the thrombosis may have preceeded the membranous nephropathy? As I recall there were some papers suggesting that the thrombosis may have produced the membranous nephropathy. Can we regard that subject closed?

COMMENT: The consensus among nephrologists as far as that particular matter is concerned as I understand, is that membranous nephropathy preceeds the thrombosis. Renal vein thrombosis can be found by means of a venocavogram, etc., and that practically in all instances, as you mentioned, it's of no significance, it's just a curiosity. It does not cause problems.

QUESTION: Changing the subject, is there any real advantage in using the more specific beta-blockers in general and in some particular situations?

RESPONSE: I don't know. The beta-one, beta-two selective blockers, I have no personal experience with; I don't know. I think that a recent review shed some doubt on the validity of selective beta-one, beta-two blockade. I have no experience and I am not a pharmacologist. I think they said that high enough doses of beta-one blockers block beta-two,and beta-two blockers block beta-one; it was a dose related phenomenon. I can't answer your question more specifically than that.

COMMENT: If we stay now on the subject of hypertension, I think this question just opened such discussion. When Captopril becomes available to you, how would you fit it in a scheme of decision making as to which drug should be used for each situation?

RESPONSE: I think its obvious use would be in patients with either renal artery stenosis who have very high renin levels or in the ten percent of renal failure patients who have very high levels. In those patients, it could even be the initial drug to be used just like propranolol. As far as the high renin and essential hypertensives,I have to defer that to my colleague. I would think, from my experience, that it would be relatively limited to the patients who have high renin levels.

COMMENT: If I may, I would like to ask the members of the panel if they care to postulate an explanation for the fact that a definite percentage of patients with proven minimal change nephrotic syndrome at the onset have hypertension?

RESPONSE: I have often wondered about that also. I've pondered over that for many hours unsuccessfully. Obviously, when they are volume depleted they are going to be poorly perfusing their kidneys and turn on renin. Then, renin raises blood pressure but as a compensatory mechanism because they are hypotensive in the first place. Rarely do compensatory mechanisms overshoot. So, blood pressure should be just raised up towards normal by that mechanism;so why patients are hypertensive with nephrosis, a small percentage, I don't know.

MODERATOR: How often do you see that? What would be the guess of the panelists as to how often they see hypertension in their own practice? We don't see, practically ever, hypertension in our nephrotic patients.

Whenever we see it, we get concerned and look for an explanation as happened recently with a patient who came from Curacao. We evaluated the patient, thinking that she may have a glomerulopathy other than minimal change but we did not find it. The biopsy revealed normal glomeruli without proliferation of any cells and without deposits. The figure of up to 25% was quoted in the literature; this was surprising to us. Would you comment on that?

COMMENT: I have seen with certain frequency this hypertension at the beginning of the nephrotic syndrome when they are very edematous. This is a very transient hypertension and not very severe. As far as I know, nobody has found the mechanism involved in these cases. This hypertension subsides almost at the same time that the edema decreases. It never has been of any clinical importance.

MODERATOR: Would you call that a nephritic component? In other words, do you find any other indicator of a nephritic component added to a nephrotic syndrome, a mixed picture? It's just a transient hypertension which usually is mild and does not require treatment?

RESPONSE: Right. I'm referring to those cases in which there is no nephritic component; the ordinary nephrotic syndrome with some mild hypertension, very transient, but not with other components.

MODERATOR: I raised that question on purpose because in that particular patient, presented at our Grand Rounds, the statements were made that this would be called a "nephritic component" and we did not agree with this. For the record, I wanted to have that point clarified.

QUESTION: We have seen patients with hemolytic uremic syndrome with a very persistent and resistant hypertension. We found in these children high renin plus very increased uric acid. How would you treat these patients?

RESPONSE: First of all I would like to expand on it. I agree. I think hemolytic uremic syndrome is the renal disease which has the highest incidence and the highest levels of elevated blood pressure. The boy I showed on dialysis who required bilateral nephrectomy had hemolytic uremic syndrome. I think a renin-suppressing drug makes sense. Propranolol is a fairly effective drug, suppressing renin and lowering blood pressure, but it is not tremendously effective in patients with really high renin levels and really high blood pressure. Captopril would certainly be the drug to use but it's not available to you. So, we go back to nonspecific therapy. If I had tried the other drugs and they didn't work, I would use Minoxidil alone or in combination with propranolol and a diuretic.

MODERATOR: I would like to ask you to give us your own approach to the management of hypertension in patients who are on dialysis --without telling us that you are doing the best or the most logical thing. It would be interesting to us to know how you actually manage those situations.

RESPONSE: To begin with, we often do measurements of extracellular fluid volume from bromide space to try to get some idea of dry weight but I don't think that's necessary to do. I think your dry weight is really a clinical determination which the nurses know as well or better than I do. We do the same thing that probably everyone else does. We limit salt intake. Our standard is no added salt diet which comes out to be 2-3 grams of sodium. We usually do not limit water intake because we feel that water usually goes with sodium and if they don't take in sodium, they won't take in water. Patients with high renin may be an exception because renin has a direct effect on the thirst mechanism of the brain to stimulate to drink water. In that case water restriction may be necessary but in more than 90% of patients, salt restriction alone is necessary. Then we do ultrafiltration. We try to get a maximum ultrafiltration during dialysis. That's a bag of worms. We sometimes use the method with pure ultrafiltration for the first hour and then solute removal for the next three hours. That has not been tremendously successful in our hands. Maybe we just haven't perfected it enough. Then many of the patients, despite salt restriction, despite ultrafiltration during dialysis, do require anti-hypertensive medicines. Those are the ones we have talked about already. We always withhold the last dose of the drug so that the patients don't receive any on the morning of dialysis. We want the blood pressure to be fairly high when going into dialysis so that it will be supported while we filter and take off the excess fluid which is the cause of the hypertension in the first place. So, just to reiterate: salt restriction, ultrafiltration, and anti-hypertensive drugs but no drug the morning of dialysis.

MODERATOR: Do you have a drug that you prefer to use in those patients because of the ease of dialysis removal or because of the lack of complications? Do you know of antihypertensive drugs that you would stay away from because of the fact that they are not dialyzable or will facilitate the occurrence of hypotension or other problems?

RESPONSE: I think hydralazine is a fairly short-acting drug so if you don't give any hydralazine the morning of dialysis, give them the last dose the previous evening,that drug will be gone by the time of the hemodialysis. So, that's a good drug to use because you don't want the drug effect during dialysis. Methyldopa is a longer acting drug so, to that extent, hydralazine probably is a better drug to give to dialysis patients than methyldopa is. In practice, however, we use methyldopa, hydralazine, and of course, propranolol especially in patients who have high renin levels.

MODERATOR: Does anybody want to add a comment? Basically, we follow similar approaches and try to use hydralazine (Apresoline) as much as possible. Regarding hydralazine, you did recommend rather high dosages; we have used these doses at times and have not found any problems. At the same time, the clinical pharmacologists have warned us that they have seen myocardial infarctions in patients with tachycardia and who receive hydralazine in high doses. Do you have any word of caution? Have you seen that complication? If you started with a patient with tachycardia, would you use hydralazine, or hydralazine plus propranolol, or hydralazine plus reserpine, or no hydralazine?

RESPONSE: First of all I would like to say something which maybe I didn't stress enough earlier. That is that as a nephrologist, most of the patients I see with hypertension have very severe hypertension and I use high doses of drugs. Some of the doses I use certainly are higher than you would use in practice with patients who have mild hypertension. I just don't see mild hypertension, unfortunately. I have not seen any of those complications with hydralazine. It just gets back to the fact that in pediatrics we are lucky that we are dealing with children with good cardiovascular systems who don't have atheromata and who are not prone to myocardial thromboses. I think that that certainly is a word of caution which we should take and think about, even though in pediatrics it is not a problem. Have they seen it in children or was it in adults?

MODERATOR: I believe that they saw it in older children around ten or teenagers. But, those are sometimes comments not well documented; still, it has remained as a worry in my mind-- something that we may need to keep as a possibility. Therefore, my approach is, whenever we have a patient with tachycardia, administer small doses and maybe add propranolol or reserpine before we increase the hydralazine dose.

RESPONSE: Yes, I would definitely add propranolol. I have no experience with reserpine.

MODERATOR: Any other comments?

QUESTION: Is there any practical way to assess total exchangeable sodium? Another question related to that, you reported three or six patients who had high renin and high extracellular fluid volume. What is your approach to those patients?

RESPONSE: First, of course total exchangeable sodium has to be measured by using radioisotopes, which we don't like to do in children. Bromide space should yield somewhat similar information. However, there is evidence that bromide does permeate somewhat in the cells in patients with renal failure. People who have shown that, have some doubts on using the bromide space in patients with renal failure. In that case, how one should assess volume status is a little bit unclear. Patients could have both renin dependent hypertension and volume dependent hypertension. If they are massively overloaded with fluid, I think it behooves you to take off fluid and the blood pressure will come down. You may reach a certain point where they have come down from a very volume-expanded stage to a normal volume stage. In a small percentage of patients with high renin, if you lower their volume a little bit more than that, you may precipitate hypertension. It's hard to know when you are going to get to that state. But that is a very unusual occurrence. In most patients with high renin and expanded volume, it is appropriate to ultrafiltrate and take off volume. Only a few patients in a few specific circumstances ever get an overshoot of blood pressure.

MODERATOR: In terms of the management of the hypertensive emergency, you mentioned two drugs which most of us use, namely, diazoxide and sodium nitroprusside. I would like to ask you about your experience with diazoxide and its use not as a bolus injection but as a continuous drip. We have had some experience, occasionally even before the drug was approved for clinical use, and had no problems except that of sodium retention. Since then some occasional comments, brief reports have appeared here and there. I would like to know your thoughts on that. Regarding sodium nitroprusside, would you be kind enough to comment on the combined use of sodium nitroprusside for several days and dialysis; we proposed the latter to remove fluid and the metabolic products of nitroprusside.

RESPONSE: I have no experience with slow drip diazoxide so I would have to rely on the literature. You know better than I do. I cannot comment on that.

MODERATOR: You do not foresee any real problems if diuretics were to be added to counter the sodium-retaining properties of diazoxide-- just empirically.

RESPONSE: No, not in general. I think, as we mentioned before, there have certainly been reported cases of severe hypotension from diazoxide since it's such an effective drug. If you happened to be giving a lot of furosemide, you might get into that problem more often. But again, a severe hypotension is pretty rare. Usually we are still trying to get the blood pressure down to normal; we are not worrying about overshooting to get hypotension. I wouldn't think empirically that a diuretic should be used.

MODERATOR: That is the rationale we followed for the drip-- that we could control the situation better than giving a fixed dose. Once the bolus injection is in the circulation, you have no way of retrieving it. What about dialysis and sodium nitroprusside?

RESPONSE: You are doing the dialysis to get off the metabolites of nitroprusside. Is that right?

MODERATOR: And to help in the management of the hypertension. This was a very severe problem --a patient who had uncontrollable hypertension and was barely manageable with sodium nitroprusside. We basically started to remove the metabolic products but in the process, accomplished the other goal which also was very desirable - the removal of fluid and with that, control of the hypertension.

RESPONSE: I would think that that would be a very unusual circumstance because, as we mentioned before, more frequently than not, in hypertensive patients on hemodialysis, you try to keep them a little bit hypertensive so you can remove the fluid. In fact, some people even give pressor drugs during dialysis to increase blood pressure so they can remove the excess fluid. I think it would have to be an awfully hypertensive patient that would withstand both pharmacological reduction of hypertension and fluid removal during dialysis at the same time and be able to sustain the blood pressure enough so that you could remove fluid. I think that your patient must have been an awfully hypertensive, sick patient.

MODERATOR: Yes. The patient had a cardiac arrest and so on and was really a challenge. If I may take the last few minutes, what about the point you just made about maintaining blood pressure in patients from whom you need to remove fluids. Do you have any approach that you would recommend to be followed? We attempted at one time to do that with various drugs and had the rather horrifying experience of the coils exploding--we were using coils at that time--when we were maintaining artificially high blood pressure. The patient had severe bleeding and cardiovascular problems but fortunately he proceeded to do well. Do you have any approaches or words of caution on that?

RESPONSE: I don't think we do anything substantively different from anyone else. We have not used any vasopressors to maintain pressure while we take off fluid. Occasionally, in patients who were hypoalbuminemic we would infuse a vial or two of serum albumin during dialysis to try to pull fluid from the interstitial to the intravascular spaces and then be able to take it off with the dialyzer. Of course, patients who need a transfusion, on the day that you give the transfusion, you are sustaining their circulation by that method. Then you can crank up your negative pressure and take off a lot more fluid on those days. So, those are little tricks you can occasionally use but you are not going to give a patient a transfusion every day so you can take off more fluid.

MODERATOR: Based on that very bad experience we had and other attempts in that same patient, I think that we all here would agree that the use of hypertensive drugs would not be desirable. At that time we were having quite a bit of hypertension in our patients. Would any one of our group like to mention the type of approach we have followed so successfully in the recent past?

RESPONSE: Maybe we are more careful in assessing the transmembrane pressure required by a certain patient. The speed, how we try to get that ultrafiltration pressure probably is another variable. Certain patients don't tolerate going too rapidly to the expected or calculated ultrafiltration pressure. They drop their blood pressure and then the blood pressure is more difficult to control. We have also changed, practically moving all the patients to the hollow fiber type of dialyzer that has less compliance and therefore, we can control better the variables of dialysis than with the coil or the parallel plate dialyzers. We have not been requiring any vasopressor drugs.

QUESTION: Have you had to use much hypertonic saline?

RESPONSE: We don't use nowadays 5% or 15% saline. All we tend to do really in those patients is just as you commented; we use ultrafiltration for the first hour and then clearance by regular hemodialysis. Occasionally we infuse albumin in hypoalbuminemic patients.

COMMENT: Raising the sodium content of the bath may help the hypotensive patient.

MODERATOR: Is that agreeable?

RESPONSE: I haven't done it but I have heard other people say the same thing.

MODERATOR: Thanks to the panel and to the hearty registrants who have participated to the end. With this, we conclude Pediatric Nephrology Seminar VIII.

V

WORKSHOP

WORKSHOP: CLINICO-PATHOLOGICAL CORRELATIONS

José Strauss, M.D., Moderator

MODERATOR: We have four cases for your consideration, and will appreciate as much audience participation as possible. We also have a set of distinguished presentors. We shall start with Dr. Michael Freundlich who is a member of the Division of Pediatric Nephrology at the University of Miami School of Medicine. He is Clinical Assistant Professor of Pediatrics and will present the first case. This case will be discussed by Dr. Victoriano Pardo who is Professor of Pathology and Director of the Electronmicroscopy Laboratory at the Veterans Administration Medical Center.

DR. FREUNDLICH: The first case is a 13 year old girl with an initial complaint of vomiting and diarrhea for several days and a sore throat for two weeks. She was given a one week course of ampicillin. She had no urine output for the 24-hours prior to admission. On the initial P.E., she was an obese female with no acute signs of dehydration; the thyroid was symmetrically enlarged. The heart rate was regular with a II/VI systolic murmur at the apex. The rest of the P.E. was normal. It is not known if she had any urinalysis prior to the admission one and the past history was unremarkable. The initial laboratory data were as follows: U/A: 3+ protein, 3+ blood, pH 6, SG 1035, 100 WBC's, 10-25 RBC's, 3-8 granular casts and 2-6 hyaline casts. Hb 12.3 g/dl, Hct 25%, Na^+ 136 mEq/L, K^+ 2.2 mEq/L, Cl 96 mEq/L, CO_2 25 mm/L, Anion Gap 15 mEq/L, BUN 40 mg/dl, serum creatinine 2.4 mg/dl, ESR 30 mm/hr, ASO 500 U throat culture negative for streptococcus, ANA and CRP both negative. Stool culture negative. C'3 90 mg/dl, C'4 31 mg/dl. Repeated ASO 10 days after admission was 1250 U Parameters of thyroid hormone activity indicated overt hyperthyroidism. Monospot, hepatitis B surface antigen and PPD were negative. During the first two weeks of hospitalization her clinical course was complicated by: protracted hypertension predominantly systolic, premature ventricular contractions, hyponatremia of 125-131 mEq/L range (with concomitant low urine-sodium concentration of 10 mEq/L), hypokalemia in the 2.5 mEq/L range (with UK^+ of 25 mEq/L) and marked azotemia with BUN climbing to 198 mg/dl with a concomitant serum creatinine value of 1.5 mg/dl and oliguria. Additional lab data included: albumin 2.8 g/dl, antithyroid antibodies negative, Ca 7.4 mg/dl, P 4.6 mg/dl, daily protein excretion 1.6 gm, blood volume determination by Cr^{51} and I^{125} injection was normal 1 month after admission. She was treated with propranolol, propylthiouracil as well as dopamine infusion at the rate of 2 μg/kg/minute to try to improve renal blood flow.

The patient progressively improved, urine output increased, and the BUN and serum K^+ levels returned to normal limits. The dose of propranolol required to control her hypertension was 40 mg QID and the propylthiouracil was kept at 100 mg BID.

A percutaneous renal biopsy was performed 5 weeks after admission. It revealed a picture of membrano-proliferative glomerulonephritis. The patient was discharged from the hospital after a 6 weeks stay in good general condition, with mild edema and controlled hypertension, with BUN of 30 mg/dl and creatinine of 0.7 mg/dl.

DR. PARDO: Figure 1 is the light microscopy of the biopsy, a representative glomerulus. In the glomeruli it is difficult to see clear features. The first impression is that there is a lot of proliferation and occasionally one can see that the mesangial areas are prominent with the loops hanging outside. In another portion of the glomerulus there is quite a marked intracapillary proliferation. There is no interstitial fibrosis or tubular atrophy. There is a splitting of the basement membrane. The whole picture is a bit confusing because there is also a lot of "train track" appearance. That is, there are some transverse anastomoses between the parallel lines of the basement membrane. The appearance is consistent with a mesangiocapillary process.

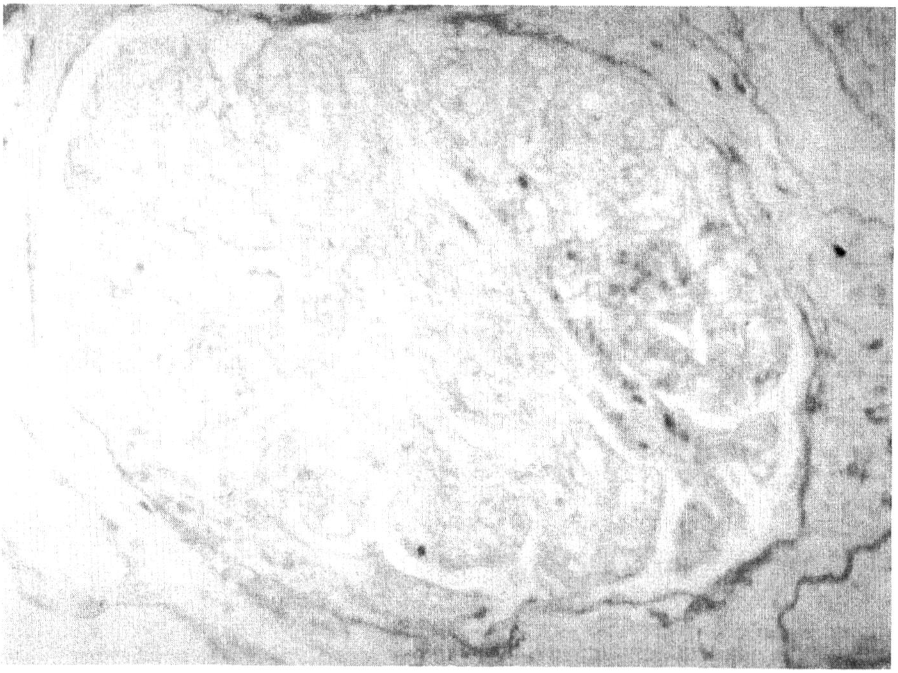

FIGURE 1

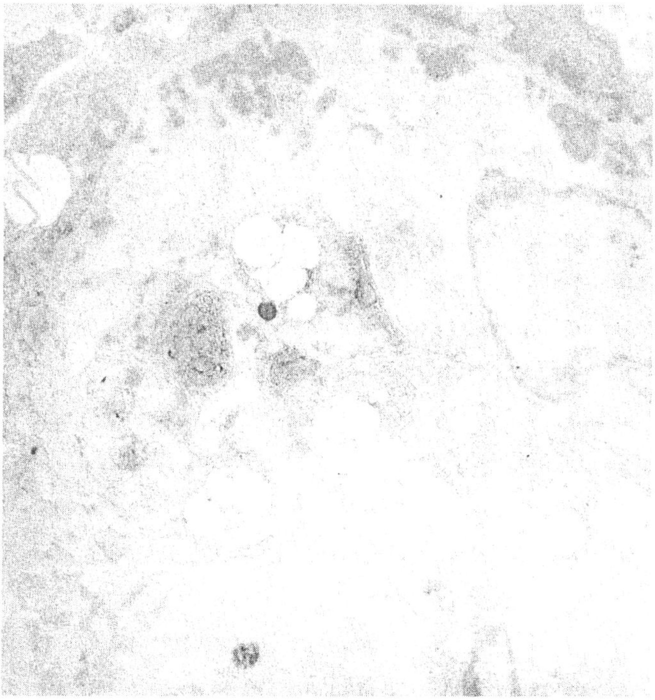

FIGURE 2

Figure 2 is the electron microscopy of the glomerulus that we selected. It is not the best for identification of the membrano-proliferative or mesangiocapillary features because there is a lot of intracapillary proliferation also. There are some foam cells and one can see some subendothelial and some subepithelial deposits; some of the latter appear to be a little bit transparent and give the appearance of membranous changes, that some of the deposits are being reabsorbed. On higher magnification we saw that the deposits are subendothelial and subepithelial.

There was not a lot of immunofluorescent material. There was mainly IgG and C'3 deposited in the peripheral loops. I believe this appearance does not correspond to any of the classical mesangiocapillary glomerulonephritis: type one that has subendothelial deposits or type two with intramembranous dense deposits. This appears to be a type three or mixed type variety, a combination of membranous and mesangio-capillary diseases, in the manner described by Burkholder. It doesn't correspond with the type three described by others.

MODERATOR: Any questions for Drs. Freundlich or Pardo regarding the history or the biopsy?

QUESTION: Were there any polymorphonuclear leukocytes? Any exhudation at all on the microscopy slides?

RESPONSE: There were a few but they were not dominant. I would not say that there was a clear-cut exudative component.

QUESTION: Could you please clarify when you say it was not a typical type three, what do you mean?

RESPONSE: Yes. The type with fragmentation of the basement membrane or rupture of the basement membrane.

QUESTION: Are there any features of the biopsy that would make you think that it is a post-infectious glomerulonephritis?

RESPONSE: That's a very good question. I always have lots of problems differentiating acute post-infectious and membranoproliferative or mesangiocapillary glomerulonephritis. Some of the pictures that other authors show as mesangiocapillary, for example, I would diagnose as post-infectious. The Mexicans have numerous cases of post-infectious glomerulonephritis that go into mesangiocapillary changes. That's a very difficult diagnosis.

MODERATOR: There is a Mexican at this Seminar. Maybe he would like to comment on that point; any other point he may want to make would be welcomed.

RESPONSE: I was disappointed with the preparation. I wanted to look at something more clear. It's not clear for post-streptococcal glomerulonephritis or for membranoproliferative. Then, I was expecting tc see something in the immunofluorescence since it is so important, but it was very, very poor. From the clinical point of view, it doesn't seem to me that this is a mesangiocapillary glomerulonephritis because I haven't seen such a case starting in that way with acute renal failure. Of course, here we have a component of diarrhea, vomiting, and dehydration, all of which raise the question if this is a functional oliguria or is this Acute Renal Failure. Anyway, the results of the biopsy confused me. I would rather prefer to think in terms of acute glomerulonephritis, the usual type, but...I am confused because of the results.

MODERATOR: Did you mean that the preparation was not clear or you thought that the results were not right for a diagnosis? Would you have wanted to see more findings or a different stain or a different preparation?

RESPONSE: It's the same. If you don't see clear findings you cannot give a clear diagnosis.

MODERATOR: But when you said that the immunofluorescence was "poor", what did you mean?

RESPONSE: Well, I cannot see deposits in the immunofluorescence; I don't know why.

DR. PARDO: I want to clarify the "poor" point. There were not many deposits but the deposits, I believe, are there. The reason why we take pictures on all our cases is because then we can review them. I would say there is a minimum amount of deposits but they are there. We can dim the lights and we will see them. Concerning the problem of mesangiocapillary glomerulonephritis, I believe we all agree it is a histologic diagnosis and the clinical manifestations may vary a lot. You have our cases of sickle cell anemia that show a histologic picture that is typically a mesangiocapillary type one but the clinical manifestations are completely different. If I try to make a diagnosis of mesangiocapillary just on the basis of the clinical presentation, I would be lost. I would agree, it is a very difficult diagnosis. We experienced this when we reviewed our cases of sickle cell anemia. Some of these patients have intercurrent, acute post-infectious glomerulonephritis. In the biopsies sometimes you see acute post-infectious nephritis with peripheral mesangial extension and it looks like mesangiocapillary. It may be a very difficult diagnosis. At least tentatively my working diagnosis would be mesangiocapillary glomerulopathy of the variety that is not clear, the type three, because it has membranous features. Now if you want to call it in some other way, I would agree but we have to have a common ground for discussion.

MODERATOR: Before we leave that subject. Histologically, would you agree that it is mesangiocapillary or would you say that the clinical part is not correct? Would you clarify that for us, please?

RESPONSE: The clinical part doesn't fit very well but when you don't have a very clear clinical pattern, if you have a clear histo-pathological pattern then you can make the diagnosis. If you don't have a clear histo-pathological pattern, then it's very confusing.

COMMENT: It's interesting to comment on the urine specific gravity of 1035 in that a high specific gravity is characteristically described as occurring in post-infectious nephritis, for whatever value that might have. I do not know what the specific gravity is in the acute exacerbation of membranoproliferative nephritis.

MODERATOR: With protein in the urine, right?

RESPONSE: With protein in the urine. The other comment would be something about the complement. If this is indeed membranoproliferative nephritis, the serum complements that we have here are normal. Of course, somewhere between 10 and 20% of cases do have normocomplementemia and the question that would arise is what has happened to these complement levels six weeks, 12 weeks, later on.

MODERATOR: Again, it's important that we clarify that Dr. Pardo, Dr. McIntosh, and myself among the original groups described a membranoproliferative histological picture in patients with sickle cell anemia and also in a patient with sickle cell trait who were not hypocomplementemic. So it's important to separate the clinical from the histological picture. This is the reason why I was asking the clarification. Dr. Freundlich, can you tell us whether we have repeated the complements?

RESPONSE: Yes, and they are about the same.

MODERATOR: Complements are unchanged.

COMMENT: To my mind this is not a typical MPGN. Did you do silver impregnated electron microscopy?

RESPONSE: No.

COMMENT: Some authors seem to use that as a criterion for defining type III MPGN. In other laboratories who don't do it, it becomes a somewhat nebulous issue.

RESPONSE: I was referring to a different type III membranoproliferative GN. This doesn't seem to be it. There are some features of membranous GN in some loops. Therefore, this is eliminated without silver impregnation.

COMMENT: It's clearly not type one or two, either. This individual has a number of atypical features which are hard to explain--curious hypokalemia and there seems to be a rather profound dissociation of BUN and serum creatinine at one point, which is a curiosity but which I don't think has much bearing on what the patient has. I believe that the patient has a primary renal disease. What is it, then? It doesn't seem to fit typical post-infectious GN. There are a few reports of immune complex disease associated with thyroid disease in which thyroid antibodies and antigens are demonstrable in the glomerulus. So, since she had clinical thyroid disease, I wonder if it is related to that. Despite the absence of certain antithyroid antibodies.

MODERATOR: Right. That was our concern or question also. Could hyperthyroidism be responsible for a hypercatabolic state where you have excessive losses of potassium and some of the other findings? But we never could really explain the clinical picture either. That's the reason we are presenting her here. If she were a simple case, she wouldn't be presented.

COMMENT: Is it possible that you can explain her hypokalemia on the basis of secondary hypermineralocorticoidism with vomiting and some other things going on?

MODERATOR: But of this severity? It was really very impressive! I forget the actual numbers involved but she received large amounts of potassium without her serum potassium being corrected.

COMMENT: If her urinary potassium was 25 mEq/L it should not have taken extraordinary amounts of potassium supplement to keep up with those losses. How high could her urinary losses have been?

RESPONSE: That was one of the confusing items we dealt with. She remained hypokalemic despite administration of large amounts of K^+. By large I mean up to 80 mEq/day. She remained with protracted oliguria and hypokalemia for two weeks (serum K^+ in the 2.3 - 2.4 mEq/L range). Another not very clear picture was that, despite her hypokalemia, the kaliuresis remained in the 25 mEq/L range. Not very appropriate for low serum potassium. We also were disturbed by the high BUN, out of proportion to the relatively modest elevation of serum creatinine. We couldn't find a clear cut explanation for it. But once urinary flow increased, probably related in some way to the relative better control of her hypertension and the infusion of dopamine, her urinary flow increased and her BUN rapidly decreased. So, we weren't very sure about what we were dealing with; but certainly, there were some atypical features,as you can appreciate.

QUESTION: Do you think you reversed her acute oliguria with dopamine?

RESPONSE: I don't know if that is the sole reason for the reversion. As I mentioned, she was started on propylthiouracil also for a couple of days before her urine output picked up. So, there were several events concurring chronologically, i.e. control of hypertension, propylthiouracil, large administration of potassium and dopamine. So, I don't know. She was very sick, very, very sick. Amazingly, she is doing beautifully now.

MODERATOR: We have time for two questions more. Short ones to be followed by short answers, please.

QUESTION: Was there any disagreement or discussion about proceeding with the renal biopsy when it was done? Did the potassium rise with the propranolol treatment?

RESPONSE: As a matter of fact, the decision about a renal biopsy was not an easy one for several reasons. First, we obviously would have loved to perform the renal biopsy at the height of her disease but we didn't do that for obvious reasons. She was extremely sick and she was very hypertensive. She was having PVC's constantly and she was overtly disequilibrated from a fluid and electrolyte point of view. So, we left our intellectual curiosity for a later date. Indeed, there was a lot of debate. Once her hypertension became under control and clinically she was more stable, we went ahead and did the biopsy.

QUESTION: What I really wanted to know is, was anybody of the opinion that renal biopsy was not necessary or that it was inappropriate at that time with good history and laboratory support for post-infectious glomerulonephritis?

RESPONSE: The only paraclinical evidence we had for post-streptococcal glomerulonephritis was the finding of a rising ASO titer. That was the only relatively clear-cut evidence for post-strep GN. For the rest, we didn't believe there was evidence for post-strep GN. It is known that high ASO titers, first of all, might be prevalent in a high percent of the population and, second, that it might certainly be associated with other nephropathies, causally or not. We didn't believe that the sole increase in the ASO titer would be conclusive for post-strep GN. Regarding the second question ("Did the potassium come up with the propranolol administration?"), as I said, with propranolol and high doses of K, dopamine and everything was instituted at once so I'm not sure that we can answer that question. Too many things (high doses of K^+, dopamine, etc.) were done to the patient at about the same time.

QUESTION: Is the serum potassium up now?

RESPONSE: Oh yes. It is normal now, but we cannot ascribe that to any treatment, either.

COMMENT: Regarding the biopsy, I think the usual game plan that most of us have is that if it is a typical post-infectious glomerulonephritis in which the acute signs reverse within the first week or so, a biopsy is completely unnecessary. But where there is persistence of oliguria or azotemia or some atypical features, many of us would do a biopsy.

MODERATOR: We have the unwritten rule of two weeks. Whenever there is symptomatology or abnormal blood findings (besides hypocomplementemia) for two weeks, we do a kidney biopsy. We biopsy all patients with so-called post-infectious glomerulonephritis who have normocomplementemia.

QUESTION: If this is a post-infectious glomerulonephritis nonstreptococcal would you not have expected to have a higher C_3 level? The C_3 level that we are seeing now is actually low.

RESPONSE: My experience with C_3 levels is, they don't have an extremely high precision in the sense of being variable and having a very broad latitude of normal range. Take a normal C_3 and put two standard deviations around it and I think it might be hard to discern whether it is clearly going up or going down.

MODERATOR: We must go to the next case now. Dr. Richard Zakheim is going to present this patient. He is director of the Division of Pediatric Cardiology at Variety Childrens Hospital in Miami. The histopathology is going to be presented and discussed by Dr. Juan Peyser who is Associate Pathologist at Variety.

DR. ZAKHEIM: This was a nine year old girl, referred from Costa Rica, an American girl whose parents were missionaries. The chief complaint was convulsions associated with hypertension which occurred two weeks prior to her admission to Variety Childrens Hospital. She had generalized tonic-clonic convulsions and it was noted during the episode, according to people at that time, that her blood pressure was 140/100 mm Hg. She had been complaining prior to admission and actually immediately preceeding the convulsions, of vomiting and headaches. Prior to that, she had been a perfectly healthy nine year old girl. There is no family history of hypertension. On admission her blood pressure was somewhat variable. Her diastolic was always at least 100 mm Hg; sometimes it hit pressures as high as 160/120 mm Hg. On admission, it was 140/100 mm Hg. Her weight was 46 pounds. Her height, 46 inches. She was alert, cooperative, in no distress. Her chest was clear. Examination of her heart was normal, femoral pulses were normal. Bruits over the abdomen and the flank were listened to carefully and there weren't any. The neurologic examination,aside from some weakness, was essentially normal. Her fundi to the neurologist appeared normal. There was certainly no papilledema. She had numerous laboratory values. Urinalysis: specific gravity varied on occasion but on admission was 1.003 (she had other ones with higher specific gravity); urine pH was not remarkable. Most of her urinalyses had no protein; an occasional casual urinalysis did have 1+ protein. On the Addis Count she had 1.6×10^6 RBC's and 8×10^5 WBC's/12 hrs. Her serum sodium was 134 mEq/L. Her potassiums were consistently low. She had several of them, some as low as 2.8 mEq/L. BUN was 15 mg/dl, creatinine 0.3 mg/dl, hemoglobin and white cell count were not remarkable. Urine cultures were negative. The electroencephalogram showed mild, nonspecific abnormalities. She was on phenobarbital when she came. She had a blood aldosterone level of 64 ng/100 ml (normal 4-31). She had two casual renins: one getting up first thing in the morning, and one after walking around for about four hours. The values were 51 ng/ml and 31 ng/ml. Intravenous pyelogram revealed a small right kidney. An arteriogram identified a right renal artery stenosis. At the time of the arteriogram she had renal vein renins done, the results of which are shown schematically in Figure 3.

It can be seen that the renal vein renins from the right kidney were consistently higher than the rest and following lasix, this difference was even more marked. Another interesting part of the clinical picture, she complained of weakness and this was relieved by potassium supplements. In addition, she received Inderal and Apresoline. After about a week in the hospital, she had a right nephrectomy performed following which her blood pressure over the next week gradually returned towards normal. The family subsequently moved to Salt Lake City, Utah. We spoke with them a couple of weeks ago to find out how the child is doing. She is doing fine and is off of all medications now. Her blood pressure is fine and her electroencephalogram is now back to normal.

FIGURE 3. Renal Vein Renins

QUESTION: What are the upper limits for renins in your hospital lab?

RESPONSE: Normal was 4.5. The blood was sent out to Bio-Science Laboratory.

QUESTION: Was a voiding cystourethrogram done?

RESPONSE: No, it wasn't done.

QUESTION: Was this a nephro-ureterectomy or just a nephrectomy?

RESPONSE: It was a nephrectomy as far as I know.

QUESTION: What did the chest X-ray show?

RESPONSE: She had left ventricular hypertrophy on the electrocardiogram and on her chest X-ray which I imagine indicated she had the hypertension for some time.

MODERATOR: Do we have any more questions about the clinical material or radiological aspects?

QUESTION: Was the opposite kidney large?

RESPONSE: Yes. It looked like it was twice the size of the right kidney, probably even larger than a normal kidney.

COMMENT: My reason for asking is that this is twice as large as that which you would expect if the patient had been born with a congenital small kidney on the opposite side. It may have a different implication as to what might be the etiology of the renal lesion in the small kidney. If the stenosis developed eight months before you saw the patient, you wouldn't expect the opposite kidney to be as large as in the unilateral congenitally small or absent kidney.

COMMENT: Was the creatinine clearance actually calculated? Because .3 mg/dl serum creatinine for a nine year old is a low value.

RESPONSE: As far as I know, a creatinine clearance wasn't done.

MODERATOR: Thank you, Dr. Zakheim. Now Dr. Juan Peyser will discuss the histopathology.

DR. PEYSER: This was *the* case for me. Through the entire process of going through the specimen for the histology, I learned, I learned. Maybe now we will learn more about it. The specimen that we received fresh was a kidney that measured .5 x 4 x 3 cm. There was attached a piece of renal artery that measured approximately 1.5 cm. After fixation, the surface had a kind of geographical pattern of retraction and discoloration, reddish in some places, yellow in others (Figure 4). The parenchyma, except for an area that was thinner in the cortex, appeared grossly to be normal. When we came to the section of the artery, there was a point in which there was an occlusion, a stenotic area that was practically with no lumen at inspection. We took sections

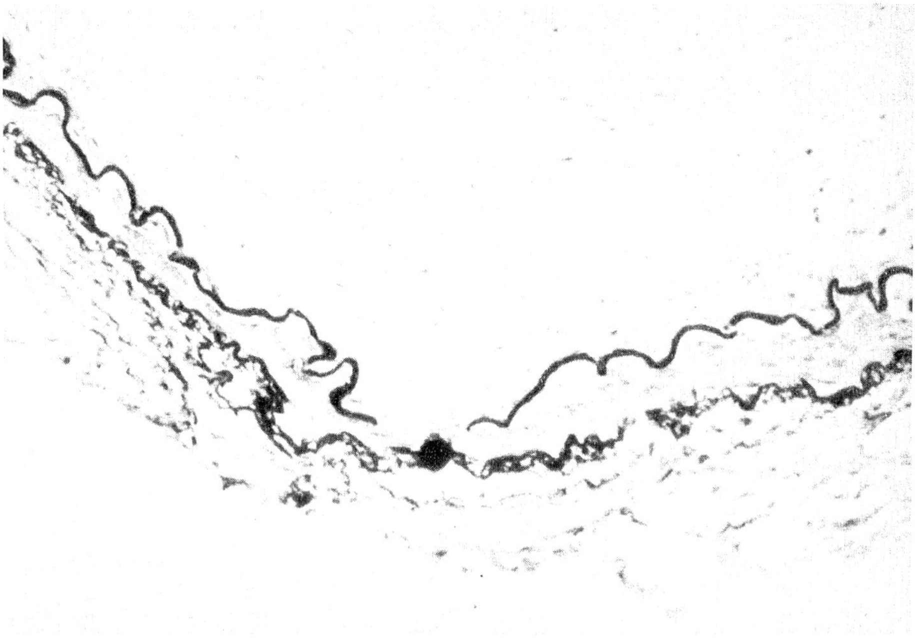

FIGURE 4

FIGURE 5

from this area; at low magnification, the lumen was almost completely occluded by proliferation of fibrous tissue that left a very little ring of lumen inside. Since some of this could have been an artifact from the formalin fixation, we obtained an elastic stain. It showed that the intima had a tremendous proliferation of fibrous tissue with some recanalization or vascularization. The media showed a kind of coiling and fragmentation of elastica. The intima, in addition to the proliferation, had a little focal area of mononuclear cell infiltrate, particularly lymphocytes. The internal lamina showed fragmentation. The parenchyma showed extensive areas in which there was a fibrous replacement particularly below the capsule with some degree of dilatation of blood vessels. The glomeruli were fairly preserved in the adjoining area (Figure 5). In the trichrome stain, we saw the well-delimited area in which there was fibrosis with some spared glomeruli. Another finding was the presence of areas of mononuclear cell infiltrate, lymphocytes and some histiocytes; this was present throughout the sections. Some glomeruli showed a type of fibrous capsule around them but with the glomeruli themselves preserved.

Essentially we considered this to be a problem of renal artery obstruction. A stenosis of the renal artery that was segmental, that did not repeat itself in other small arteries. It was the only lesion we could find. We dissected everything inside the parenchyma of the kidney trying to follow and see if this phenomenon repeated itself in other areas. This was not the case. Therefore, we concluded that the problem was displastic changes of the intima which, considering its histological location, we called Intimal Fibroplasia, primary type.

MODERATOR: Any questions?

QUESTION: I wonder if this is not a case of renal segmental hypoplasia. There are very definite changes in the parenchyma; there is a clear-cut separation of the area which is affected and the one which is preserved. In the area with the damage, the glomeruli are scarred and there are very clearly atrophic tubuli. This is what Renée Habib calls Renal Segmental Hypoplasia. Again, what was said before, the difference between the two kidneys was very, very striking. We have here a small kidney and the other is a big kidney. Of course, with the renal arterial stenosis we see a difference but this is a very striking difference. Ordinarily, with renal artery stenosis we do not see such a big difference in size. I looked in the X-rays, but I couldn't see any of the alterations in the renal contour like those we see in the kidney with segmental hypoplasia. I didn't see the scars but of course it was only one X-ray picture. So, from the histopathological point of view I think it is Renal Segmental Hypoplasia. It fits with the clinical picture also. I wonder if a voiding cysto-urethrogram (VCU) was done to see if there was vesico-ureteral reflux.

MODERATOR: Was a VCU done?

RESPONSE: One was done and there was no reflux.

DR. PEYSER: I would like to clarify one thing. From the point of view of the pathologist, the gross findings had the kind of lesion that you would expect in areas of infarct that are old in the sense that there was fibrosis, there was retraction, and they were triangular with the base to the capsule and the vertex to the artery. We thought of segmental hypoplasia but we ruled that out because we had a clear cut stenosis in the renal artery (that evidently is there and in no other place). We thought that this could explain the ischemic changes which happened in progressive form and what we found was the scar of the ischemic lesions. Dr. Pardo, do you have any opinion about that?

DR. PARDO: I saw the slides. I was thinking of the criteria for segmental hypoplasia that Habib has established. There are three main criteria: First, deformity of the papilla (not present here); second, thyroid appearance of the parenchyma (not present here); third, a mass of fibrous tissue with glomeruli very difficult to identify (not present here). So I don't think that, histopathologically, we can maintain the diagnosis of Renal Segmental Hypoplasia if we follow Habib's criteria.

QUESTION: Out of curiosity, were there any blood pressure measurements two years, four years, six years before this child was seen? Do you have any idea of how long the blood pressure was elevated? What about the history of headaches?

RESPONSE: The history of headaches was relatively acute. Besides the fact that we knew the child was generally healthy, there were no blood pressure measurements. She had not started complaining of anything until within the month prior to hospitalization. She complained of headaches a few days before she had the convulsion.

MODERATOR: From the histological pictures shown, this case to me does resemble those cases that Dr. Habib has presented here and in other places as Focal Segmental Hypoplasia. What about the concept that this diagnosis could be made with the renal arteriogram? Can we say anything from the arteriogram that we saw?

RESPONSE: Having reported many cases in which the autopsy reveals a renal artery stenosis without the patient having had hypertension, I want to emphasize the fact that finding a renal artery stenosis present does not make it the cause of the hypertension. I insist that what was shown to us (the histological alterations in the renal parenchyma) has many alterations that we recognize as Renal Segmental Hypoplasia.

MODERATOR: When you mention renal artery stenosis, do you only refer to the main renal artery? What about the renal artery branches? Whenever we have looked for Renal Segmental Hypoplasia, we have expected to get some changes in the branches that may give us supplemental information that a flat X-ray does not give us. Is that a mistaken concept? Do you think that you can support or rule out the diagnosis with the arteriogram, especially if there is no main renal artery stenosis?

RESPONSE: I don't know.

MODERATOR: You do not use the renal arteriogram in the cases in whom you suspect Renal Segmental Hypoplasia?

RESPONSE: No, because if we find in the simple X-ray the alterations in the renal contour and then if we have in the IVP more of these changes (the renal scars, etc.), then I think that that is enough. We don't have arteriograms in most of our cases with Renal Segmental Hypoplasia.

COMMENT: From a pathological perspective, how does this differ from what you would see in reflux nephropathy?

RESPONSE: In fact, there is not any difference. I think it is the same entity, only that Dr. Hodson calls it Reflux Nephropathy and Renée Habib calls it Renal Segmental Hypoplasia. But they are the same thing from the histological point of view. They are the same thing from the radiological point of view. Now, again, some of these cases are without any vesicoureteral reflux and the people who defend the reflux as pathogenesis say that there was reflux during intrauterine life and that it disappeared later on. They say that it is not necessary to have the reflux at the time of the diagnosis.

COMMENT: The only comment I have is that at least in adult medicine, being a high grade renal artery obstruction, there should be some collateral circulation. That is strikingly absent here. There is no collateral circulation.

COMMENT: I notice that everybody has been avoiding commenting on the renins from the renal veins. Can anybody explain why they are so much lower than those from the peripheral veins or why the superior vena cava values are lower than the inferior vena cava and lower than the unaffected side?

RESPONSE: Of course, the ones that were done peripherally were done at different times--like a week before. As everybody knows, these renin values are very treacherous. Ideally you would want to sample both renal veins at the same time which was not done here. Only one catheter was used and each one was done in sequence. Although she seemed to be in a pretty stable state and the whole sampling procedure was done within minutes, there could have been changes due to the different sampling times. I don't have a vast experience on this but actually it struck me that the values seemed more clear-cut than most other values you would get. At least, there was always the right kidney that had the higher values and after Lasix it had a 2:1 ratio when compared to the left kidney.

COMMENT: A couple of comments about the renins. When you did the renal renins, was the child on treatment or not?

RESPONSE: She was on treatment.

QUESTION: On what medication?

RESPONSE: She was getting Apresoline and Aldactone.

COMMENT: It's possible that some of the difference in renin might be one, position; two, time of day; three, therapy. At least in our laboratory, the reproducibility of renin measurements is approximately 15% and if you take that out to three standard deviations, you get to 50% difference between right and left. Before we feel comfortable in saying that there's lateralization of renins ... if you look at them before Lasix, one does not see the 50% difference. This may be because the kidney is small and it's secreting per minute not all that much renin but when stimulated you now see the difference because you get further suppression of the contralateral side. Laragh has a scoring index for recognizing differences that indicate curability. One of them is the difference,with the renins higher on the involved side. Another criterium--which we really don't talk about much but which this child demonstrates--is suppression of renin on the opposite side. At least after Lasix the values on the left side were the same if not less than in the inferior vena cava after figuring in variability. So, you've got elevation on one side and suppression on the other side. The usual renal arterial-venus difference is 25% if one samples the arterial tree and the renal vein because of renin secretion by the kidney. You certainly have suppression demonstrable. I think these criteria tend to fit those which suggest curability as defined by Laragh. Certainly, you had the result from your nephrectomy. The question I would ask is if you didn't do the Lasix stimulation test and you had only the results before Lasix (which is what you will find--no Lasix administration, certainly in a number of institutions), would you still have taken out the kidney? One more point or question: did you do a renal scan of the total function? How much function was there on the right side?

RESPONSE: They did do a renal scan and it was qualitative not quantitative. There seemed to be good blood flow to the right kidney, which was surprising. It filled at the same time as the left kidney. But, there was not anything quantitative about it. As you know, kidneys like this, assuming that we forget about the Lasix, occasionally have been taken out and there is a certain percentage of success in any event--sometimes even without the lateralization for reasons which I don't understand. It would have made it pretty tough. Although you are looking at a kidney that is small with a clear renal artery stenosis in a child that's got hypertension. I think it would probably be worth...the procedure is relatively low risk and the chances are at least fair that it would be successful.

QUESTION: It was mentioned that it took about a week for the blood pressure to go down. We've had a similar patient, only the blood pressure ranged from 190/120 mm Hg with very marked renin changes. After the kidney was removed for about a month the blood pressure didn't change and we were very frightened. A month later it dropped and it has remained normal for three or four years. If this is renin dependent, then what's the mechanism of that blood pressure staying high?

RESPONSE: I don't have a definitive answer. We, too, have seen it. One of the things that people have thought about it is that if you have elevated blood pressure for a period of time, some of the vascular walls imbide something; you increase the sodium content of the vessel wall itself and after removal, whatever the process is, it takes a number of months for the blood pressure to return to a normal level. I know that others have had similar experiences. We have seen it a few times.

COMMENT: In the Goldblatt model, high renin levels and increased total peripheral resistance are relatively early phenomena. Then later, increased cardiac output becomes part of the picture. It may be that the persistent hypertension may have something to do with increased cardiac output which persists for a while.

MODERATOR: We shall go now to Case #3. Dr. David Jaffe, Instructor of Medicine, Division of Nephrology, will present the case.

DR. JAFFE: The patient we are discussing is a 21 year old female. It's an interesting problem which you might see in younger age groups as well. She was in good health until three years prior to her last admission to Jackson Memorial Hospital, in 1977. At that time, she was seen by a local physician, complaining only of fatigue and weight loss. We don't have any information from that period; it is currently not available even from the physician. However, she was diagnosed as having Systemic Lupus; I have to presume that the criteria of the American Rheumatological Society were followed. She was placed on prednisone, 80 mg/day. At that time, there are questions as to whether pericardial effusion and "renal failure" were present. There is indication from the patient that she describes both of these; however, we have no documentation, and from talking with her further, it does not sound from the clinical information that either of these were present. Two years prior to her last admission, she was admitted to Jackson Memorial Hospital for the first time. At that time, she had an intrauterine pregnancy of 24 weeks. The physical examination, other than being pregnant, was unremarkable. From laboratory studies obtained on that admission she was found to be anemic with a hematocrit of 23.2%. She had an elevated Erythrosedimentation Rate (138 mm hr). VDRL and FTA were both positive. She had a urinary protein excretion of 5 mg/dl and the remainder of the urinalysis was unremarkable with the exception of 10-15 white cells/HPF. Her platelet count was 115,000/ml. Her renal function seemed to be good; she had a BUN of 8 mg/dl and a serum creatinine of 0.5 mg/dl. At this time, her ANA was positive with a titer of 1:2048. Her anti-double stranded DNA was also positive with a titer of 1:640. Serum complement (C_3 53 mg/dl and C_4 8 mg/dl) was below the normal limits for our laboratory. On a 24-hr urine specimen, creatinine clearance was 103 cc/min on a specimen containing 700 mg creatinine for 24 hrs. At that time there were two other creatinine clearances attempted both of which yielded values of 40 ml/min but were less than adequate collections. So, throughout her entire case history there has been some questions as to her clearances but still this is as close to being accurate as possible.

At that point in time she was still on 80 mg prednisone/day. She signed out against medical advice and was readmitted three weeks later. She self-tapered the corticosteroids from 80 to 40 mg/day for no apparent reason. At this time, ANA was positive only to a titer of 1:128, C_3 and C_4 were still depressed. She had two more creatinine clearances which yielded values of 40-45 ml/min and a third value of 151 ml/min which was felt to be more accurate. The remainder of her pregnancy was unremarkable except for an episode of herpetic vulvovaginitis which responded to treatment locally and she delivered a healthy female infant by cesarean section in February, 1980. The remainder of this hospital course was uncomplicated. She was subsequently re-admitted for several days with a wound infection. At this time, her BUN was 10 mg/dl, serum creatinine 0.8 mg/dl, and corticosteroids subsequently were discontinued. She had no evidence of any manifestations of lupus and throughout the entire number of hospitalizations,at this point had not been noted by any examiner at anytime to be hypertensive.

In August of 1980, she was noted to be hypertensive. She went to one of the Jackson Memorial Clinics and diastolic blood pressure of 96 mm Hg was obtained. At that time, she also complained of some arthralgias. Active lupus was diagnosed and the patient was placed on Aldomet, 500 mg BID and prednisone in a dose between 60 and 80 mg/day was reinstituted.

In September of 1980, she was admitted to Jackson Memorial Hospital Medical ICU with acute onset of seizures and what was diagnosed as malignant hypertension as manifested by the seizures, diastolic blood pressure of 130 mm Hg, evidence of fundoscopic changes grade III and evidence of left ventricular hypertrophy. At this admission, her BUN was noted to be 60 mg/dl, and serum creatinine, 3.0 mg/dl. A 24 hr creatinine clearance felt to be accurate was 25 ml/min. She was placed on prednisone, 80 mg/day, and for treatment of her hypertension, Inderal, 240 mg twice daily and then a variety of medications including 300 mg of Apresoline which was discontinued at our advice because of the question of active lupus and its interfering with our determinations. She was placed on minipress in less than therapeutic doses. When we were first consulted during this admission, we suggested increasing both minipress and adding clonidine to her regimen. None of these measures succeeded in bringing her diastolic blood pressure to any point below 120 mm Hg. We ultimately made a suggestion that the patient receive minoxidil and she was started on 5 mg twice a day with a reduction of her blood pressure. During this hospitalization the patient underwent a percutaneous renal biopsy the results of which you will see. While awaiting the results, at the recommendation of the Rheumatology Service, she received 3 g boluses of methylprednisolone. During this hospitalization her blood pressure did finally return to a diastolic of 90 mm Hg with treatment. However, there was no change in the renal function, no change in the creatinine clearance. Subsequent to this admission, she has been followed in the Rheumatology and Renal Clinics with no further improvement in her renal function.

MODERATOR: I have a question about biopsy in a patient with hypertension. We recently reported (with Dr. Elberg as the senior author) a project using sodium nitroprusside to perform a kidney biopsy in a hypertensive patient fearing complications like excessive bleeding. Did you have any problems with that?

RESPONSE: No, but I must admit also that at the time of her biopsy, arterial blood pressure was being controlled by Minoxidil. I didn't add into the presentation the possibility of a CNS lesion. Since we didn't see her first, when she came to us she had had a lumbar puncture which was negative, a CT scan which was also unremarkable, and an EEG which revealed no focal abnormality. Her renal evaluation prior to a renal consultation included a renal scan which revealed poor function bilaterally but equal blood flow and an abdominal ultrasound which did not reveal any difference in kidney size.

MODERATOR: Thank you, Dr. Jaffe. Dr. Pardo will now present the histopathology.

DR. PARDO: I was very surprised when I looked at the biopsy because it seemed to be a mesangial type of lupus. Usually I associate hypertension with a more active form of disease--a diffuse glomerulonephritis. It can be seen that the lesions are mainly in the mesangial area with an increase in matrix and increase in number of cells. Usually you have no more than three mesangial cells together. Looking at the periphery, the capillaries are completely clean (Figure 6). The prominent finding was a complete obliteration of the arterioles by connective tissue. In Figure 7, an arteriole can be seen coming into the glomerulus; I don't know for sure whether it is afferent or efferent, but probably it is an afferent arteriole because the wall is somewhat thick. There probably is an organized thrombin in the arteriole. Again, the glomerulus itself shows only changes of mesangial proliferation. Looking at the parenchyma, one can see that there is an increase in interstitial fibrous tissue with wrinkling and thickening of the basement membrane of the tubules. This is consistent with tubular atrophy; that means probably that the renal insufficiency is irreversible. The degree of interstitial fibrosis and tubular atrophy (more than 30% of the parenchyma in this case) has one of the best histological correlations with chronic renal failure. Some glomeruli showed fibrinoid changes, probably remnants of an acute process or something acute super-imposed, but still not well controlled.

QUESTION: I notice the FTA was positive. No comment is made on treating the patient for syphilis.

RESPONSE: Throughout multiple hospital admissions, the FTA was noted to be positive. She received treatment on a number of occasions.

QUESTION: I was wondering about electron microscopy.

RESPONSE: By electron microscopy there were mesangial deposits. Those pictures were not very helpful.

QUESTION: The latest creatinine clearance was on September 1980. Do you have any latest renal function studies?

RESPONSE: Yes. It is virtually the same as it was then.

QUESTION: Did you consider a second drug for active lupus?

RESPONSE: Based on what I saw on the biopsy, and since the patient had been on adequate doses of cortico-steroids for an extended period of time, except for treatment of hypertension, I wouldn't treat her with anything.

MODERATOR: Somebody in the audience reviewed for us Systemic Lupus Erythematosus at one time. He has a large number of patients of his own. I'm sure he has something to say about this subject.

RESPONSE: In the biopsy, you see the typical picture of nephrosclerosis. Arteriosclerosis was very definite in this case. It is hard for me to believe the sudden change of almost normal renal function to a state in which the renal function came down with not too much of glomerulosclerosis. The glomeruli seem to be more preserved. With these changes in arterioles and other vessels which correspond to active lupus nephropathy, I don't know if you need to consider this case as end-stage lupus nephropathy. Maybe with more active treatment something still can be done.

MODERATOR: Would you agree that time would have done as much as treatment? By the criteria you use, was the treatment indicated? Would you have used other drugs?

RESPONSE: It has been demonstrated that they don't do any better with combinations of other drugs in addition to corticosteroids. I wouldn't give other drugs.

DR. PARDO: I believe that the best correlate with renal failure more than the glomerular lesion is interstitial fibrosis and tubular atrophy. I would also like to know your opinion concerning the so-called lupus arteritis. Every time I see a lupus patient with so-called arteritis and fibrinoid changes in the vessels, the patient has had malignant hypertension. So, I think one has to be very careful to recognize proper lupus vasculitis and the effects of malignant hypertension in the kidney. I believe that some of the reported lupus vasculitis or lupus arteritis are the effects of malignant hypertension on the kidney. In addition to that, I wonder if the treatment with corticosteroids or other treatment may activate a mesangial lupus and produce the vascular lesion. This is just speculation.

COMMENT: I don't know that steroids would activate lupus.

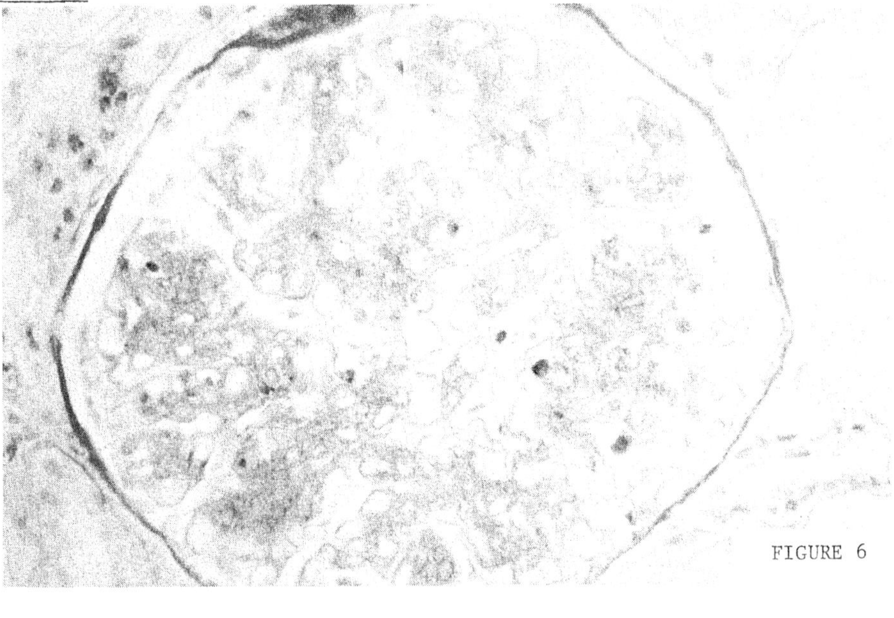

FIGURE 6

RESPONSE: In the sense of the vascular lesions. Something happens in there that does not fit.

COMMENT: Some workers in New York have shown some data that corticosteroids sensitized vascular receptors to angiotensin II. This could be used to explain the hypertension of Cushings syndrome as well as hypertension of corticosteroid therapy. In this context, corticosteroids may promote some vascular diseases. This patient had substantial doses of prednisone.

COMMENT: There are occasional patients with lupus who appear to have primary tubulointerstitial component with dense deposits in tubular basement membrane and positive immunofluorescence. I assume that there was none of that.

DR. PARDO: No. There was very little. From the point of view of the histology, it was a mesangial lupus. This is the third case I've seen of this type.

COMMENT: Wouldn't she be a good one in whom to consider using converting enzyme blocker if she's on steroids, in light of what you just said -- steroids increasing the vasculitis or vascular responsiveness? Particularly if she has high renin and angiotensin levels.

RESPONSE: They were not done.

COMMENT: Converting enzyme inhibitors have become increasingly associated with a nephropathy. I would be reluctant to use it in a nephrotic syndrome patient who probably has an immune complex disease. I don't know if there is any practical way to control the angiotensin component of her hypertensior at this point.

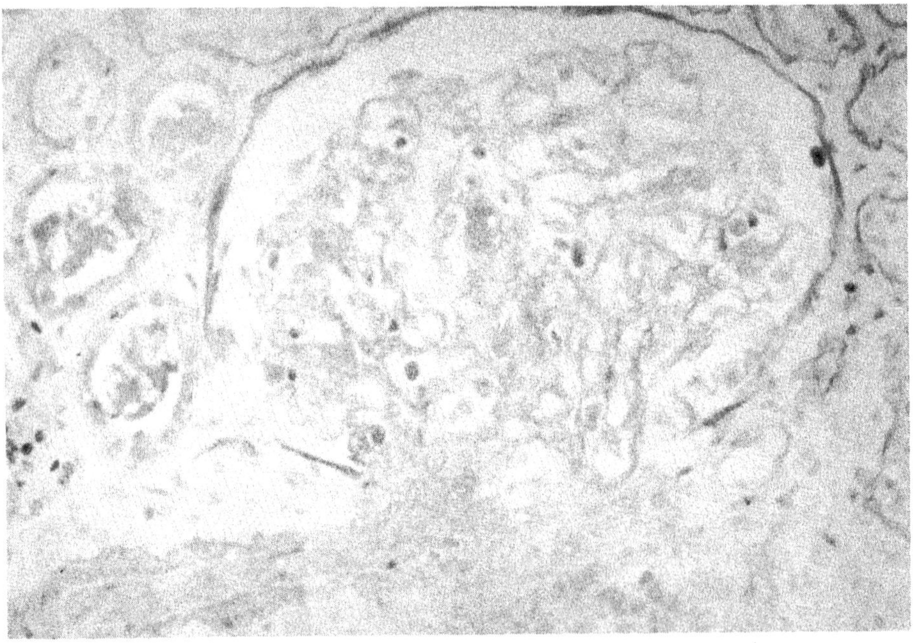

FIGURE 7

COMMENT: A question that we always toss around is whether or not to give Apresoline to somebody with systemic lupus because of Apresoline's ability to cause a lupus like syndrome. We also use it in our children with lupus (as you have done) but I think it's something worth mentioning in passing. Now, there are other good alternative drugs available.

MODERATOR: Any other comment on that point? I guess the concept is well accepted. We shall go now to the last case. Dr. Helen Gorman who is Clinical Assistant Professor of Pediatrics and a member of the Division of Pediatric Nephrology, is presenting this case.

DR. GORMAN: This is the case of a white young man who will be 19 in February. He first came to our attention in October, 1974, at the age of 12 with presentation of a history of abdominal pain, arthralgia, purpuric rash on lower legs and oliguria, impetigo four weeks previously, followed by fever treated with an antibiotic. BUN 60 mg/dl, serum creatinine 8.0 mg/dl, ANA negative, serum C'3 normal. Urinalysis with proteinuria and hematuria. Initial diagnosis: Henoch-Schonlein purpura with nephritis and Acute Renal Failure. Hemodialysis was instituted, and a renal biopsy obtained. Treatment was then started with prednisone, cyclophosphamide and heparin. Within a few days, renal function began to improve. Concurrently, severe hypertension with associated encephalopathy and congestive cardiac failure developed. To control arterial blood pressure, diazoxide, sodium nitroprusside, then Minoxidil with Propranolol and furosemide were required. After three weeks, hemodialysis and heparin were discontinued. Cyclophosphamide was given for two months, intermittently because of periodic leukopenia. Prednisone therapy was tapered to 20 mg daily at time of discharge, when renal function was almost normal with insignificant proteinuria, and hypertension moderately controlled with Minoxidil 60 mg, Propranolol 320 mg and furosemide 160 mg daily. Subsequent course: Continuing brittle hypertension aggravated by episodes of fluid retention. November 1975: Creatinine clearance normal; peripheral renin activity 30.7 ng/ml/hour, with 160 mEq Na^+ excretion/24 hs. March 1976: Generalized tonic convulsion; E.E.G. diffusely abnormal; treated with phenobarbital. August 1977: Echocardiogram showed marked concentric hypertrophy of left ventricle. December 1978: E.E.G. improved; occasional spike-wave discharges of right hemisphere. August 1979: Echocardiogram improved.

Clinically, there has been gradual improvement of hypertension with reduction of anti-hypertensive medication. Infrequent episodes of intercurrent infection resolved without complication; growth and development have been normal. No further seizures have occurred. He is now going to college. Current medications: Minoxidil 30 mg, Propranolol 120 mg, furosemide 100 mg/day, prednisone 15 mg every other day.

MODERATOR: Any questions? Nobody is going to challenge the various drugs used in the past and even currently used?

QUESTION: Actually, I was going to ask that. Could you please explain the initial therapy for Henoch-Schönlein Purpura and continuation of prednisone for the past five years?

RESPONSE: This is rather difficult to explain. When I came upon this case, the other two medications (cyclophosphamide and heparin) had been stopped and he was on prednisone. It was not by default but I think because he was doing extremely well. We had no hard data upon which to base continuation of treatment but on the other hand there have been anecdotal reports of improvement with immunosuppression in the particular disease he had which you will hear about in a minute. We opted to continue it on perhaps somewhat slender grounds. I'm not sure. Perhaps this will come up in the discussion to follow the histological presentation.

MODERATOR: This was an extremely sick child.

QUESTION: Do you have an ASO titer level or any of the streptococcal enzymes antibodies?

RESPONSE: ASO titer -- at the beginning he did have apparently a documented streptococcal infection before admission. I don't have the titers here.

QUESTION: His rash was typical of HS purpura originally?

RESPONSE: According to my understanding from the chart. I didn't see it myself.

MODERATOR: That was not the diagnosis of the Division of Pediatric Nephrology. It was a clinical impression in the floor or the referring physician's statement. It's hard to recall the details because we have been carrying him as a typical "something else" (to be clarified hopefully after the histology is shown). I don't recall that at any time we considered that diagnosis seriously.

DR. PARDO: This is another puzzling case. When one looks at this patient's biopsy and knows the initial diagnosis, the first impression one gets is that this is a typical case of Schoenlein-Henoch Purpura with mesangial proliferative glomerulonephritis. One can see the clear look in the glomerular periphery and some mesangial proliferation, perhaps some intracapillary extension. This case does not show any crescents or morphological manifestations that would suggest that this is a serious disease. So, the glomerular lesion was quite benign at least morphologically. There were large deposits of IgA in the mesangium, in the pattern you see in Henoch-Schoenlein, in IgA nephropathy and systemic lupus. So, I think that the histology and the immunofluorescence were quite consistent with Henoch-Schoenlein Purpura. But there were many areas where the vessels had practically disappeared. In Figure 8 we see the lumen of a vessel but in the wall, practically you cannot identify any muscle. It's an explosion of inflammation, necrosis, fibrinoid necrosis, lymphocytes, plasma cells, and granulocytes (some of them eosinophils). These findings were present in 4 or 5 arterioles studied and are typical of periarteritis because there is inflammation around the vessels. In other areas you could see the muscle, the interna elastica and rupture of the elastica with fibrinoid changes. That is the hallmark of necrotizing arteritis of the polyarteritis nodosa variety. I was even more surprised when I took a look at the electron microscopy. In Figure 9 you can see the typical subepithelial humps and the epithelial side with some microvilli degeneration probably secondary to proteinuria.

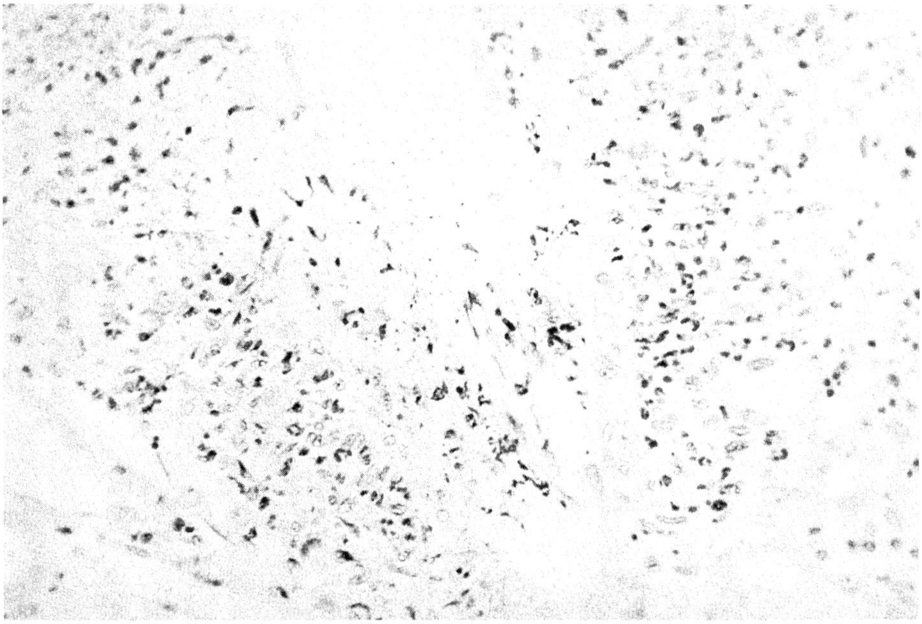

FIGURE 8

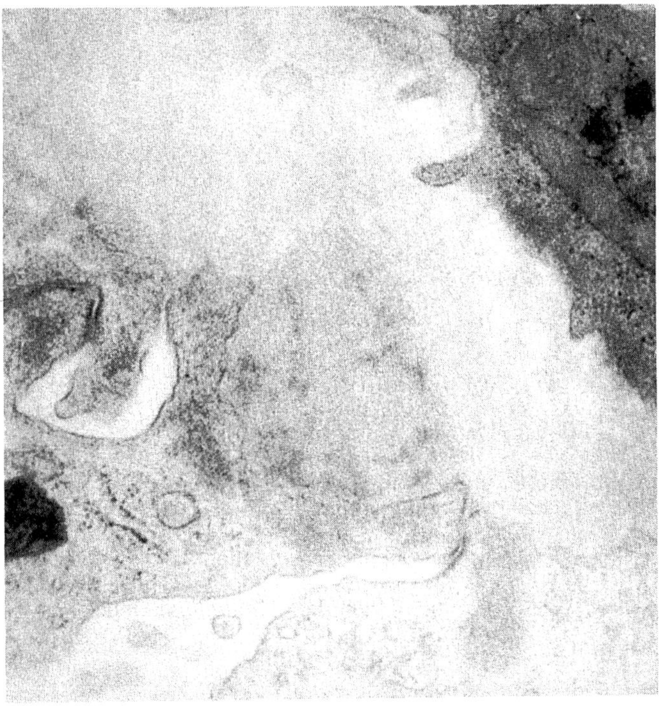

FIGURE 9

In summary, this is a case which histologically fits the glomerular lesion of Henoch-Schoenlein Purpura, has a polyarteritis and has the EM features for Post-infectious Glomerulonephritis.

COMMENT: I have seen case reports of the whole panoply that has just been pointed out--Post-infectious Glomerulonephritis periarteritis and HS purpura.

QUESTION: Any idea as to what is the antigen or about antigen-antibody complexes?

ANSWER: Circulating immune complexes were negative.

COMMENT: When I see the onset of Acute Renal Failure with this clinical picture of purpura and so on, I think about Polyarteritis Nodosa because it is one of the ways it may present. Now, the histopathology that we saw is compatible with lesions for Polyarteritis Nodosa. I'm not very happy about all the other findings. I mean, I don't pay too much attention to the humps because they are not pathognomonic. Not from the point of view of excluding the diagnosis of Polyarteritis Nodosa. I don't think you can exclude this because you find these humps. I'm not very happy about the findings in the immunofluorescence.

MODERATOR: The IgA deposits in the mesangium?

COMMENT: Only IgA!

COMMENT: There was only a bit here and there. But, it was IgA, no question.

COMMENT: We have seen a case of what looks like Post-infectious Nephritis which has the changes of polyarteritis such as you have described here. We haven't seen HS Purpura on top of the IgA deposits that you have here. The IgA deposits are rather strange. Of course, there is now a lot of discussion about HS Purpura and IgA Nephropathy perhaps being an extension of the disease. But then, that doesn't fit in with the post infectious aspect. It's a rather remarkable and I think unique constellation of findings.

MODERATOR: For whatever it is worth, Dr. Elberg (when he was with us) shared this case with one of our distinguished visiting pathologists; this person was satisfied that it was Polyarteritis Nodosa and was surprised that the patient was still alive.

COMMENT: As I recall, somewhere around 1974-75 we had three, four or five cases that looked like they had a purpuric rash and something that looked like renal periarteritis which we treated with corticosteroids for a year or so and seemed to have gone away. Nothing like this whole constellation but it is interesting that since then, we haven't seen much like this. Have you seen anything like this since then?

MODERATOR: This was a very sick child. We did not hesitate to use all this blind combination of drugs. It was a time when readily we were treating the so-called Rapidly Progressive Glomerulonephritis with triple therapy, whether we helped him or not, we don't know, but he did very well. We have not had another patient like him ever.

COMMENT: I've never seen a patient who had fairly moderately advanced renal insufficiency who did not have crescents. If the patient does not have crescents, then I look for something else in the picture like vasculitis.

MODERATOR: The interesting thing is that his renal function has remained at quite an acceptable level. His problems subsequently have been hypertension and the iatrogenic problems which developed from the many therapeutic agents used.

COMMENT: Reviewing the pathology literature, even in Heptinstall's book in the chapter on Henoch Schonlein Purpura, it is mentioned specifically that some of these cases may show arteritis but does not go any deeper at all. I reviewed two papers that perhaps may be pertinent. One is from the Hospital Necker in France; they reviewed 100 cases of Henoch Schonlein Purpura and found two cases of vasculitis with fibrinoid changes; they did not find inflammation. I don't know if you can compare these cases. The other is a paper by Cameron and his group; I have only read the abstract since I have been unable to get the paper published in Histopathology in 1977. He describes humps in Henoch Schonlein Purpura.

COMMENT: I have seen a fatal case of a teenage boy who presented as a Rapidly Progressive Glomerulonephritis and did not have crescents; he had titers elevation suggestive of recent streptococcal infection and he had abdominal pain, arthralgias, purpura and Polyarteritis Nodosa picture on post mortem. So, he showed elements of a post-infectious picture with severe vasculitis.

QUESTION: I was wondering if you don't think it could be a case of Thrombotic Thrombocytopenic Purpura? We see cases like this in Hemolytic Uremic Syndrome in which we were able to describe the arteritis plus the humps.

COMMENT: I think the presence of IgA is a very strong argument in favor of Henoch Schonlein Purpura. Usually you don't see IgA in massive amounts in those three entities: IgA Nephropathy, Systemic Lupus, and Henoch Schonlein Purpura. I think that the immunofluorescence is crucial.

QUESTION: Did you have a platelet count?

DR. GORMAN: Yes. It was normal.

COMMENT: My reason for asking is that we recently saw a child who came in with what looked like malignant hypertension who had a blood smear that looked like the Hemolytic Uremic Syndrome with a microangiopathic hemolytic anemia, but had a normal platelet count. The latter helped us, at least in our own thinking, to separate out Thrombotic Thrombocytopenic Purpura and Hemolytic Uremic Syndrome from some other processes.

MODERATOR: This patient was initially worked up with Pediatric Hematology, so I would imagine that both the Hemolytic Uremic Syndrome and TTP were carefully ruled out.

QUESTION: Has this patient had a complete recovery of renal function?

RESPONSE: Yes.

QUESTION: Why do you think the patient is still having so many problems with hypertension?

MODERATOR: We would like to get a repeat biopsy. I was very courageous when he first came. Since then, I have become a bit older and more cautious. So we should repeat the biopsy one day and see what those vessels look like.

QUESTION: Has he had any renal scan recently? You might be able to get some information that way--in terms of perfusion patterns.

RESPONSE: That's a good suggestion.

COMMENT: Or residual Polyarteritis Nodosa lesions by renal arteriogram. That's fairly non-invasive and it's carrying it a long way but he still has persistent hypertension.

QUESTION: Has his echocardiogram returned to normal or is that still abnormal?

ANSWER: It's improved. We haven't had one since August '79. It did show marked improvement. Also, his electrocardiogram has shown marked improvement.

COMMENT: One of the long term issues in terms of repeat biopsies, etc. is, what is ultimately going to happen to the patient. In this child's case, is hypertension what ultimately will destroy him? Is there anything that can be done? Probably not, even with another biopsy. But the question remains.

QUESTION; Could I ask this question again about corticosteroid treatment? I would like to know what members of the panel feel about continuing this rather low dose of prednisone on alternate days for this long period of time. I wonder if we are doing anything or not, in a way perpetuating his hypertension.

COMMENT: I don't think that 15 mg every other day is going to worsen his hypertension. I also don't think it is doing very much for his underlying lesion. Other people might have other views. The children that we have treated, we've sort of quit therapy after a year or two unless there was some evidence of re-exacerbation of the disease. Again, a repeat biopsy would be helpful in this regard.

QUESTION: Does he have a normal urinalysis?

RESPONSE: Yes, he has no proteinuria and no hematuria at this time.

MODERATOR: Would biopsy of some other area less invasive than the kidney be sufficient? We always run into that problem. Dr. Pardo did some muscle biopsies for diabetic patients with no complications; valuable data was gathered in this manner.

RESPONSE: You have to know where the eggs are. You have to go to the kidney. One thing I wanted to mention even though it is anecdotal. Lately I have seen three or four cases of this type of patient with hypertension, renal disease and some type of vasculopathy. They have renal failure due to the vascular component. One of them underwent bilateral nephrectomy. I knew it was a case of polyarteritis. I had to do special stains to find one vessel that showed the ruptured elastica. All the others showed concentric arterioles with nephrosclerosis.

MODERATOR: She progressed very rapidly and went into End-Stage Renal Disease in a matter of weeks.

COMMENT: I have seen a couple of Hemolytic Uremic patients with a hypertensive component. The glomerular lesion is quiet. But they are doomed because of the vascular component. You cannot cure those vessels. They are completely destroyed. The only thing left is tissue replaced by a fibrous string. That's all. It's extremely optimistic to say that you can cure that type of lesion.

COMMENT: More than fifteen years ago I saw a child with the same clinical picture as this one. It was a Polyarteritis Nodosa. I treated him for three months with prednisone and then the proteinuria disappeared, all the urinary sediment alterations became normal, and the renal function also became normal. The hypertension subsided and then I stopped the treatment. One year later there was some relapse. He was treated again with prednisone and I repeated the biopsy. The arterial lesions, the arterioles, were almost normal. Now, fifteen years have passed and he has normal pressure and normal renal function. No alterations. We follow this patient every year, check all these things, and he is doing very well.

MODERATOR: This patient has had other problems and has persisted with hypertension, some cardiovascular problems, some cerebral problems which could be related to the treatment or the hypertension but our concern was that this was a systemic arteritis for which we may need to continue treatment.

COMMENT: We don't have much evidence that you need to continue treatment. Again, long treatment may help to sustain the symptomatology.

MODERATOR: So, is it the recommendation of the panel to discontinue prednisone? We feel that the anti-hypertensive medication is needed. We have not had any hypotension while on treatment. We have had problems in maintaining at times, even rather recently, the blood pressure from hypertensive levels down to within normal ranges. Since things have been rather quiet, we could try gradually to discontinue all medications.

COMMENT: In my experience, Polyarteritis Nodosa is not a protracted disease. I would expect that the vasculitis is burned out; there is really no reason to stay on prednisone.

COMMENT: One other comment about corticosteroid therapy, even though it may not have relevance to this particular patient. At the International Pediatric Nephrology Symposium, the comment was made that giving a little more prednisone than the International Collaborative Study Group may perhaps explain the better results of one group than of others treating Membranoproliferative Nephritis. Of course, this disease may have a hypertensive component. That group is giving at least 60 mg per meter square every other day which is substantially more than the 15 mg of the other groups. If you were to translate this to another disease, it would seem that you would have to give more prednisone (if what was said is correct) in order to have a meaningful effect although it is pure speculation at this time.

COMMENT: I think it is very important that the patient was also treated with cyclophosphamide. At the time (1975) cyclophosphamide was not well known as to its effects in vasculitis. You may wonder how much of the improvement was due to prednisone or to cyclophosphamide.

MODERATOR: What about that point? What about the comment that the arteritis may have run its course?

RESPONSE: Yes, I agree. I think it's a one chance affair. At least the variety one usually sees.

MODERATOR: Well, unfortunately our time has also run out. We must end our Workshop here. Thanks are due to all the participants (faculty and registrants) for their participation.

APPENDIX

CLINICAL RESEARCH AND THE REVIEW PROCESS: AN INTRODUCTION

Antonia C. Novello, M.D.

The mission of the National Institutes of Health (NIH) is to improve the health of the American people by increasing our understanding of the processes underlying human health and by acquiring new knowledge to help prevent, detect, diagnose, and treat disease. To accomplish this mission, the NIH has intramural research and clinical programs, supports research extramurally in universities and medical schools, trains promising young researchers, and helps to develop and maintain research resources. In these times of budgetary constraints and intense competition for the available funds, it would be useful for new researchers to know how the system operates so that they can handle the review process efficiently and with less anxiety.

MECHANISMS OF SUPPORT

The most common mode of competing for research funds is through the grant mechanism of which there are many types, each with specific considerations. Several of these types that are especially useful for a new investigator are discussed below, and mention will be made of the basic differences among some of the most commonly utilized types.

Research Project Grant (R01)

A research project grant supports a discrete specified project in an area representing the interest and competency of the principal investigator who is designated by the applicant institution. This is the most common mechanism for acquiring research funds.

New Investigator Research Award (NIRA or R23)

This award is designed to encourage new investigators in basic or clinical sciences (including those who have interrupted careers) to develop their interests in biomedical and behavioral research. Thus, it is aimed at bridging the transition from training status to that of established investigator, allowing for relatively inexperienced investigators to submit meritorious and original ideas. Although the review process is the same as for R01's, certain features differentiate the two support mechanisms:

1) For a NIRA, the investigator must be a citizen of the USA or a non-citizen national lawfully admitted to the US for permanent residence.

2) The NIRA investigator must have a doctoral degree (M.D., Ph.D., or D.O., etc.) or its equivalent, with at least two years of full-time research experience. In most instances, the principal investigator will have no more than five years of research experience after completion of formal training at the time the award is made.
3) The investigator for a NIRA must not have been a primary recipient of a Federally supported research grant, except for a pre- or postdoctoral fellowship or traineeship. (Exceptions may be granted only to individuals who are changing their scientific field.)
4) The applicant institution must be a domestic one.
5) The NIRA is made for up to three years and is not renewable. The requested total direct cost must not exceed $107,500 for the three years, with no more than $37,500 (including up to $25,000 salary plus applicable fringe benefits for the investigator) for any one year.
6) At least 50% of time and effort is to be dedicated to the proposed research project.
7) Since the applicant investigator is less likely to submit an application in the same depth as an experienced investigator, letters of recommendation should be sent with the application to the review unit. These will help in establishing the investigator as a potential candidate for independent research and will aid in the evaluation of the qualifications and experience of that person.

Clinical Investigator Award (K08)

This mechanism which provides salary and research support, is to develop research ability in individuals with clinical backgrounds by training with a sponsor competent to provide guidance in the chosen subject. The K08 differs from the R23 in that the applicant must hold a professional degree in the clinical sciences (M.D., D.O., D.V.M. or equivalent), and have four to seven years of postdoctoral clinical and research experience. Holders of the Ph.D. with or without accompanying health degree or comparable degrees are not eligible for a K08, nor are individuals holding associate or full professorships. The candidate is expected to spend a minimum of 75% of time and effort in research.

The award is made on an annual basis for a maximum of three years. The salary is not to exceed $25,000 each year for the three year period. Up to $20,000 will be provided for supplies, equipment, travel, etc., including technical help. Indirect cost will be reimbursed up to 8% of the total cost. (Time and amount varies among Institutes, the PI should contact the appropriate Institute, if the award is made, for further information.) The institution does not have to guarantee placement of the candidate on its permanent, full-time faculty; but the institution must provide evidence of its commitment to the candidate's research development.

Research Career Development Award (RCDA or K04)

The RCDA is designed to enhance the research capability of individuals in the formative stages of their careers who have already demonstrated outstanding potential for contributing as independent investigators to health related research. It is not intended for untried investigators, for productive, independent investigators with significant numbers of publications of high quality, or for persons of senior academic rank. The award is not intended to substitute one source of salary support for another, nor is it intended to be a mechanism for providing institutional support. Rather, this award is available for those whose research potential is apparent, but who need additional experience in a productive scientific environment conducive to the development of a career in independent research. The following criteria apply:

1) The candidate must have at least three years of relevant post-doctoral experience prior to the award. The application must document accomplishments during this period that demonstrate research potential.
2) A plan must be included for additional experience in a productive scientific environment.
3) The applicant must be nominated by a domestic non-Federal and nonprofit institution engaged in health related research.
4) The award is for a single support period of five years at a salary (up to a maximum of $30,000) for each budget period. Fringe benefits are to be available through each individual institution's policies, and indirect cost will be reimbursed up to 8%.
5) The institution must show a commitment to the candidate for five years, which should be reflected in a statement from the sponsoring official. It should allow for the candidate to spend essentially full time in the actual conduct of the research and research-related activities, and thus reduce or defer demands for teaching service or committee duties.
6) At all times the application must demonstrate that the award will make a difference in the development of the candidate as an independent investigator.

PEER REVIEW SYSTEM

Once a grant application is duly approved and signed by the appropriate officials in the principal investigator's institution, it is submitted to the Division of Research Grants (DRG). Receipt dates for all competing continuation (renewal), supplemental, new program project and center, Research Career Development Award and fellowship applications are February 1, June 1, and October 1. All new regular applications (R01, R23, RCDA) are due on March 1, July 1, and November 1. After the application has been received and processed by Branch staff, it receives a number and is coded. This number, found in the upper right hand corner of the application's face page is important, for it is the primary way of tracing the application. A sample application number is given below:

Application type	Activity code	Awarding Organization	Serial #	Suffixes Grant Yr	Other
1	R01	AM (NIADDK)	15311	05	*A1

(Competing new application) (Investigator initiated project)
*"A"-plus a number designates an amendment to the application, or a revision.
"S"-plus a number designates a supplement.

The application is then reviewed for relevance to the overall NIH mission and assigned to the appropriate Scientific Review Group for evaluation and to the appropriate awarding organization for second level program review and possible funding. The individuals responsible for assignment decisions are the Referral Officers, health science administrators, most of whom also serve as Executive Secretaries of Scientific Review groups. These assignments are based on the scientific content of the grant and the scientific expertise of the group; assignments to an Institute are based on the mission and programmatic interests of the Institute.

If the subject matter in the application overlaps the interest of two Institutes, a dual assignment may be made, with the primary assignments going to the Institute whose area receives the greatest emphasis in the application.

After the processing and assigning by Referral Branch staff, the application is sent to the appropriate initial review group. In DRG, these groups are called Study Sections. They consist of 15 to 20 members, and have as their primary function the review and evaluation of the scientific merit of the research grant applications submitted to the NIH.

Primary processing of the application, before Study Section meeting, is carried out by the Executive Secretary of the Study Section. He or she checks the application for completeness in budget, letters of recommendation when appropriate, bibliography, possible conflicts of interest, human subjects form, addendum, past, present and concurrent funding, and level of effort. Following this, the Executive Secretary assigns each application to at least two members of the review group for in depth evaluation. The applications are reviewed in detail by the assigned reviewers, at least eight weeks before the Study Section meeting, and read by the other members of the Study Section, as well as special consultants, when needed.

During the Study Section meetings which occur three times a year, and last for approximately three days, the chairperson calls upon the primary reviewers to summarize their written summary critiques. These include,

Description: A clear and concise description of the objectives and procedures of the application. For deferred, or revised applications, a description of the background and any substantive changes since the previous review are also included.

Critique: A comprehensive evaluation of the application, including the significance and originality of the proposed study in its scientific field, the validity of the hypothesis, the logic of the aims, the weaknesses and strengths and the feasibility and adequacy of the procedures.

Investigators: The competence of the principal investigator(s) and key staff to conduct the proposed research, including their academic qualifications, research experience, productivity, and special attributes.

Resources and Environment: Any special aspects of the facilities and equipment as well as the extent of departmental and interdepartmental cooperation if applicable. The availability of essential laboratory, clinical, animal, computer, or other resources is commented on.

Budget: Whether all items of the budget are realistic and justified in terms of the aims and methods. Adequate justification for each suggested modification in amount or duration of support must be made. In addition, any apparent overlap with active or pending support should be considered.

Other Considerations: a) Involvement of Human Subjects. Consideration is given to any possible physical, psychological, or social injury that individuals might experience while participating as subjects in research, development, or related activities, and whether the rights and welfare of such individuals will be adequately protected. b) Animal Welfare. If animals are to be used in a project, a consideration will be made whether the animals will be given proper care and humane treatment so that they will not suffer unnecessary discomfort, pain, or injury. c) Hazardous Materials and Procedures. Potentially hazardous materials and procedures identified and a decision as to whether the proposed protection provided by the investigator will be adequate. After the discussion is completed, a formal motion is introduced and seconded for a recommended action. Three possible alternatives, all based on scientific merit, are made: approval, with assignment of priority score; disapproval, with no priority assigned; or deferral.

Approval is recommended if the application is of sufficient merit to be worthy of support based on the applicable review criteria. The vote for approval is equivalent to a recommendation that a grant be awarded, provided sufficient funds are available. A priority rating is required. Approval can be without restriction or with recorded expression of concern to be communicated to the applicant or sponsoring institution. Approval can be made also with limitations or restrictions on the scope of the work proposed, or the elimination of objectionable procedures involving human subjects or animals.

Disapproval is recommended when the application is not of sufficient merit to be worthy of support. Disapproval may also be recommended when gravely hazardous or unethical procedures are involved, or when no funds can be recommended, as in the case of a supplement deemed to be unnecessary. No priority rating is required.

Deferral is recommended when the Study Section cannot make a recommendation without additional information. This information may be obtained by a project site visit or by the submission of additional material by the applicant. Deferred applications are normally reviewed again at the next Study Section meeting.

After the final recommended action of the Study Section, each member privately records a numerical score that will represent his or her opinion of the scientific merit relative to the particular research area. The numerical rating is based on a scale of 1.0, the best, to 5.0, the least acceptable rating, with increments of 0.1.

These reviewers' ratings are averaged and multiplied by 100, providing a three digit rating known as the priority score, which is found in the right-hand side of the written document summarizing the Study Section review, called the summary statement or "pink sheet." This priority score and the critique of the Study Section are important elements but not the only ones considered in the funding decisions. Other considerations, such as relevance of the goals of the proposed research to the mission of the Institute, program balance, duplication or overlapping support from other agencies, and availability of funds, are also part of the funding decision.

After these summaries are completed, they are forwarded to the assigned Institutes together with all other records concerning the application for a second level review by the National Advisory Council or Board of the Institute. These Councils or Boards meet three times per year, six to eight weeks after the Study Sections. They consist of approximately 12 members including scientists and non-scientists. The scientific members of these Councils have considerable experience in review and committee work and share the needs and areas of interest of the particular Institute they advise. They usually serve from three to four years and have broad functions and duties. Their recommendations are not based on scientific consideration alone, but reflect the needs and objectives of the mission of the Institute and the NIH goals.

After the application and the pertinent review materials are sent from DRG to the respective Institute, a program director or staff program administrator will be responsible for its administration in the event that an award is made. Approximately two to four weeks before Council meets, the program administrators and their staff prepare books of these materials and mail them to the Council members. These are meant to acquaint the members with all applications, especially those that will need special action at the Council meeting. Following the Council meeting, the program director notifies all applicants by mail of the final recommendation arrived at by the Council and encloses the respective summary statement. Applicants who receive priority scores in the fundable range will be informed by the pertinent program person of the specific possibility of an award.

SUMMARY

This article is designed to provide new researchers with basic information about the peer review system used at the NIH. Because of the complexity of the system, it could not be all inclusive but anyone interested in a more detailed discussion of one or more aspects of the peer review system can read selections from the bibliography given below. Single copies of most of the publications are available from the Office of Grant Inquiries, Division of Research Grants, National Institutes of Health, Bethesda, Maryland 20205.

BIBLIOGRAPHY

1. Eaves, G.N.: Who reads your project-grant application to the National Institutes of Health? Federation Proceedings 31:2, 1972.
2. Eaves, G.N.: The project-grant application of the National Institutes of Health: introduction. Federation Proceedings 32:1541, 1973.
3. Eaves, G.N.: The grant application: an exercise in scientific writing. Federation Proceedings 32:1541, 1973.
4. Eaves, G.N.: A successful grant application to the National Institutes of Health: a case history. Grants Magazine 1:263, 1978.
5. Henley, C.: Peer review of research grant applications at the National Institutes of Health. Federation Proceedings 36:2066; 2186; 2335, 1977.
6. Malone, T.E.: Preparation of the project-grant application: assistance from the institutes and other awarding units. Federation Proceedings 32:1546, 1973.
7. Merritt, D.H., and Eaves, G.N.: Site visits for the review of grant applications to the National Institutes of Health; views of an applicant and a scientist administrator. Federation Proceedings 34:131, 1975.

Orientation Handbook for Members of Scientific Review Groups, August 1981. U.S. Department of Health and Human Services, Public Health Service, National Institutes of Health.

PARTICIPANTS

Program Chairman

José Strauss, M.D., Professor of Pediatrics; Director, Division of Pediatric Nephrology, University of Miami School of Medicine, Miami, Florida, USA.

Guest Faculty

Gustavo Gordillo-Paniagua, M.D., Director, Department of Pediatric Nephrology, Hospital Infantil, Mexico City, Mexico.

Alan B. Gruskin, M.D., Professor of Pediatrics; Director, Division of Pediatric Nephrology, Department of Pediatrics, Temple University School of Medicine and St. Christopher's Hospital for Children, Philadelphia, Pennsylvania, USA.

Ronald J. Kallen, M.D., Assistant Director of Pediatrics, Mt. Sinai Hospital, Cleveland, Ohio, USA.

Antonia C. Novello, M.D., Executive Secretary, General Medicine B Study Section, Division of Research Grants, SRB, National Institutes of Health, Bethesda, Maryland, USA.

Donald E. Potter, M.D., Associate Clinical Professor of Pediatrics, Division of Nephrology, Department of Pediatrics, University of California, San Francisco, California, USA.

Juan Rodriguez-Soriano, M.D., Head, Department of Pediatrics, Hospital Infantil de la Seguridad Social, Bilbao, Spain.

Local Faculty

Eduardo Bancalari, M.D., Professor of Pediatrics; Director, Division of Neonatology, Department of Pediatrics, University of Miami School of Medicine, Miami, Florida, USA.

Jacques J. Bourgoignie, M.D., Professor of Medicine Director, Division of Nephrology, University of Miami School of Medicine, Miami, Florida, USA.

Michael Freundlich, M.D., Clinical Instructor of Pediatrics, Division of Pediatric Nephrology, Department of Pediatrics, University of Miami School of Medicine, Miami, Florida, USA.

Mary Jane Jesse, M.D., Professor of Pediatrics, Division of Cardiology; Vice Chairman, Section of Child Health, Department of Pediatrics, University of Miami School of Medicine, Miami, Florida, USA.

Victoriano Pardo, M.D., Professor of Pathology; Director, Electron Microscopy Laboratory, Veterans Administration Medical Center, Miami, Florida, USA.

Eliseo Perez-Stable, M.D., Professor of Medicine, University of Miami School of Medicine; Chief, Medical Service, Veterans Administration Medical Center, Miami, Florida, USA.

Carlos A. Vaamonde, M.D., Professor of Medicine, University of Miami School of Medicine; Chief of Nephrology, Veterans Administration Medical Center, Miami, Florida, USA.

Gaston Zilleruelo, M.D., Assistant Professor of Pediatrics, Coordinator, Dialysis and Transplantation, Division of Pediatric Nephrology, University of Miami School of Medicine, Miami, Florida, USA.

Other Contributors

*H. Jorge Baluarte, M.D., Department of Pediatrics, Temple University School of Medicine and St. Christopher's Hospital for Children, Philadelphia, Pennsylvania, USA.

*René Feiman, M.D., Hospital Infantil de Mexico, Mexico City, Mexico.

Helen Corman, M.D., Clinical Assistant Professor of Pediatrics, Division of Pediatric Nephrology, Department of Pediatrics, University of Miami School of Medicine, Miami, Florida, USA.

David Jaffe, M.D., Instructor of Medicine, Division of Nephrology, Department of Medicine, University of Miami School of Medicine, Miami, Florida, USA.

*Barry J. Materson, M.D., Associate Professor of Medicine, University of Miami School of Medicine; Assistant Chief Medical Service, Veterans Administration Medical Center, Miami, Florida, USA.

*Felipe Mota-Hernandez, M.D., Hospital Infantil de Mexico, Mexico City, Mexico.

*Ricardo Muñoz-Arizpe, M.D., Division of Pediatric Nephrology, Hospital Infantil, Mexico City, Mexico.

Juan Peyser, M.D., Associate Pathologist, Variety Childrens Hospital, Miami, Florida, USA.

*Martin S. Polinsky, M.D., Department of Pediatrics, Temple University School of Medicine and St. Christopher's Hospital for Children, Philadelphia, Pennsylvania, USA.

*James W. Prebis, M.D., Department of Pediatrics, Temple University School of Medicine and St. Christopher's Hospital for Children, Philadelphia, Pennsylvania, USA.

*Howard W. Rosenblum, M.D., Department of Pediatrics, Temple University School of Medicine and St. Christopher's Hospital for Children, Philadelphia, Pennsylvania, USA.

*Alfredo Vallo, M.D., Department of Pediatrics, Hospital Infantil de la Seguridad Social, Bilbao, Spain.

Richard Zakheim, M.D. Director, Division of Pediatric Cardiology, Variety Childrens Hospital, Miami, Florida, USA.

*Co-authors

AUTHOR INDEX

SUBJECT INDEX

GPSR Compliance

The European Union's (EU) General Product Safety Regulation (GPSR) is a set of rules that requires consumer products to be safe and our obligations to ensure this.

If you have any concerns about our products, you can contact us on ProductSafety@springernature.com

In case Publisher is established outside the EU, the EU authorized representative is:

Springer Nature Customer Service Center GmbH
Europaplatz 3
69115 Heidelberg, Germany

Batch number: 10761599

Printed by Printforce, the Netherlands